Challenges and Management of Cataracts and Glaucoma

Challenges and Management of Cataracts and Glaucoma

Edited by Leroy Campbell

STATES ACADEMIC PRESS
www.statesacademicpress.com

States Academic Press,
109 South 5th Street,
Brooklyn, NY 11249, USA

Visit us on the World Wide Web at:
www.statesacademicpress.com

ISBN: 978-1-63989-101-6

Cataloging-in-Publication Data

Challenges and management of cataracts and glaucoma / edited by Leroy Campbell.
p. cm.
Includes bibliographical references and index.
ISBN 978-1-63989-101-6
1. Cataract. 2. Glaucoma. 3. Cataract--Surgery. 4. Glaucoma--Treatment.
5. Eye--Diseases--Treatment. I. Campbell, Leroy.
RE451 .C43 2022
617.742 059--dc23

Table of Contents

Preface

Glaucoma includes a group of eye diseases which lead to damage in the optic nerve and can cause vision loss. The most common type is wide angle glaucoma, also known as open angle glaucoma, in which the drainage angle for fluid within the eye remains open. The other types of glaucoma are narrow angle or closed angle glaucoma, and normal tension glaucoma, which are less common. Wide angle glaucoma occurs slowly over time and causes no pain. A cataract is a cloudy area in the lens of one or both eyes that develops slowly and results in a decrease in vision. Its symptoms comprise blurry or double vision, faded colors, trouble with bright lights, halos around light and trouble seeing at night. This book is a compilation of chapters that discuss the most vital concepts and emerging trends in the management of cataracts and glaucoma. It will also provide interesting topics for research which interested readers can take up. Through this book, we attempt to further enlighten the readers about the new concepts in this field of research.

This book is a comprehensive compilation of works of different researchers from varied parts of the world. It includes valuable experiences of the researchers with the sole objective of providing the readers (learners) with a proper knowledge of the concerned field. This book will be beneficial in evoking inspiration and enhancing the knowledge of the interested readers.

In the end, I would like to extend my heartiest thanks to the authors who worked with great determination on their chapters. I also appreciate the publisher's support in the course of the book. I would also like to deeply acknowledge my family who stood by me as a source of inspiration during the project.

Editor

1

Analysis of the Disturbances Caused by Intraocular Forced Convection Mechanism Failure

Humberto D. Silva, Eduardo D. Silva,
Maria Tamires D. Silva, Cristiana P. Dória and
Cristiane P. Dória

Abstract

In this chapter, we show the refractive error treatment result of a patient, the first author, who restarted in 2000, after a 4-year break, at the study start. According to previous publications, the treatment consists of rehydration and elimination of agglutinated, dehydrated and deposited metabolic residues in the cornea, the trabecular meshwork, the crystalline lens and the retina, as a consequence of the failure in the mechanism of intraocular mass transfer by forced convection. However, the forced movement of the metabolic mass to rehydrate one region can cause dehydration in another region. Therefore, the patient developed posterior and capsular cataract in their respective eyes, right and left. This dehydration, during the treatment, increases the difficulties for the success of the treatment. The first part is a chronological record of the most important components of the treatment. Then, the research method and the material used are discussed. The main symptoms and signs are analyzed and correlated with the failure of the mass transfer process and the accumulation of metabolic residues. The anatomy of binocular vision is analyzed as a part of the forced convection mechanism, and in conclusion, the report shows the main oculomotor functions, topographic mapping of corneas over an interval of 17 months.

Keywords: cataract, glaucoma, saccadic movement, torsional movement, refractive error, uveitis, floaters

1. Introduction

The research began in 1996 when the first author (will be called the patient) realized that after 4 h of working on a computer, his vision was blurred and, after performing other activities, the view was retrieved. Then, the patient realized the possibility of regaining his vision, which was showing the beginning of the symptoms of presbyopia. The patient presented visual acuity OD 6/10 and OS 9/10 and corrective lenses NV, OD +0.25 and OS +0.75. Work interruption occurred in the same year due to anterior recurrent uveitis of unknown cause in the left eye, which increased the intraocular pressure to 40 mmHg in the first crisis. Two years before the start on this study, the patient had his first two cases of uveitis, but the most important crisis occurred after the study began and the patient took a few days to get medical help. To control intraocular pressure, the patient received three intraocular injection on alternate days. Even with the patient's narrative that he did not feel well, the doctor reduced the dosage of medications. The patient still felt pain when pressing the left eye in the superior nasal position through the superior eyelid. The patient returned to the doctor after 2 days, having noticed the blurred image in the left eye. The physician diagnosed the recurrence of uveitis and intraocular pressure at 40 mmHg. At the end of treatment, the pain in the sclera did not exist. Many other painful inflammations had occurred in the left eye, but at this early stage, physicians consulted in Brazil and France did not prescribe any treatment. Treatment was started the next day after uveitis was diagnosed. At that time when the pain symptom occurred in the sclera, the patient used a medication eye-drop prescribed for the treatment of uveitis to impede damage progression. A single drop once was sufficient to eliminate the symptom and avoid uveitis, but when the symptom did not go away, the patient used another dose the next day. On June 15, 1998, the patient had visual acuity 8/10, with corrective lenses. The research for vision recovery was restarted in the year 2000 after an oculomotor relaxation procedure, advised by the patient's brother, who had read in a self-help book on eyesight.

After 2009, the same ophthalmologist periodically examines the patient, but sometimes the patient looks for another professional in order to obtain information from the doctor when he first examines the patient. A posterior cataract had developed in the right eye and capsular in the left eye. **Table 1** shows the lenses prescribed by doctors. The prescribed lenses do not change the direction of the elimination treatment of the intraocular metabolic residues. In 2012, ophthalmologists informed the patient that, without surgical intervention in the left eye, the patient would have great difficulty in passing the eye examination to renew his driver's license, scheduled for 2014. So, 15 days before the date of renewal, the patient underwent 12 sessions of 30-min exercise on different days with occlusion of the right eye and added 2 days without exercises. The patient was approved in the exam.

Although the patient perceived changes in visual perception during treatment progress, however, it was not possible to establish treatment phases through these changes. The changes in visual perception depend on the element being observed. The observed element can be an object, a light source or an image, with or without letters, that is near or far, in a certain environment. The environment can be dark, or light, with or without diffused light, under the influence of various luminous intensities. In addition to the environment, visual perception is severely influenced by dehydration, agglutination and the amount of metabolic residues accumulated.

The physical characteristics of the residue disposed orally vary with the progress of the treatment of recovery of sight. Eliminated residue is the one with the least resistance to movement. The movement resistance depends on the location of the accumulation region and the

Calendar date	Rx		Spherical	Cylindrical	Axis
1975	D.V.	O.D.	—	—	—
		O.S.	—	—	—
	N.V.	O.D.	+0.25	—	—
		O.S.	+0.25	—	—
1994	D.V.	O.D.	—	—	—
		O.S.	—	—	—
	N.V.	O.D.	+2.50	0.50	35°
		O.S.	+2.50	0.50	155°
December 02, 1996	D.V.	O.D.	—	—	—
		O.S.	—	—	—
	N.V.	O.D.	+0.50	—	—
		O.S.	+0.75	—	—
1997	D.V.	O.D.	+1.50	0.50	30°
		O.S.	+1.50	0.25	140°
	N.V.	O.D.	+2.50	0.50	30°
		O.S.	+2.50	0.25	140°
1999	D.V.	O.D.	+1.50	0.50	35°
		O.S.	+1.50	0.50	140°
	N.V.	O.D.	+3.50	0.50	35°
		O.S.	+3.50	0.50	140°
July 18, 2003	D.V.	O.D.	+1.50	0.50	180°
		O.S.	1.25	—	—
	N.V.	O.D.	+2.50	0.50	180°
		O.S.	+2.50	—	—
June 20, 2006	D.V.	O.D.	+1.25	0.50	65°
		O.S.	+1.00	0.50	125°
	N.V.	O.D.	+2.75	0.50	65°
		O.S.	+2.75	0.50	125°
June 30, 2006	D.V.	O.D.	+1.25	−0.50	30°
		O.S.	+1.00	−0.50	155°
	N.V.	O.D.	+2.75	−0.50	30°
		O.S.	+2.75	−0.50	155°
March 19, 2007	D.V.	O.D.	+1.00	−0.50	35°
		O.S.	+1.00	−0.50	120°
	N.V.	O.D.	+2.25	—	—
		O.S.	−2.25	—	—

Calendar date	Rx		Spherical	Cylindrical	Axis
October 01, 2012	D.V.	O.D.	—	−0.50	100°
		O.S.	−0.50	−1.50	100°
	N.V.	O.D.	+2.50	add	—
		O.S.	+2.50	add	—
November 12, 2012	D.V.	O.D.	+0.50	−0.75	90°
		O.S.	−1.00	−0.75	105°
	N.V.	O.D.	+3.25	−0.75	90°
		O.S.	+1.75	−0.75	105°
February 07, 2013	D.V.	O.D.	−0.75	—	—
		O.S.	−2.00	—	—
	N.V.	O.D.	+2.25	add	—
		O.S.	+2.25	add	—
July 22, 2013	D.V.	O.D.	+0.50	−1.25	85°
		O.S.	−1.50	−1.00	105°
	N.V.	O.D.	+2.75	add	—
		O.S.	+2.75	add	—

Table 1. Lenses prescribed by doctors.

physical and biochemical characteristics. These characteristics are mainly associated with the compositions of their components, viscosity, dehydration, color, transparency and acidity. Some of these characteristics can be observed in oral elimination.

At the beginning of treatment, it was very easy to perceive the negative afterimage, but it has not been observed for a long time. This pathology was solved. Initially, the appearance of new floaters was observed. Then, there were floaters that changed their appearance, one divided into two, maintaining a discreet connection. The oldest floater had already added new expansion, but kept its round, black core. Sometimes after the beginning of treatment, the oldest floater changes in appearance and returns to the initial appearance.

When the light source, in a dark environment, is refracted in light rays projected on the retina, it may suggest the beginning of the residue elimination phase; the perception of the colored arc, around the light source, indicates residues with a high index of refraction, very dehydrated, with great viscosity; blurry sight can indicate residues available on the cornea for disposal.

The intraocular process of accumulation of metabolic residues, as well as its intraocular process of elimination of metabolic residues, occurs essentially through the involuntary oculomotor movement that acts with the objective of producing the best projection in the temporal retina. In the process of eliminating the accumulated metabolic residue, the patient voluntarily interferes in the oculomotor movement so that the metabolic residue interferes in the projected image in the temporal retina, and then, the involuntary movement rehydrates the accumulated residues in the region, reduces its viscosity, and produces the best projection in the temporal retina. Much attention, just as there is anterior ocular torsional movement, due to the difficulty of adaptation of the cornea, a posterior ocular torsional movement can occur, cause physical tension in the optic nerve and cause normal tension glaucoma.

2. Method

Teamwork was used to interview professionals and patients. Team studies, based on the interpretation of symptoms, among others, corneal burning, tear production and resistance to visual adaptation to a fixed target, performed through the horizontal periodic movement of the head (the duration of the exercise is within the range of 5-30 min). Studies of anatomy and biophysics of the eyes as a system of dynamic action are made. Simulation of a physical model to reproduce the studies of Scheiner, apud [1], was used to associate the main refractive errors and the patient's symptomatology. Simulation of a hypothetical mathematical model was made to study the daily intraocular pressure variation. As the main form of treatment progress evaluation, a light source, at the same distance, was initially used to measure the diameter of its dispersion, evaluated in the number of adjacent diameters of the source. At the present, a traffic light is used as the light source for measurement. Visual acuity and corrective lens parameters are not used to evaluate the reduction of intraocular metabolic residue.

3. Eyesight regeneration and analysis of symptoms and signs

3.1. Materials

In this section, the main materials used for vision recovery are listed in alphabetical order, together with a brief description of the use.

Corrective lenses, +19 D, +10 D, +5 D, +2.5 D, −5D: Negative lenses were abandoned shortly after starting treatment because they did not present difficulties during exercises. Corrective lenses have been included in vision recovery exercises because anyone, without accumulation of intraocular metabolic residue, can read a text with any corrective lens.

Cotton-polyester fabric, nylon mesh: Light obstruction acts as a load for oculomotor movement. The mesh with thicker wire requires more oculomotor effort. By having a greater aperture in its mesh, the nylon mesh interferes in the elimination of the metabolic residues that are sheltered by the shadow of the light obstructed by its wires. The cotton-polyester fabric, by having a smaller opening in its mesh, can eliminate the residuals left by the nylon mesh.

Eyewear (temporal): Occlusion of temporal visual fields to increase the power of the rectus and ciliary muscles without the help of the oblique muscles.

Eyewear (nasal): Occlusion of the nasal visual fields to stimulate the movements related to the projection of the image in the nasal retina (needed but with little use).

Pinhole glasses: Used only at the beginning of treatment as a test. The use of these glasses can cause patient well-being because it eliminates a small volume of metabolic residue, but the volume eliminated is insufficient to solve the problems of refraction error. In addition, its use is not recommended during activities involving patient control or movement, such as driving a vehicle or walking. The holes in the lenses select the visual axis direction, and Scheiner's experiment apud [1] shows that the selection of the visual direction presents to the patient's target at different distances, making it impossible to evaluate the distance of the target and cause an accident.

Sun: Treatment using sunlight has been used several times because it is a source of light with greater intraocular penetration power. It is because of its power that, when looking at the Sun, one or more regions become dark. This strong light causes movements in the dehydrated and viscous metabolic residue that becomes opaque for some time, the accumulation region. Opacity ends due to involuntary intraocular movement. It is the involuntary movement of adaptation to the dark.

Compact fluorescent lamp: Used as fixation point.

Treadmill equipment: Ocular exercise performed on a treadmill does not cause sleep. Six is a great speed for the exercises. It is necessary that there is ample front and lateral visual space.

3.2. Symptoms and signs

During the exercises, there may be, in one or both eyes, fiery sensation along with bloodshot eye. After, there may be itching. Sweat can be severe on one side of the head or on both sides. Exercises can stimulate bruxism, pain in the jaw joint, tongue, and marks on the face. Although there is no direct relationship in many cases, this takes a lot of time and effort to perform the image fusion in a certain direction, or to maintain the fusion of images during the movement of the fixation point. By carrying out the exertion for a long time, it can divert the attention of the patient and it passes on to transmit force to these other parts of the body. After the exercises, sight may become blurry or there may be some other painless modification. For a short time, there may be a foreign body sensation in the cornea or intraocular. There may be acute pain of short duration.

Auditory perception: In 2003, on routine examination, the patient became aware of the absence of 6 kHz frequency perception and the presence of permanent noise, only in the left ear. In the analysis performed by an otorhinolaryngologist, no other pathology was found. In subsequent years, the patient was evaluated to verify the evolution of auditory perception. The patient began to perceive small hearing in the frequency of 6 kHz and reduced the perception in the adjacent frequencies, including in the right ear. Currently, the patient has noticed some relationship between the exercises for recovery of sight and the perceived noise, because the noise in the right ear stops and the amplitude of the remaining noise varies with the direction of the exercise. Then, among the criteria of choice of exercises are the direction of greater variation in the amplitude of the noise and displacement of fixed images. Thus, the variation in noise should be considered, in the choice of the exercise for the eyesight recovery.

Dizziness: Exercising may cause dizziness, and in this way, the patient should hold onto the equipment support during the exercises.

Imbalance: May be perceptible or imperceptible. The imperceptible can cause the patient to knock down nearby objects, can in certain situations move one or more steps, as if drunk, for a short time, can cause pain in the sciatic nerve, and can produce dry callus on the bottom of the feet (**Figure 1**). Sometime later, they suffered fatigue in the right leg. Tiredness settled in the upper posterior region of the knee and then settled in the upper posterior region of the thigh, and the same symptom started in the left leg. This caused a great deal of suffering. It was not thought to be due to muscle strain. The hypothesis was that there was a problem of balance, since the dry callus had already been treated, and balance requires many activities of the lower limbs. Early in the morning, when the patient was seated, he began the eye exercise with eyewear (temporal), to strengthen and straighten the muscles, the symptoms immediately disappeared. The patient worked all day with the symptom of one who had walked for a long time. Two days later, the patient spent a lot of time with the symptom of muscle relaxation in both legs.

Torticollis: The most common signs are the sensation of contraction and pain on one side of the neck that can radiate to the back. It can be caused by stimuli of recurring displacement of the projected image on the retina.

3.3. Analysis of some ocular pathologies

The analysis was based on the progress of the recovery of the patient's vision, in addition to the conclusions reached in our other publications. The ocular refractive error has its origin in the accumulation, dehydration and agglutination of the intraocular metabolic residue [2] caused by the defect in the mechanical system of mass transfer in the cornea (between the corneal layers) [2–4], trabecular meshwork [5], lens [6] and retina [7, 8]. Congenital and acquired pathologies increased the mass transfer deficiency.

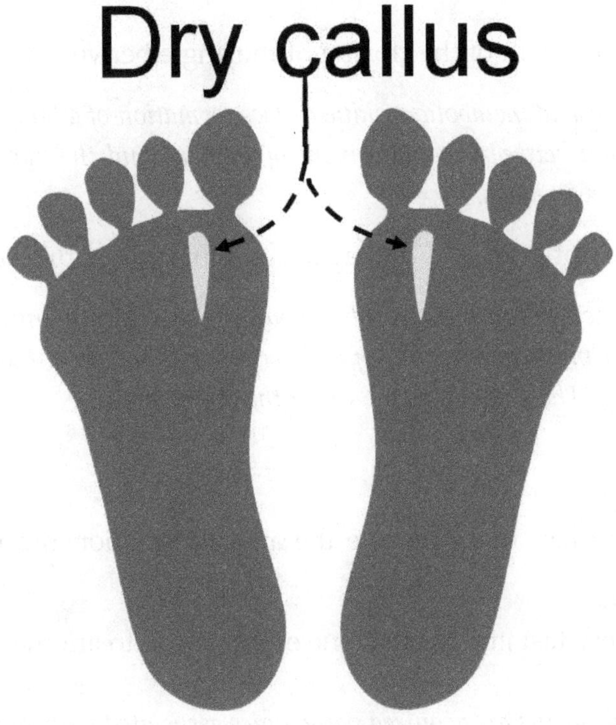

Figure 1. Diagram showing the dry callus location.

Cataract: It is the accumulation of dehydrated metabolic residue in the lens. As the residue is translucent, its dehydration is opaque.

Because it is an accumulation, it is natural to increase the volume and rigidity of the lens, as well as to associate the age of the person with its consequences, among them visual acuity. During the exercises, there may be an intraocular foreign body sensation as well as a small, rapid and uncomfortable intraocular pain because of cataracts.

Dark adaptation: The eye takes longer than 20 min to fully adapt from bright sunlight to dark [9].

The eyes are organs of the visual system. The eye transmits the luminous image to the retina that, through electrochemical impulses, transmits to the brain. The image interpretation can trigger a physical protection action, that is, the person through the image can move the hand or foot to perform a body protection action. The hand and foot take well less than 20 min to make the maximum displacement. So "the eye is a radar that spends 20 minutes to identify an attack, and in defence, it can trigger a missile attacking the target in a minute, so this radar is not for this operation." This means a serious visual impairment. A person without accumulated intraocular metabolic residue can look at the sun and then read a text written in black ink on white paper. In the appendix, it is shown that the adaptation time to the dark is not greater than 0.24 s (Eq. 7).

Glaucoma:

- **Open-angle:** It is caused by slow obstruction of the trabecular meshwork, resulting in increased eye pressure.

In Ref. [5], *it shows how the metabolic residues coming from the cornea can slowly obstruct the trabecular meshwork, increasing the resistance of the aqueous humor and, consequently, increasing the intraocular pressure.*

- **Angle-closure:** It is the result of the closing of the angle between the iris and the cornea.

The accumulation of dehydrated metabolic residue causes formation of a large refractive error and may cause defective coordination between the movement of the lens and the movement of the oculomotor muscles. See in keratoconus analysis.

- **Normal-tension:** The optic nerve is damaged without the eye pressure being too high [5].

The accumulation of intraocular metabolic residue modifies the shape, volume and mass of the eye, and as a result, the oculomotor muscles move out of their ergonomic movement and change the position of the eye in the ocular cavity. These changes can strain the optic nerve.

Eye movements [10]:

- **Conjugate:** They are those that preserve the angular relationship between the right and left eyes.
- **Saccadic:** They are very fast jumps from one eye position to another.

Saccadic and vergence movements are acquired pathologies associated with agglutinated metabolic residues. These clusters form intraocular lenses, which project images into the retina, in different places.

In 1619, Scheiner described these images apud [1]. *Then, when the visual axis changes agglutination, the image of interest jumps from the fovea to another location. This jump causes a rapid movement of the eye in the opposite direction (saccadic movement) to transfer the image to fovea. If the jump of the eye causes the return of the visual axis to the anterior agglutination in order to cause recurrent periodic movement, then it can cause photosensitive epilepsy* [2].

- **Vergence:** Eye movement for fusion of retinal images and obtaining binocular vision.

Floaters: These are deposits of metabolic residue, in the cornea or lens, with various sizes, shape, consistency and refractive index and can be transparent, translucent or opaque.

During treatment, the oldest floater is opaque, but on many days, it presents itself in different forms and opacity. Another floater was divided in two and maintained connection between both.

Headache: This is a warning symptom of a greater problem that is occurring in the body.

You should not take medicine and you should do exercises. If you delay in taking action, the treatment is much longer. Precisely, on the day that the writing of this work is being finalized, the right eyeball of the patient presented a pain sensation, similar to the occurrence, shortly after the injection in the left eye of the same patient. It is probable that the right eye has performed movements that cause mechanical tension in the optic nerve. If immediate corrective action is not provided, it can cause glaucoma with normal pressure. In both cases, the treatment is the same given in relation to the imperceptible imbalance of the body, motor coordination and increase of the power of the rectus muscles.

Keratoconus: Changes of the cornea to a cone-like shape and its thickness reduction.

The torsional accommodation of the cornea is a movement of variation of the radius of its curvature. This may be caused by personal habits and ocular structure, which can progressively increase the radius of curvature, causing keratoconus, or by modifying its cylindrical periphery to the conical shape, blocking the drainage of the aqueous humor, causing angle-closure glaucoma. **Figure 2** *shows the two possibilities.*

Ocular dominance: This is the fixation of the eye with less movement (called the dominant eye) on the target and the adjustment of the contralateral one.

In Ref. [4], *it is treated as visual impairment.*

Phosphene: This can be directly induced by retina mechanical stimulation. It is easy to check when rubbing or applying pressure to closed eyes.

In Ref. [7], *it is written without naming the acquired pathology. "The metabolic secretions are accumulated in the retina forming clusters without any regularity therefore when the eyes are pressed on*

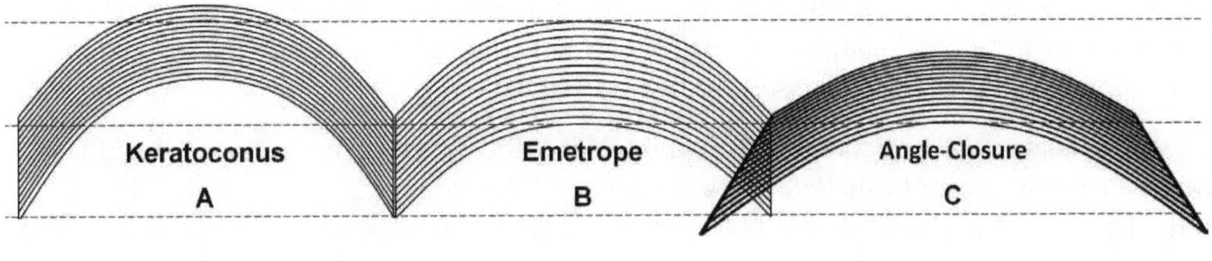

Figure 2. Scheme of the formation of keratoconus, and the angular closure.

by the hands, the photoreceptors are also pressed, and the process affects its biochemical transduction that produces an electrical signal to the brain which interprets it as a light signal." At the present, only, some blue dots are still perceived.

Photophobia: It is a symptom of abnormal light sensitivity.

When the iris fails to reduce interference from the brightness of the incident light to improve the sharpness of the temporal retinal projection. This is one of the effects of accumulation of intraocular metabolic residue. If the physician needs to use different corrective lenses between the exams with and without dilated pupils, it is necessary to verify the need to eliminate the stagnant metabolic residues in regions that are not usually used to design images in the retina.

Refractive error

- **Myopia:** When there is a need for the use of concave lens, to correct the convergence of light rays.
- **Hyperopia:** When there is a need for the use of convective lens, to correct the convergence of light rays.
- **Presbyopia:** When there is a need for the use of bifocal or progressive lens, to correct the convergence of light rays.
- **Astigmatism:** When there is a need for the use of cylindrical lens, to correct the convergence of light rays.

In Ref. [2], *it is shown that refractive error causing myopia, hyperopia, presbyopia and astigmatism has the same origin: dehydration and agglutination, intraocular, of accumulated metabolic residues.*

4. Binocular vision anatomy

Binocular eyesight uses the image fusion for greater visual accuracy. **Figure 3** shows, schematically, the main elements to explain the oculomotor control mechanism, obtained from the images projected on the retina.

Binocular vision of the fixation point on a screen (F in **Figure 3**) occurs when the visual axes of the eyes converge at this point. The F-point protrudes into the central fovea at points F_R and F_L (**Figure 3**), respectively, in the right and left eyes. The two visual axes define the visual plane. The visual plane intercepts the retina in both eyes on two anatomical horizontal meridians, in the right and left eyes. Each anatomical horizontal meridian has two sides, the temporal and the nasal. The nasal anatomical horizontal meridian includes a segment, corresponding to the optic disc, which does not send an image to the brain.

The nasal anatomical horizontal meridian intercepts the neural communication periphery of the optic nerve, closer to the left fovea, at the P_{LL} point (**Figure 3**). In the right eye, the P_{LR} retinal point is the closest to the fovea, obtained by the interception of the temporal anatomical horizontal meridian with the corresponding neural communication periphery of the

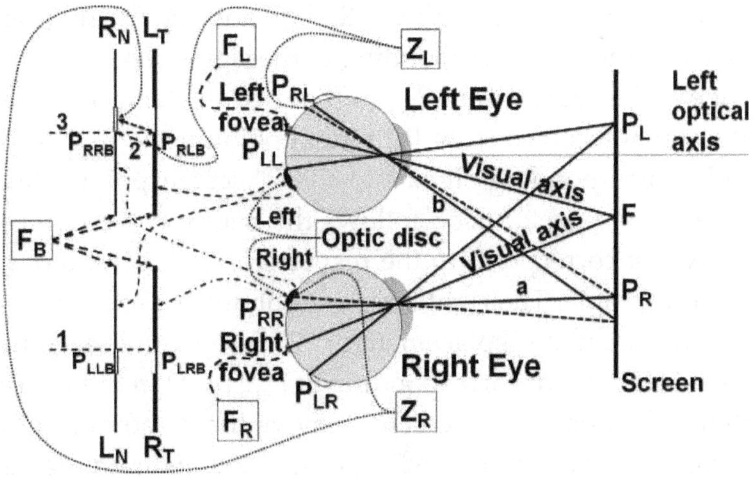

Figure 3. Binocular vision representation scheme.

contralateral optic disc (projection of the contralateral blind spot periphery). If the P_{LL} and P_{LR} retinal points are the neurologically corresponding signals to the P_L screen point retinal projections, the image fusion is perfect. The projection on the right temporal anatomical horizontal meridian, containing the P_{LR} point, sends the visual signals to the ipsilateral cerebral hemisphere in the R_T line (right temporal side), shown in **Figure 3**. The projection on the left nasal anatomical horizontal meridian, containing the P_{LL} point, sends the visual signals to the contralateral cerebral hemisphere, in the L_N line (left nasal side), shown in **Figure 3**. In the L_N line, there is a small segment for the optic disc representation. The arrow "1" locates in the brain at the intersection with the L_N line and the neural point P_{LLB} (left horizontal nasal anatomical meridian) corresponding to the signal received from P_{LL} retinal point and reaches the R_T line at the neural point P_{LRB} (right horizontal temporal anatomical meridian) corresponding to the signal received from P_{LR} retinal point. If the P_{LLB} and P_{LRB} neural points are the neurologically corresponding signals to the P_L screen point retinal projections, the images fusion is perfect, that is, the horizontal diameter of the contralateral blind spot is projected on the R_T line white highlight, indicated by "1" arrow.

The nasal anatomical horizontal meridian intercepts the neural communication periphery of the optic nerve, closer to the right fovea, at the P_{RR} point (**Figure 3**). In the left eye, the P_{RL} retinal point is the closest point of the fovea, obtained by the interception of the temporal anatomical horizontal meridian with the neural corresponding of communication periphery of the contralateral optic disc (projection of the contralateral blind spot periphery). If the P_{RR} and P_{RL} retinal points are the neurologically corresponding signals to the P_R screen point retinal projections, the image fusion is perfect. In this case, retinal points are not the neurologically corresponding signals to the P_R screen point retinal projections; therefore, there is no fusion of images, and there is binocular diplopia. The projection on the left temporal anatomical horizontal meridian, containing the P_{RL} point, sends the visual signals to the ipsilateral cerebral hemisphere in the L_T line (left temporal side) shown in **Figure 3** diagram. The projection on the right nasal anatomical horizontal meridian, containing the P_{RR} point, sends the visual signals to the contralateral cerebral hemisphere in the R_N line (right nasal side) shown in **Figure 3** diagram. In the R_N line, there is a small segment for the optic disc representation. Arrow "2" locates in the brain at the intersection with the R_N line and the neural point P_{RRB} (right horizontal nasal anatomical meridian) corresponding to the signal received from P_{RR} retinal point and reaches the L_T line at the neural point P_{RLB} (left horizontal temporal anatomical meridian) corresponding to the signal received from P_{RL} retinal point. If the P_{RRB} and P_{RLB} neural points are the neurologically corresponding signals to the P_R screen point retinal projections, the image fusion is perfect. The image fusion follows the neural correspondence shown by the "3" arrow, which does not correspond to the respective P_R screen point retinal projections; thus, there is binocular diplopia. The right superior oblique muscle action can accommodate the cornea to perform the angular displacement of "2" arrow until reaching "3" arrow (make the Z_L point coincide with P_{RL} point corresponding to P_{RLB} point in brain). That is, intersect "a" line (**Figure 3**) with the "b" line on the screen, or move the Z_R point (**Figure 3**), projected on the optic disc of the right eye, to overlap the P_{RR} point or P_{RRB} in brain. As the control is contralateral, the right superior oblique muscle action moves the Z_L point until it coincides with the P_{RL} point, that is, the horizontal diameter of the contralateral blind spot is projected on the LT line white highlight, indicated by "3" arrow.

5. Conclusion

As is well known, the brain is "cross-wired" with body movement control and superior oblique muscle but is ipsilateral to the other oculomotor muscles. For the reception of visual signals, the brain is ipsilateral to the projection in the temporal retina and contralateral to the projection in the nasal retina. In the binocular limit of lateral vision, the nose contralateral shadow is the contralateral temporal projection, so that the ipsilateral nasal projection is the only contralateral control signal of the third and sixth cranial nerve functions. Therefore, contralateral ocular movement occurs only under the influence of the projections in the ipsilateral eye. The image fusion influences only the contralateral movement of the superior oblique muscle to avoid binocular diplopia. In summary, the ipsilateral and contralateral nasal projections form the contralateral oculomotor control signals, and the ipsilateral temporal projection transmits, for the brain, the reference signal in motor control of the contralateral superior oblique muscle. In addition, the inferior oblique muscle can correct some angular deviation of ipsilateral temporal projection, without any influence of control of the superior oblique ipsilateral muscle (it does not have a reference image for motor control). In this way, it is easy to understand the contralateral influence resulting from a monocular stimulus.

Rectus muscles: Its main function is to maintain the designed fixation point in the fovea centralis. The superior and inferior rectus muscles avoid and stabilize the vertical displacement of the ipsilateral retinal projection, and the lateral and medial rectus muscles avoid and stabilize the horizontal displacement of the ipsilateral retinal projection. Maintaining eyesight at a fixation point is extremely important for proper accommodation of the crystalline lens and cornea. The fixation point can be a light source or not, and it can be fixed or movable and can be in an ambience with or without changing the lighting level. Vision may be with or without ocular occlusion, may be with or without corrective lenses and may or may not be through a mesh. The head may have a rotating, extension and flexing motion, or it may remain motionless. These are possible combinations that depend on the goal to be achieved. Exercise can cause itching in the sclera nasal region.

Ciliary muscle: It has the main function of maintaining and stabilizing the projection in the ipsilateral temporal fovea and giving it the same dimension as in the contralateral nasal fovea image. These muscles also have the ability to correct the distance from the fixation point, which may be invisible to the eye and act as a mass transfer mechanism by forced convection in the lens.

Superior oblique muscle: It has the main function of enlarging or reducing the projection in the horizontal nasal anatomical meridian, so that the same projected image in the periphery of the optical disc is the same projected image in the corresponding neural region of the periphery of this optic disc, in the contralateral temporal retina. The deviation in the ipsilateral temporal projection causes a force antagonistic to the superior obliquus muscle movement.

Inferior oblique muscle: It has the main function of correcting the angular deviation of the projection in the temporal retina in relation to the projected image in the contralateral nasal retina. The torsional accommodation of the cornea is a joint action of the oculomotor muscles to obtain fusion of the temporal and contralateral nasal images, in addition to varying the intraocular pressure. This accommodation is the mechanism of forced convective mass transfer on the cornea and retina, and it may be inferior, cylindrical or superior, but the difficulty in twisting the cornea may cause twisting of the eyes. Because of the cornea torsional accommodation, a circle in the binocular view can project with the same radius in the retinas of the eyes, with duplication of the monocular vision information, adjustable, and able to obtain a much greater mathematical precision than the accuracy of monocular vision, in accordance with human perception.

Iris: It is a thin circular structure with the main function of reducing incident light when this brightness interferes with the sharpness of the temporal retinal projection as well as diaphragmatic action, to avoid the aqueous humor return, when the pressure in the anterior chamber is greater than the pressure in the posterior chamber due to corneal accommodation.

Eyelid movement: It has the main function of mechanical transport of nutrients and metabolic residues, in addition to being able to reduce the ocular opening voluntarily or involuntarily, when the iris reaches the minimum limit of its opening. The eyelid, on a regular basis, spreads tears, for rehydration and entrainment of the metabolic residue throughout the anterior ocular surface. Tears and metabolic residues are drawn into the puncta (an opening near the nasal bridge) by capillary action and conducted to lacrimal sac through the lacrimal canaliculi and then to the nasal cavity through the nasolacrimal duct. In the nasal cavity, the tear goes out through the nose or the metabolic residue can dehydrate; the resulting mucus accumulates in the nasal cavity; or the viscous residue passes through the throat and is eliminated orally or through the digestive tract. Elimination of the metabolic residue during sleep can cause a very inflamed throat, which may be accompanied by hoarseness for a few days. Cough and sneezing may occur with the expulsion of metabolic residue. Shedding of tears (or eye discharge) of one or both eyes may occur in response to the elimination of metabolic residue from the corneal epithelium, and it can last more than a day. The elimination of metabolic residue in the cornea can be accompanied by the sensation of foreign body in the eye.

Because of the personal habits, the mobile intraocular mass may remain stagnant for a long time, so the metabolic secretions of this medium can dehydrate by decantation, increasing its viscosity and, consequently, increasing the absorption and refraction of light penetrating the eyes. This is the process of accumulation of metabolic residues in the cornea, the trabecular meshwork, the lens and the retina, causing the most known intraocular problems such as refractive errors, keratoconus, glaucoma, cataract, retinal detachment, retinitis pigmentosa and macular degeneration among other problems, which may be added with other factors. Involuntary oculomotor movement exists to reduce the refractive error of the projected image in the temporal retina. However, this involuntary movement can add other problems such as change in the volume and shape of the eyeball, cornea and lens. However, this same involuntary movement can be used to rehydrate and remove the intraocular metabolic residue, in the form of solution or suspension.

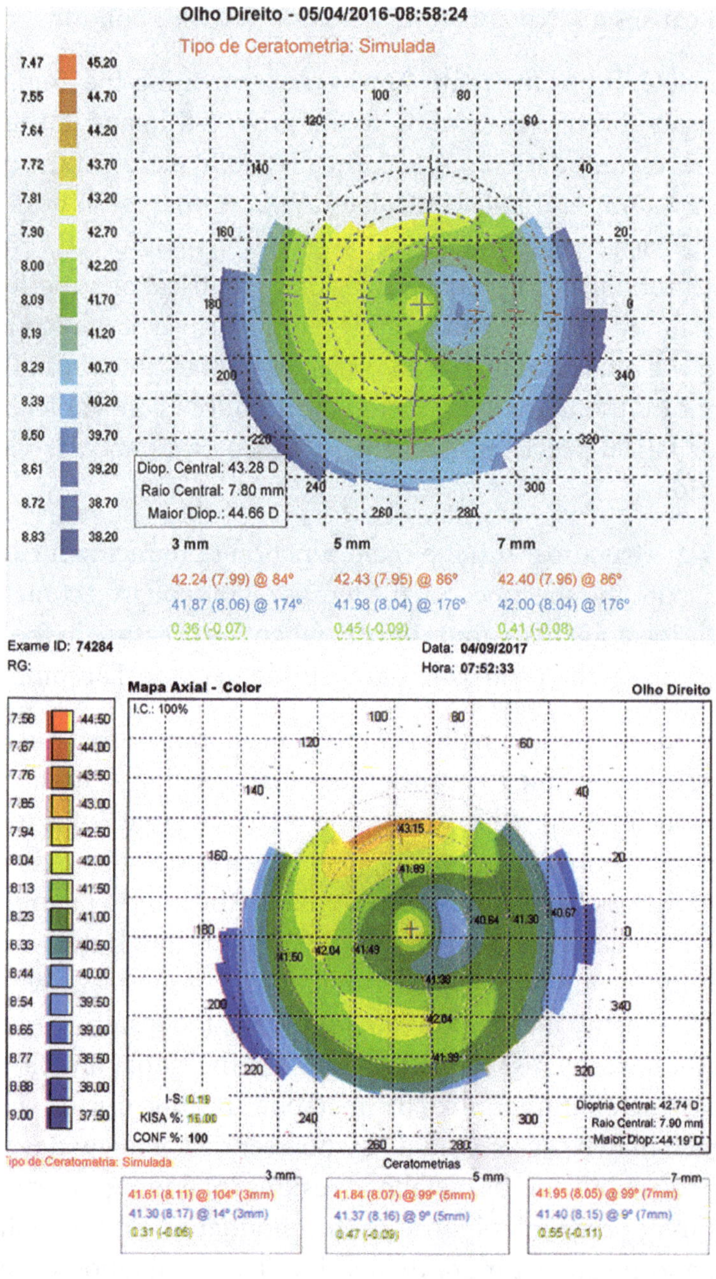

Figure 4. Corneal topography of the right eye performed on April 04, 2016, and September 05, 2017.

From the examinations performed on the patient, only a computerized corneal topography could provide some information to evaluate the progress of the treatment. For each eye and in both, it was necessary to add, on examination, the complementary volume, surplus volume and volume to be distributed, to obtain a uniform corneal lens. At the end of the work, these volumes will be null. **Figure 4** shows the corneal topography of the right eye performed on April 04, 2016, and September 05, 2017, and **Figure 5** shows the result of the same exam for the left eye. Visually, it is possible to verify the progress of the work performed, but there is no measure that can evaluate the volume of metabolic mass moved in the cornea, during 17 months. The region of the left cornea, with the most dehydrated metabolic mass, is indicated in the last examination, shown in **Figure 5**. This region has lower diopter and higher viscosity. Its rehydration causes a foreign body sensation in the cornea, but because of cataract, it can cause foreign body sensation intraocular.

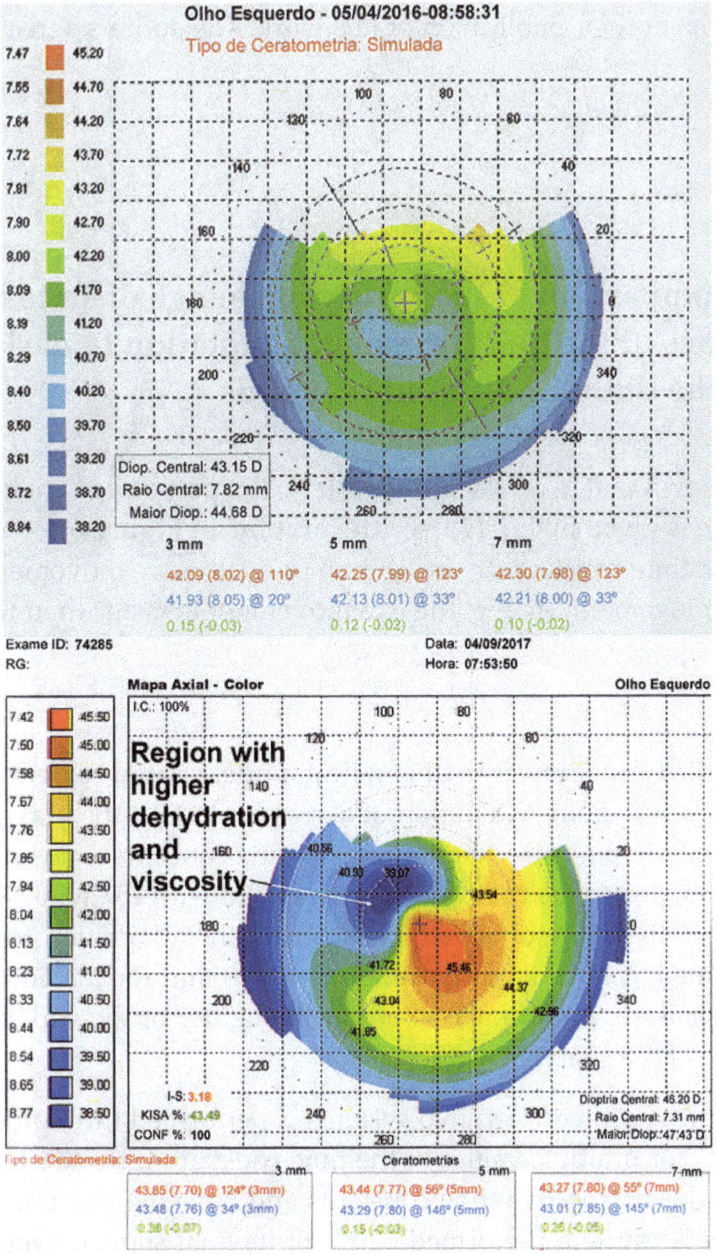

Figure 5. Corneal topography of the left eye performed on April 04, 2016, and September 05, 2017.

Acknowledgements

To God for having helped the first author, in troubles during many years of suffering that led him to become an analytical observer of events in his own body, because of his mother, under the doctor's permission, 15 days before the birth of the first author, traveled by plane. In addition, by helping us to coexist, long ago, with the harms of internal political and economic decisions. For Marcos, brother of the first two authors, who showed in 1999, in a self-help book, the importance of oculomotor relaxation for the eyesight treatment. To colleagues, of the first two authors, ANDES-SN Sindicato Nacional members, and its Seção Sindicato ADUFEPE members, who, during the intervals of some of the societies' meetings, provided with important scientific information for the study. To those who were interviewed to friends, colleagues and family members who directly or indirectly have contributed to this work. There was no public or private financial participation for publication of this work. The authors agree with the individual mentions.

A. Appendix

A.1. Dynamic comparison of the agility of change of state among different activities of the body, eyesight adaptation to dark and movements of the limbs and superior eyelids

In Ref. [5], it was shown that in a first-order system, the percentage change of the final state from an initial state is given by Eq. (1) (see the graphic in **Figure 6**), where $e = 2.71828$, t is the time and τ is the time constant. In the human body, the eye movement has less constant time than the arm movement, that is, the eye movement is faster than the arm movement.

$$f(t) = 100 \cdot (1 - e^{-t/\tau}) \tag{1}$$

In this appendix, a first-order linear mathematical model is used to determine the time constant (numerical value of agility evaluation of a system) to find the maximum displacement time of the upper limbs in personal defense, considering concepts exposed and the maximum time with eyes closed, due to the movement of the eyelid with 287 winks per minute [5]. The result is compared to the value obtained, considering the adaptation to dark with 20 min. With the data obtained, it is verified that the time of 20 min for the adaptation to the dark is unacceptable, because it would have to admit the agility of the superior members much greater than the one of the vision.

The verification of the speed between two systems is performed through the percentage execution of the activity for multiple values of the time constant. If two systems named "A" and "B" with τ_A and τ_B their respective time constants and have the relation $\tau_A = 2\tau_B$, then, when time is equal to τ_A, "A" system performed 63.2% of its final state; however, "B" system has

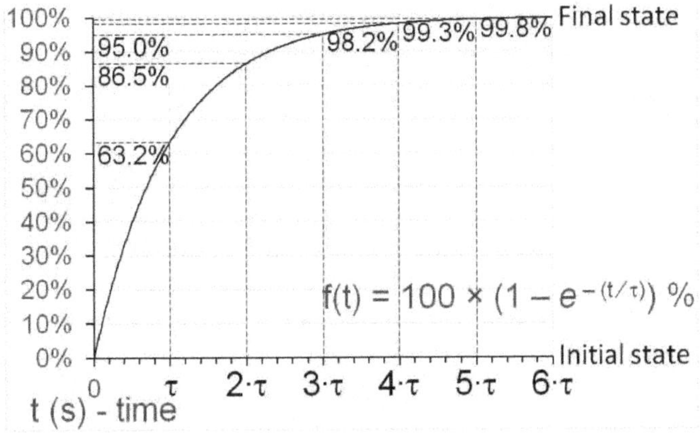

Figure 6. Graph of the function $f(t) = 100 \cdot (1 - e - t/\tau)$.

already achieved 86.5%. Therefore, the system with the shortest time constant is the fastest, in this case the "B" system.

a. **Eyelid**—287 flashes per min [5]

To simulate the movement of the eyelid, you should consider the maximum distance traveled by the eyelid should be considered as 100%. In the initial state, the eyelid is closed (or open) when the instantaneous time is equal to zero and, in the final state, the eyelid is open (or closed) when the instantaneous time is equal to τ_e, $2\tau_e$, $3\tau_e$, $4\tau_e$, $5\tau_e$, $6\tau_e$ or more, depending on the accuracy.

When t is equal to τ, the system executes 63% of the activity. When t is equal to 2τ, the system executes 86% of the activity. When t is equal to 3τ, 4τ or 5τ, the system executes 95, 98 or 99% of the activity, respectively.

Eq. (2) gives the time t_{oc} that the eyelid passes to open or close the eye, in seconds.

$$t_{oc} = 60/(2 \cdot 287) = 0.10453\ \text{s} \tag{2}$$

If **0.10453** represents 99% of the opened or closed eyelid, then the minimum time constant is $\tau_i = 0.10453/5 = 0.02091\ \text{s}$ and, if 95% of the maximum time constant is $\tau_a = 0.10453/3 = 0.03484\ \text{s}$, then the eyelid time constant τ_e is in the range $0.02091\ \text{s} \le \tau_e \le 0.03484\ \text{s}$. Eq. (3) gives the eyelid mean time constant τ_{em}.

$$\tau_{em} = (0.02091 + 0.03484)/2 = 0.02788\ \text{s} \tag{3}$$

Thus, the eyelid system completes its activity between $3\tau_{em}$ and $5\tau_{em}$, so its average time is $4\tau_{em}$, and the eyelid opens or closes the eye with time t_e given by Eq. (4), which is considered the transition time for the state change (from opened or closed eye to closed or opened eye or from light to dark).

$$t_e = 4 \cdot 0.02788 = 0.1115\ \text{s} \tag{4}$$

The neural system of reception and comprehension of the retinal image spends the same eyelid time t_e, to complete the whole process, after the conclusion of the eyelid movement, so that the total processing time t_{na} is given by Eq. (5), for the situation **a** (eyelid—287 flashes per minute).

$$t_{na} = (1+1) \cdot t_e = 2 \cdot 0.1115 = 0.223\,\text{s} \tag{5}$$

If the neural system has the completion time t_{na}, its time constant varies between $\tau_{nia} = 0.223/5 = 0.0446\ \text{s}$ and $\tau_{naa} = 0.223/3 = 0.07433\ \text{s}$ and then the neural time constant τ_{na} is in the range $0.0446\,\text{s} \le \tau_{na} \le 0.07433\,\text{s}$. Eq. (6) gives the neural mean time constant τ_{nma}, for the situation **a** (eyelid—287 flashes per minute).

$$\tau_{nma} = (0.0446 + 0.07433)/2 = 0.05947\,\text{s} \tag{6}$$

The neural system completes its activity between $3\tau_{nma}$ and $5\tau_{nma}$, so its average time is $4\tau_{nma}$, and the image interpretation occurs with time t_{na} given by Eq. (7), which is considered the transition time for the state change (the time of interpretation of the retinal image).

$$t_{na} = 4 \cdot 0.05947 = 0.23786\ \text{s} \tag{7}$$

The superior limb movement system, to reach the maximum displacement, takes twice the time t_{na} of the reception and comprehension of the retinal image process, after its completion, so that Eq. 8 gives the total processing time t_{sa}, that is, slightly less than one second for superior limb maximal displacement.

$$t_{sa} = (2+1) \cdot t_{na} = 3 \cdot 0.23786 = 0.71359\ \text{s} \tag{8}$$

b. Dark adaptation—30 min [9]

If the neural system has the completion time $t_{nb} = 20.0\ \text{min}$ (in Ref. [9] cites 30 min), its time constant varies between $\tau_{nib} = 20/5 = 4.0\ \text{min}$ and $\tau_{nab} = 20/3 = 6.66667\ \text{min}$, that is, $4.0\ \text{min} \le \tau_{nb} \le 6.66667\ \text{min}$. Eq. 9 gives the neural mean time constant τ_{nmb}, for the situation **b** (dark adaptation—30 min [9]).

$$\tau_{nmb} = (4.0 + 6.666)/2 = 5.33333\ \text{min} \tag{9}$$

The neural system completes its activity between $3\tau_{nmb}$ and $5\tau_{nmb}$, so its average time is $4\tau_{nmb}$, and the image interpretation occurs with time Eq. (10), which is considered the transition time for the state change (the time of interpretation of the retinal image).

$$t_{nb} = 4 \cdot 5.33333 = 21.33333\ \text{min} \tag{10}$$

The movement system of the superior limbs takes twice the time, t_{nb}, to reach the maximum displacement of the reception and comprehension of the retinal image process, after its completion, so that Eq. 11 gives the total processing time t_{sb}, that is, slightly more than an hour for superior limb maximal displacement.

$$t_{sb} = (2+1) \cdot t_{nb} = 3 \cdot 21.33333 = 64.0 \text{ min} \tag{11}$$

Thus, the mathematical model and its parameters have shown that if the measured eyelid movement, 287 flashes per minute [5], is considered as a reference, it obtains, for the displacement of the upper limbs, the time $t_{sa} = 0.71359$ s, compatible with the reality. However, if the time of 20 min (30 min [9]) is considered as a reference for adaptation to the dark, it obtains, for the displacement of the upper limbs, the time $t_{sb} = 64$ min, incompatible with reality.

The exposed model does not consider dead time (the time lag between the beginning of stimulus given to a system and the beginning of resulting response); however, it is possible to adopt $t_{na} = 0.23786$ s and $t_{nb} = 21.33333$ min as the dead time in the respective simulations. In this case, the dead time, considering the eyelid movement, is compatible with reality and confirms the simplified representation of the event, whereas for the second case, the waiting time is incompatible for the defense of the body, therefore, or the parameter adopted is incompatible or the model chosen is not applicable. This work adopted the first alternative.

Author details

Humberto D. Silva[1]*, Eduardo D. Silva[1], Maria Tamires D. Silva[2], Cristiana P. Dória[2] and Cristiane P. Dória[2]

*Address all correspondence to: hdoria@ufpe.br

1 Universidade Federal de Pernambuco, Recife, Brazil

2 Independent Professional, Recife, Brazil

References

[1] Werner L, Trindade F, Pereira F, Werner L. Physiology of accommodation and presbyopia. Arquivos Brasileiros de Oftalmologia. 2000;**63**:503-509. DOI: 10.1590/S0004

[2] Silva HD, Dória LCP, Dória CP, Dória CP, Silva MCTD, Silva HD Jr, MTD S. Simulation of the Errors of Refraction in the Human Eye. In: Öchsner A, da Silva LFM, Altenbach H, editors. Analysis and Design of Biological Materials and Structures. Berlin, Heidelberg: Springer Berlin Heidelberg; 2012. pp. 187-200. DOI: https://doi.org/10.1007/978-3-642-22131-6_15

[3] Silva HD, Dória LCP, Dória CP, Dória CP, Silva Md CTD, Júnior HDS, Silva MTD. Nutrients and metabolic secretions transfer in cornea. Defect and Diffusion Forum. 2011;**312-315**:737-742. DOI: 10.4028/www.scientific.net/DDF.312-315.737

[4] Silva HD, Dória LCP, Dória CP, Dória CP, do Carmo M, Silva TD, Silva HD Jr, Silva MTD. Analysis of failure mechanism of forced convection in the cornea of the human eye. In: Öchsner A, da Silva LFM, Altenbach H, editors. Characterization and Development of Biosystems and Biomaterials. Berlin, Heidelberg: Springer-Berlin-Heidelberg; 2013. pp. 217-226. DOI: http://www.springer.com/materials/biomaterials/book/978-3-642-31469-8

[5] Silva HD, Dória LCP, Dória CP, Dória CP, Carmo M, Silva TD, Silva HD Jr, Silva MTD. Simulation of variation of intraocular pressure. In: Öchsner A, da Silva LFM, Altenbach H, editors. Characterization and Development of Biosystems and Biomaterials. Berlin, Heidelberg: Springer-Berlin-Heidelberg; 2013. pp. 235-253. DOI: http://www.springer.com/materials/biomaterials/book/978-3-642-31469-8

[6] Silva HD, Dória Silva E, Dória LCP, Dória CP, Dória CP, Silva Md CTD, Júnior HDS, Silva MTD. Forced convection mechanism failure in the eye can cause cataract. Defect and Diffusion Forum. 2013;**334-335**:225-229. DOI: 10.4028/www.scientific.net/DDF.334-335.225

[7] Silva HD, Dória LCP, Dória CP, Dória CP, Silva Md CTD, Júnior HDS, Silva MTD. Mass transport mechanism in the retina of the human eye. Defect and Diffusion Forum. 2012;**326-328**:18-23. DOI: 10.4028/www.scientific.net/DDF.326-328.18

[8] Agarwal M, Ulmer JL, Chandra T, Klein AP, Mark LP, Mohan S. Imaging correlates of neural control of ocular movements. European Radiology. 2016;**26**:2193-2205. DOI: 10.1007/s00330-015-4004-9

[9] Bye LA, Modi NC, Stanford M, editors. Basic Sciences for Ophthalmology. 1st ed. United Kingdom: Oxford University Press; 2013. 288 pp. 0191004073, 9780191004070

[10] Silva HD, Dória Silva E, Dória LCP, Dória CP, Dória CP, Silva Md CTD, Júnior HDS, Silva MTD. Forced convection mechanism failure in the eye can cause macular degeneration. Defect and Diffusion Forum. 2013;**334-335**:230-234. DOI: 10.4028/www.scientific.net/DDF.334-335.230

2

Newer Intraocular Pressure Measurement Techniques

Maria Letizia Salvetat, Marco Zeppieri and Paolo Brusini

Abstract

An elevated intraocular pressure (IOP) has been shown to be one of the major risk factors for glaucoma. It is of utmost importance to obtain accurate and precise IOP when dealing with patients with ocular hypertension and glaucoma, especially patients who have undergone ocular surgery. Goldmann applanation tonometer (GAT) was first introduced in the 1950s and is still currently considered as the gold standard to measure IOP. Although the reproducibility of GAT has shown to be quite good, its accuracy provides several limitations. In particular, IOP measurements taken with GAT have been demonstrated to be influenced by many corneal parameters, including central thickness, curvature, astigmatism and biomechanics. Other disadvantages of GAT include the need for local anesthetic drops, for fluorescein and for a slitlamp. Several different methods have been proposed to overcome the disadvantages found in GAT. The newer devices used as alternative tonometric methods include the iCare rebound tonometer, the BioResonator applanation resonance tonometer, the Pascal dynamic contour tonometer, the ocular response analyzer, the Corvis ST pachy-tonometer and Ocuton S. The precision and accuracy of these alternative tonometric methods in comparison with GAT have been reported and discussed.

Keywords: tonometry, intraocular pressure, precision, accuracy, central corneal thickness, corneal biomechanical properties

1. Introduction

1.1. Importance of the intraocular pressure (IOP) measurement

Accurate and reproducible IOP evaluation is crucial with regard to the classification, management and follow-up of patients with ocular hypertension and glaucoma, and in patients that have undergone ocular surgical procedures.

Elevated intraocular pressure (IOP) has been shown to be one of the major risk factors for glaucoma [1]. Although the vulnerability of the optic nerve can vary among patients, longitudinal randomized controlled population-based trials have provided strong evidence that the reduction in the mean IOP of only 1 mmHg is significantly effective in preventing the development [2] and in delaying the progression [3] of the glaucomatous damage. Goldmann applanation tonometer (GAT) has been considered as the clinical gold standard for IOP measurement since it was introduced in the 1950s [4]. Although the reproducibility of GAT has shown to be quite good, its accuracy provides several limitations. In particular, IOP measurements taken with GAT have been shown to be influenced by many corneal parameters, including central thickness, curvature, astigmatism and biomechanics. Other disadvantages of GAT include need for local anesthetic drops, fluorescein and a slitlamp. Several different methods have been proposed to overcome the disadvantages found in GAT. The newer alternative tonometric methods include the iCare rebound tonometer, the BioResonator applanation resonance tonometer, the Pascal dynamic contour tonometer, the ocular response analyzer and the Corvis ST pachy-tonometer.

The purpose of this chapter is to discuss the advantages, disadvantages, precision and accuracy of the "newer" alternative tonometric methods.

Newer tonometers covered in this chapter include the following:

i. ***Rebound tonometry***

ii. ***BioResonator applanation resonance tonometer (ART)***

iii. ***Pascal dynamic contour tonometer (DCT)***

iv. ***Ocular response analyzer (ORA)***

v. ***Corvis ST pachy-tonometer***

vi. ***Ocuton S***

I. Rebound tonometry

Rebound tonometry, also known as "impact" or "dynamic tonometry," was first introduced by Obbink about 60 years ago [5]. In 1997, Kontiola introduced an improved and simpler new rebound tonometer, better known as an induction-based impact tonometer [6], that became commercially available as the iCare tonometer in 2003 (**Figure 1**). The method is based on the use of a moving probe that collides with the eye: the motion parameters of the probe, which vary according to eye pressure, are monitored and used in the calculation of IOP [6].

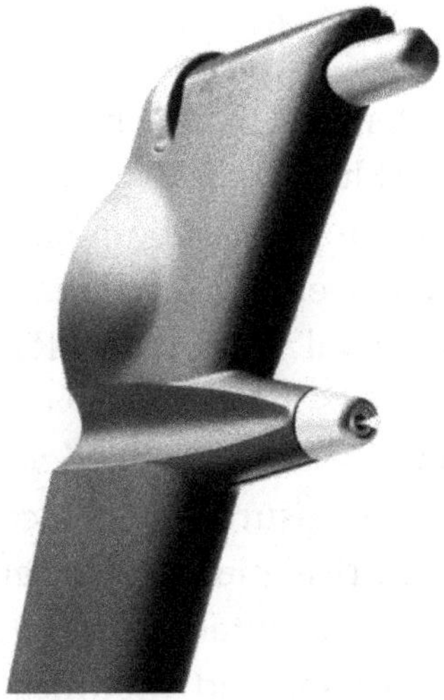

Figure 1. The iCare rebound tonometer.

The iCare (Tiolat Oy, Helsinki, Finland) is routinely used in clinical practice in several clinics nowadays. The device is handy and light-weighed (250 g) [7]. It is composed of a small disposable thin metal probe (about 5 cm in length and 1 mm in diameter) and a solenoid and magnet housed in a metal case. The tonometer is placed in front of the eye, using the forehead to properly position the tip of the probe about 5 mm from the central cornea. The button is pressed in taking IOP measurements, which activates an electric signal that is sent to the solenoid and magnet to move the probe forward. The tip of the probe hits the cornea, rebounds and induces a voltage in the solenoid, which amplifies the signal to a microprocessor. It is advisable to take at least six readings, so that a mean IOP can be calculated by the built-in software [7].

The iCare PRO is a new version, which provides advantages not offered in the previous model, such as measuring IOP also in a supine position, thus useful in bedridden and surgical patients. The iCare one is a simplified version, which has recently been introduced. It can be used independently by patients for at-home autotonometry [8].

The iCare tonometer has shown good reproducibility [9] and correlation with GAT and other tonometers in healthy and glaucomatous eyes [9], and in eyes after keratoplasty [10]. A tendency of the iCare to overestimate the IOP measurements taken with GAT, with a similar trend at different IOP levels, has been reported by several authors [11, 12].

Although iCare was designed not to be influenced by corneal properties, studies have shown that CCT and other corneal structural characteristics affect IOP readings [9, 10, 13]. The iCare tonometer appeared less influenced by corneal edema when compared to GAT [10, 14].

The main advantages of this tonometric method are that the instrument is small, lightweight and portable, easy to use; slitlamp, local anesthesia and fluorescein are not required; IOP is taken in a comfortable sitting position and with the iCare PRO also in the supine position; the rapid measurement enables monitoring in noncompliant subjects. The probes are disposable, and thus, the risk of microbiological contaminations is avoided.

II. BioResonator applanation resonance tonometer (ART)

The applanation resonance tonometer (ART) is a new tonometer based on the resonance technique (**Figure 2**) proposed by Eklund et al. in 2003 [15]. The ART estimates IOP by combining simultaneous continuous sampling of both parameters considered in the applanation principle, which include the force needed to applanate the cornea and the corresponding contact area [15]. The current commercial version of ART, known as the BioResonator ART (Medical sensors and Instruments, BioResonator AB, Sweden), has been recently released and is available in a manual and automatic servo-controlled version [16]. The instrument is made up of a sensor and transducer that can measure the contact force in a continuous manner. The resonance sensor is made up of a cylindrical piezoelectric element that has a known resonance frequency. When the sensor is brought in contact with the cornea, the acoustic impedance of the cornea mechanically loads the sensor and modifies the resonance frequency, with a frequency shift, which is proportional to the contact area between sensor and cornea [15]. IOP is calculated from the slope of the relationship between force and frequency evaluated in a specific frequency shift interval corresponding to an interval applanation area between 4.9 and 11.0 mm^2 [15]. The sensor module of the ART is attached to a standard slitlamp in a similar position as the GAT probe. The ART probe is disinfected with 70% ethanol before each subject, and local anesthetic drop (0.4% benoxinate hydrochloride) is required before IOP measurements. ART is available in two versions: the manual one (BioResonator ART manual), in which the sensor is manually pushed toward the cornea, and the automatic servo-controlled version (BioResonator ART servo), in which a small motor provides the sensor movement. The device provides the median of repeated IOP values, in addition to a Quality Index (QI >2 should be excluded) that reflects the standard deviation of the data. The ART is self-calibrated.

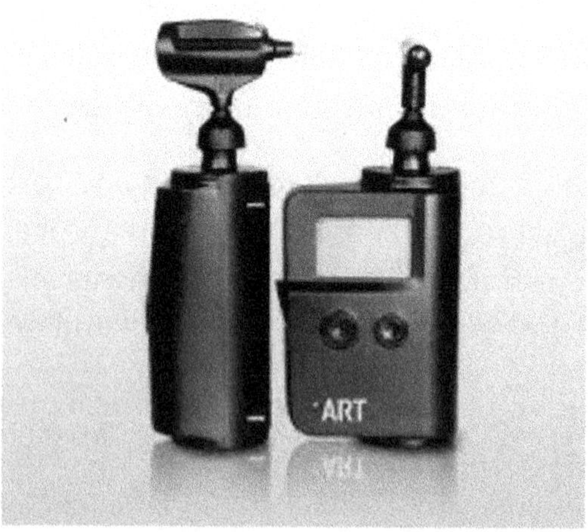

Figure 2. The bioresonator applanation resonance tonometer (ART).

BioResonator ART IOP measurements have been demonstrated to be affected by CCT [15, 17]. The overestimation of the IOP measurements obtained with ART relative to GAT has been demonstrated in previous studies [17].

III. Pascal dynamic contour tonometer (DCT)

The pascal dynamic contour tonometer (DCT) (**Figure 3**), developed by Kaufmann et al. [18], is not based on corneal applanation. It has a concave measuring tip, which is applied on the corneal surface to provide a "contour matching" with the aid of a built-in sensor, which is representative of the pressure inside the eye. The Pascal DCT should be therefore less influenced by corneal properties. Previous studies have shown that there is a good concordance between Pascal DCT and GAT in eyes with normal corneas [19]. In eyes that have undergone laser *in situ* keratomileusis (LASIK), the Pascal DCT appears to provide a more reliable measurement of IOP than GAT, which tends to measure artificially lower IOP values [20].

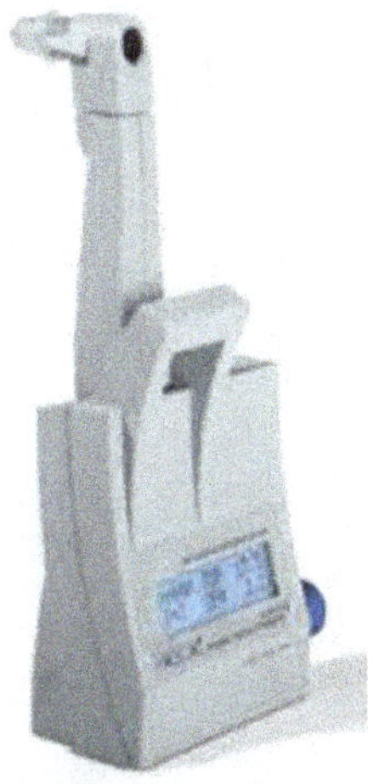

Figure 3. The pascal dynamic contour tonometer (DCT).

The Pascal DCT (SMT Swiss Microtechnology AG, Zurich, Switzerland) [18] is slitlamp mounted and is calibrated automatically. The tonometer has a 10 mm concave radius tip and a built-in 1 mm sensor. The device beeps when the correct position on the corneal surface is obtained. The instrument measures IOP with the use of anesthetic drops in about 5 s and provides digital outcomes in addition to ocular pulse amplitude and quality score (Q that ranges from 1 to 6) data. Acceptable data are defined as Q < 4.

The Pascal DCT has shown high reproducibility [21]. As reported by several authors, the Pascal DCT measurements tend to be higher than GAT readings [22].

The Pascal DCT measurement seems to be not significantly affected by CCT [19]. Moreover, studies conducted on cadaver eyes and in patients who had undergone LASIK showed a significantly lower correlation of CCT with measured IOP values with Pascal DCT than with GAT [18].

IV. Ocular response analyzer (ORA)

The ocular response analyzer (ORA) (**Figure 4**) was introduced by Luce in 2005 [23]. It is an air-puff tonometer that, in addition to the traditional IOP measurement supplied, further indents the cornea with air pressure and measures the point at which the cornea recovers from applanation. This device is based on the principle that information on corneal biomechanics can be obtained by measuring the corneal deformation in response to an air impulse. The ORA uses an electro-optical infrared system to monitor the 3-mm central cornea [23]. The puff of air moves the cornea in an inward fashion, which is considered as the first inward applanation creating a mild concave form. As the force generated by the air decreases, the surface of the cornea takes on the normal convex form in this second outward applanation phase.

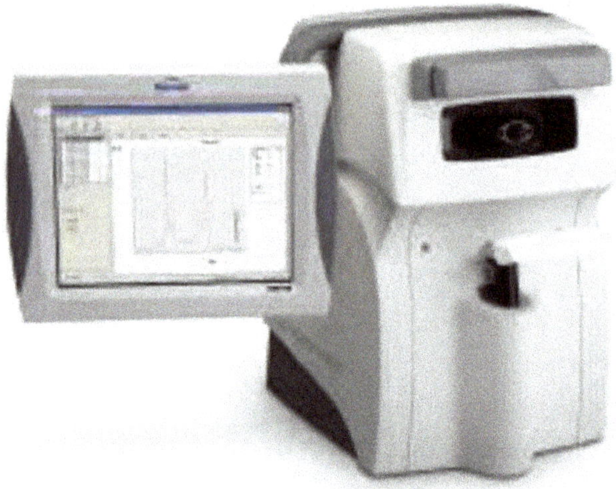

Figure 4. The ocular response analyzer (ORA).

The ORA provides interesting information on the biomechanical characteristics of the cornea. The rapid deformation of the cornea during the air impulse absorbs energy that causes a time delay in the occurrence of the applanation events that are the result of viscous damping in the corneal tissue. The difference between two independent pressure values derived from the two applanation events is defined as "hysteresis" (CH). The instruments provide the corneal compensated IOP (IOPcc) that utilizes information of individual corneal biomechanics, and it is reported to be less affected by corneal properties, such as CCT, in comparison with GAT [23].

Previous authors demonstrated that the ORA significantly overestimated IOP compared with GAT, especially at high IOP levels. Moreover, ORA IOP readings have been demonstrated to be affected by CCT [24].

V. Corvis ST

The Corvis ST (Oculus, Wetzlar, Germany) (**Figure 5**) [25] is a current used instrument that utilizes air-puff noncontact technology with built-in ultra-high-speed Scheimpflug technology. This instrument provides IOP measurements in addition to optical pachymetry data and *in vivo* corneal biomechanical parameters. The device measures corneal biomechanics data based on corneal deformation due to an applied force of air.

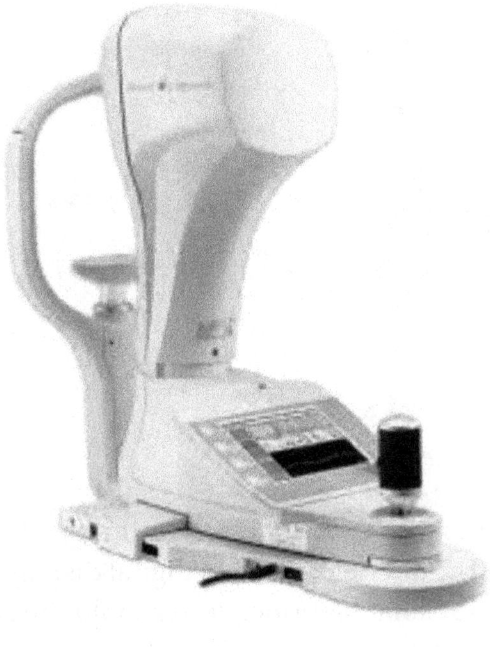

Figure 5. The Corvis ST pachy-tonometer.

The Corvis ST (Oculus, Wetzlar, Germany) released in 2013 [25] uses a quick burst of air (with a Gaussian distributed intensity and duration of 25 ms) on the center of the cornea that causes the initial inward applanation. The cornea then returns to a normal convex shape as the force of the air decreases to provide outward applanation. The Scheimpflug camera precisely records the corneal movements and records more than 100 images in about a half of a second with a resolution >600 × 400 pixels, for a central corneal surface of about 8.5 mm. The numerous corneal scans without the influence of the air puff are used to provide pachymetry readings. The first applanation phase is used to determine IOP measurements, which is not corrected for CCT and corneal deformation parameters (CDPs). The Corvis ST printout provides IOP and CCT measurements and 10 numerical corneal deformation parameters (CDPs), whose importance remains to be fully elucidated. They have been demonstrated to be highly sensitive to IOP that suggests their variation in relation to normal and pathological short- and long-term IOP fluctuations [26]. On the other hand, they are also known to be affected by IOP-independent variables, including patient age, CCT, corneal hydration, corneal stiffness and boundary conditions related to the sclera and the ocular muscles [26].

The precision of Corvis ST has been demonstrated to be excellent for the IOP and CCT values, but decreased for the CDPs [26]. The Corvis ST showed a tendency to underestimate IOP readings compared to GAT in some studies [25, 26]. IOP readings taken with Corvis ST seem to be significantly affected by CCT [25, 26].

VI. Ocuton S

The Ocuton S (EPSa GmbH, Saalfeld, Germany) (**Figure 6**) [27] is a handheld self-tonometer that works according to the principle of applanation tonometry established by Goldmann.

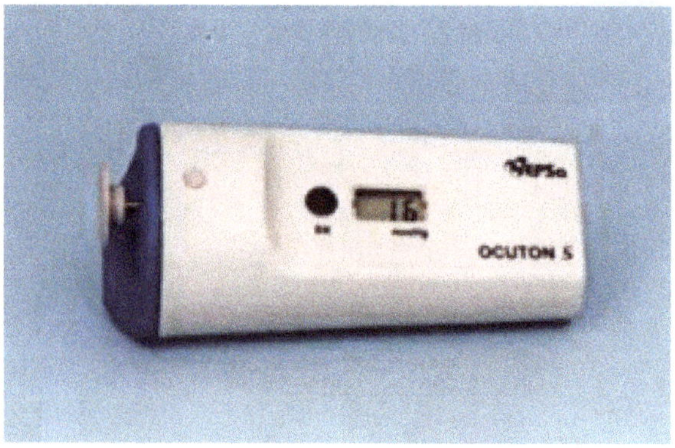

Figure 6. The Ocuton S self-tonometer.

After applying topical anesthesia, the patient holds the tonometer and applies the measuring prism directly to his cornea. The device provides a digital display of his IOP. Considering that the Ocuton S is based on the applanation principle, it should thus be influenced by the corneal thickness, although it is still unclear whether this influence is of a similar extent to that in Goldmann applanation tonometry [28].

The newer version Ocuton S*TT-MV automatically verifies the applanated area. Lanfermann and coworkers showed that the Ocuton S*TT-MV improves measuring accuracy significantly and approaches the accuracy achieved using GAT [29].

There is no "perfect" tonometer till date, and the clinicians must choose a tonometer wisely, balancing precision, accuracy, convenience and cost. IOP is a widely varying physiologic parameter; therefore, a series of IOP measurements should be taken, and the IOP data should only be used in the context of the overall clinical picture.

Author details

Maria Letizia Salvetat[1*], Marco Zeppieri[2] and Paolo Brusini[3]

*Address all correspondence to: mlsalvetat@hotmail.it

1 Department of Ophthalmology, Azienda Ospedaliero-Universitaria "Santa Maria degli Angeli", Pordenone, Italy

2 Department of Ophthalmology, Azienda Ospedaliero-Universitaria "Santa Maria della Misericordia", Udine, Italy

3 Glaucoma Unit, "Città di Udine" Health Center, Udine, Italy

References

[1] Coleman AL, Miglior S. Risk factors for glaucoma onset and progression. Surv Ophthalmol 2008;53:S3–S10.

[2] Kass MA, Heuer DK, Higginbotham EJ, Johnson CA, Keltner JL, Miller JP, Parrish RK 2nd, Wilson MR, Gordon MO. The Ocular Hypertension Treatment Study: a randomized trial determines that topical ocular hypotensive medication delays or prevents the onset of primary open-angle glaucoma. Arch Ophthalmol 2002;120:701–713.

[3] Heijl A, Leske MC, Bengtsson B, Hyman L, Bengtsson B, Hussein M. Early Manifest Glaucoma Trial Group. Reduction of intraocular pressure and glaucoma progression: results from the Early Manifest Glaucoma Trial. Arch Ophthalmol 2002;120:1268–1279.

[4] Goldmann H, Schmidt T. Ueber applanationstonometrie. Ophthalmologica 1957;134:221–242.

[5] Obbink J. Onderzoek naar het verband tusschen inwendigen oogdruk en ballistische reacties. Thesis, Utrecht, The Netherlands, 1931.

[6] Kontiola AI. A new electromechanical method for measuring intraocular pressure. Doc Ophthalmol 1997;93:265–276.

[7] Kontiola AI. A new induction-based impact method for measuring intraocular pressure. Acta Ophthalmol Scand 2000;78:142–145.

[8] Halkiadakis I, Stratos A, Stergiopoulos G, et al. Evaluation of the Icare-ONE rebound tonometer as a self-measuring intraocular pressure device in normal subjects. Graefes Arch Clin Exp Ophthalmol 2012;250(8):1207–1211.

[9] Martinez-de-la-Casa JM, Garcia-Feijoo J, Castillo A, Garcia-Sanchez J. Reproducibility and clinical evaluation of rebound tonometry. Invest Ophthalmol Vis Sci 2005;46:4578–4580.

[10] Salvetat ML, Zeppieri M, Miani F, Tosoni C, Parisi L, Brusini P. Comparison of iCare tonometer and Goldmann applanation tonometry in normal corneas and in eyes with automated lamellar and penetrating keratoplasty. Eye (Lond) 2011;25(5):642–650.

[11] Cook JA, Botello AP, Elders A, et al. Systematic review of the agreement of tonometers with Goldmann applanation tonometry. Ophthalomology 2012;119:1552–1557.

[12] Johannesson G, Hallberg P, Eklund A, Linden C. Pascal. ICare and Goldmann applanation tonometry—a comparative study. Acta Ophthalmol 2008;6:614–621.

[13] Brusini P, Salvetat ML, Zeppieri M, Tosoni C, Parisi L. Comparison of ICare tonometer with Goldmann applanation tonometer in glaucoma patients. J Glaucoma 2006;15:213–217.

[14] Neuburger M, Maier P, Böhringer D, Reinhard T, Jordan JF. The impact of corneal edema on intraocular pressure measurements using goldmann applanation tonometry, Tono-Pen XL, iCare, and ORA: an *in vitro* model. J Glaucoma 2013;22(7):584–590.

[15] Eklund A, Hallberg P, Linden C, Lindahl OA. An applanation resonator sensor for measuring intraocular using combined continuous force and area measurement. Invest Ophthalmol Vis Sci 2003;44:3017–3024.

[16] Johannesson G, Hallberg P, Eklund A, Linden C. Introduction and clinical evaluation of servo-controlled applanation resonance tonometry. Acta Ophthalmol 2012;90:677–682.

[17] Salvetat ML, Zeppieri M, Tosoni C, Brusini P. Repeatability and accuracy of the applanation resonance tonometry in healthy subjects and patients with glaucoma. Acta Ophthalmol 2014;92(1):e66–e77.

[18] Kaufmann C, Bachmann LM, Thiel MA. Intraocular pressure measurements using dynamic contour tonometry after laser *in situ* keratomileusis. Invest Ophthalmol Vis Sci 2003;44:3790–3794.

[19] Pache M, Wilmsmeyer S, Lautebach S, Funk J. Dynamic contour tonometry versus Goldmann applanation tonometry: a comparative study. Graefe's Arch Clin Exp Ophthalmol 2005;243:763–767.

[20] Park HJ, Uhm KB, Hong C. Reduction in intraocular pressure after laser *in situ* keratomileusis. J Cataract Refract Surg 2001;27:303–309.

[21] Wang AS, Alencar LM, Weinreb RN, et al. Repeatability and reproducibility of Goldmann applanation, dynamic contour, and ocular response analyzer tonometry. J Glaucoma 2013;22(2):127–132.

[22] Salvetat ML, Zeppieri M, Tosoni C, Brusini P. Comparison between Pascal dynamic contour tonometry, the TonoPen, and Goldmann applanation tonokmetry in patients with glaucoma. Acta Ophthalmol Scand 2007;85(3):272–279.

[23] Luce DA. Determining in vivo biomechanical properties of the cornea with an ocular response analyzer. J Cataract Refract Surg 2005;31:156–162.

[24] Matinez-de-la-Casa JM, Garcia-Feijoo J, Fernandez-Vidal A, et al. Ocular Response Analyzer versus Goldmann applanation tonometry for intraocular pressure measurements. Invest Ophthalmol Vis Sci 2006;47:4410–4414.

[25] Reznicek L, Muth D, Kampik A, et al. Evaluation of a novel Scheimpflug-based non-contact tonometer in healthy subjects and patients with ocular hypertension and glaucoma. Br J Ophthalmol 1013; 97: 1410–1414.

[26] Salvetat ML, Zeppieri M, Tosoni C, Felletti M, Grasso L, Brusini P. Corneal deformation parameters provided by the Corvis-ST Pachy-Tonometer in healthy subjects and glaucoma patients. J Glaucoma 2015;24(8):568–574.

[27] Draeger J, Schwartz R, Deutsch C, Groenhoff S. Clinical and experimental results with a new fully automatic self-tonometer. Fortschr Ophthalmol 1991;88(3):304–307.

[28] Sacu S, Vass C, Schemper M, Rainer G. Self-tonometry with the Ocuton S: evaluation of accuracy in glaucoma patients. Acta Ophthalmol Scand 2004;82:405–409.

[29] Lanfermann E, Jürgens C, Grossjohann R, Antal S, Tost F. Intraocular pressure measurements with the newly reconfigured Ocuton S*TT-MV self-tonometer in comparison to Goldmann applanation tonometry in glaucoma patients. Med Sci Monit 2009 Nov; 15(11):CR556–562.

3

Conventional Intraocular Pressure Measurement Techniques

Umit Yolcu, Abdullah Ilhan and Ahmet Tas

Abstract

Determining the intraocular pressure (IOP) is a part of routine ophthalmic examination. Elevated IOP is a risk factor for glaucoma, and reducing the IOP is the only way to halt or dampen glaucoma progression. Therefore, precise measurement of IOP is critical in glaucoma management. Tonometry is the procedure of determining IOP using various techniques. Various devices are available in the market for determining IOP. Each one works with different principles. Different methods have been introduced and some of them in development, but there is still no perfect clinical method for exact measurement of IOP. This chapter aims to explore various tonometry devices available in the market while explaining their working principles, features, advantages, and disadvantages. Clinicians must choose proper technique balancing the accuracy, convenience, and cost of the tonometers. Estimation values of tonometers should be used with clinical aspects of patients.

Keywords: tonometer, intraocular pressure, Goldmann applanation tonometer, Tono-Pen, Schiotz, rebound tonometer, pneumotonometer, manometry, noncontact tonometer

1. Introduction

Fluid pressure inside the eyeis responsible for maintaining the shape of the globe as known as intraocular pressure (IOP). Since Bannister described the relation between blindness and firmness of the eye in the sixteenth century, IOP has been regarded as a vital parameter of the eye. Accurate measurement of IOP with proper technique is crucial in diagnosis and management of glaucoma and related conditions. Increased IOP is known to be associated with progressive optic nerve damage [1]. Currently, lowering IOP is the only way to control glaucoma and prevent optic nerve damage. Secretion of aqueous humor and regulation of outflow are critical in maintaining the normal IOP. Aqueous humor is produced in posterior chamber, passes through the pupil into the anterior chamber, and leaves the eye via trabecular meshwork and uveo-scleral pathway. The balance between production and outflow determines the level of IOP, which is approximately 16 mmHg [2]. Age, surgery, trauma, medication, and various diseases may affect production or outflow of the aqueous humor and result in changes in IOP [3].

Tonometers are the instruments used for obtaining IOP. Measurements of an ideal tonometer should be accurate, reproducible, and repeatable. It should be portable, easy to use, simply calibrated, and standardized. Despite all the technological advances since sixteenth century, we still do not have a perfect method to measure IOP in clinical practice. Most of the currently available tonometers are used over cornea, which is only available and accessible structure for estimating IOP. All current clinical measurement techniques are affected by ocular and non-ocular factors and provide us with an estimate of the IOP [4].

Perceiving the working principles of tonometers and the factors affecting their measurement results would help examiners to choose the most proper technique.

The "conventional" tonometers covered in this chapter include:

1. Indentation tonometry: Schiotz tonometer
2. Applanation tonometry: Goldmann applanation tonometer
3. Noncontact tonometer
4. Pneumotonometer
5. Mackay-Marg tonometer and Tono-Pen tonometry
6. Transpalpebral tonometry
7. Manometry

2. Indentation tonometry: Schiotz tonometer

Schiotz tonometer works with *"indentation"* principle, which implies that higher IOP requires higher weight or force to indent. It measures the depth of corneal indentation by a plunger carrying a known weight. The body of the tonometer consists of a curved footplate that rests on the cornea and a known weighted plunger moving freely within a shaft in the footplate. When measuring the IOP, the subject must be positioned in supine position and topical anesthetic drops should be applied. After placing the footplate on the cornea perpendicularly, the plunger moves in an amount depending on the IOP. Movement of the plunger is indirectly proportional to the IOP. A scale on the plunger gives a reading of the movement amount (**Figure 1**). The reading is converted to IOP in mmHg using a conversion table.

This is a mechanical method hence not very reliable in all cases. Conversion Table assumes an average coefficient of ocular rigidity. Therefore, in case of a change in ocular rigidity, blood volume alteration during the measurement and alterations in corneal properties such as steep

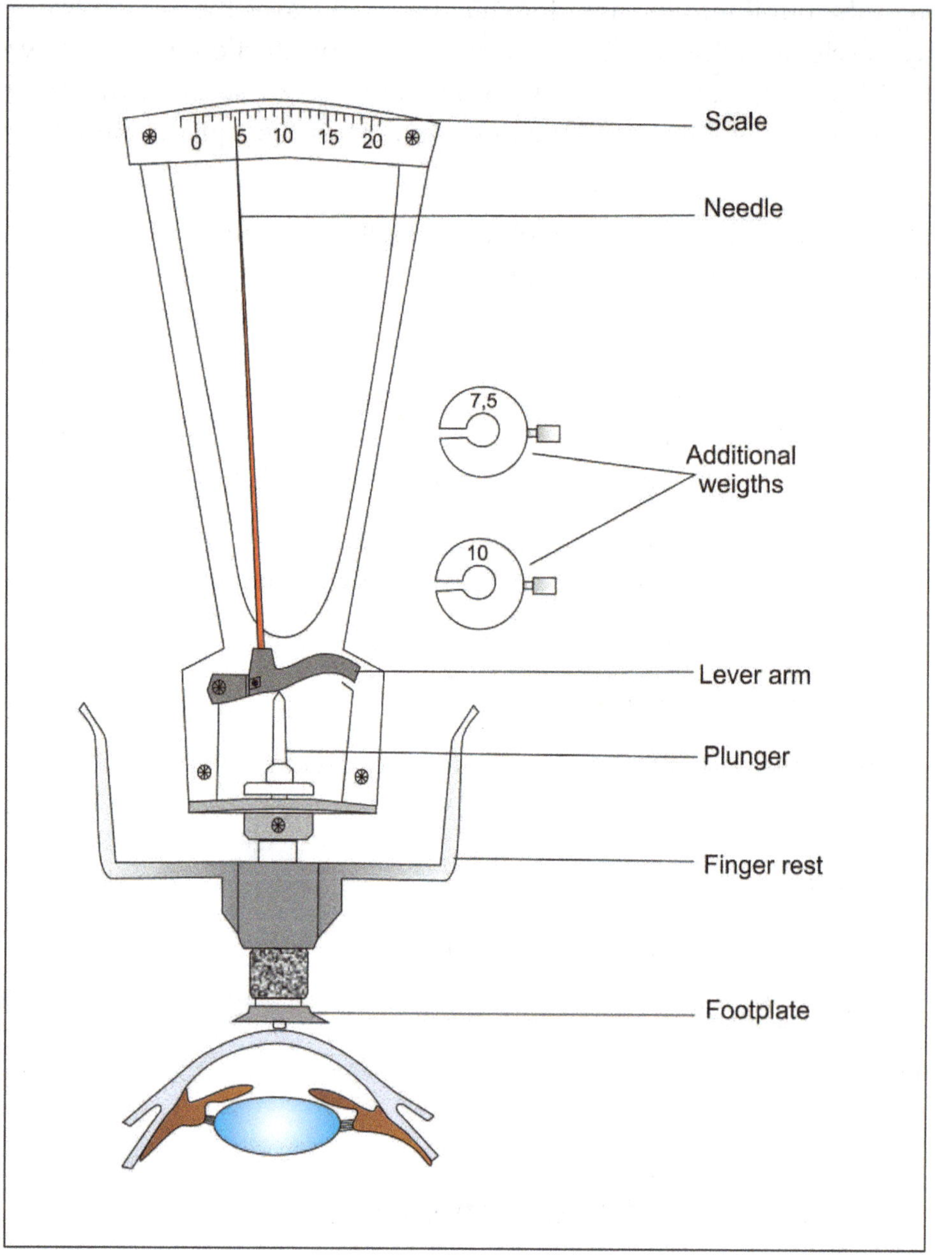

Figure 1. A schematic representation of Schiotz tonometer.

and thicker cornea can cause faulty IOP measurement results. Footplate must be sterilized either with alcohol swap or soaking with 1:1000 merthiolate solution. Schiotz tonometer is considered obsolete in many centers in the developed world but still is an important tool on peripheral centers across the developing nations.

3. Applanation tonometry: Goldmann applanation tonometer

Goldmann applanation tonometer (GAT) is the most widely used method and regarded as the reference standard. It was introduced in the mid-1950s and works based on the *"Imbert-Fick principle,"* which states that the pressure (P) inside a sphere equals the force (F) necessary to flatten its surface divided by the area (A) of flattening, P = F/A [5]. According to Imbert-Fick principle, eye must be perfectly sphere, dry, perfectly flexible, and indefinitely thin. But cornea is aspheric, wet with tear film, not perfectly flexible or thin. To overcome these limitations, Imbert-Fick law was modified. The tip to flatten the cornea was calculated, and a tip with a fixed area with a diameter of 3.06 mm (7.35 mm^2) to minimize the impact of ocular rigidity and surface tension of the tear film was chosen. GAT measures the required force to flatten an area of the cornea of 3.06 mm diameter (**Figure 2**). The force in grams required for applanating this specific area multiplied by 10 equals the IOP in mmHg.

In this method, the instrument is mounted on a slit lamp and the examiner looks at the center of the plastic prism tip, through the slit lamp microscope (**Figure 3**). Then, with the forward movement of the microscope, the tip is contacted slightly to the cornea. Local anesthetic and fluorescein drops are applied before the measurement. Fluorescein dye highlights the tear film when a cobalt blue light is used. Internal prisms of the tip divide the fluorescein meniscus into the superior and inferior arc. When the internal edges of arcs are aligned properly by adjusting the tension knob, a circular area of cornea in 3.06 mm diameter has been flattened at the apex, and examiner can read the IOP from the scale on the adjusting knob directly in mmHg by multiplying 10. After the procedure, it must be disinfected properly. Tip of the tonometer can be disinfected by 70% isopropyl alcohol wipes or soaking 3% hydrogen peroxide solution. The GAT provides an average of IOP between diastolic and systolic pressure.

According to the inventors, optimal IOP measurement can be achieved if the central corneal thickness is approximately 0.5 mm with a well-calibrated GAT [6]. Ehlers et al. reported that GAT most accurately measures intracameral IOP if the central corneal thickness was 520 μm. Variations in corneal thickness and elastic properties have a significant effect on applanation readings of GAT [7, 8]. Thicker corneas can cause overestimation of IOP, and thinner corneas

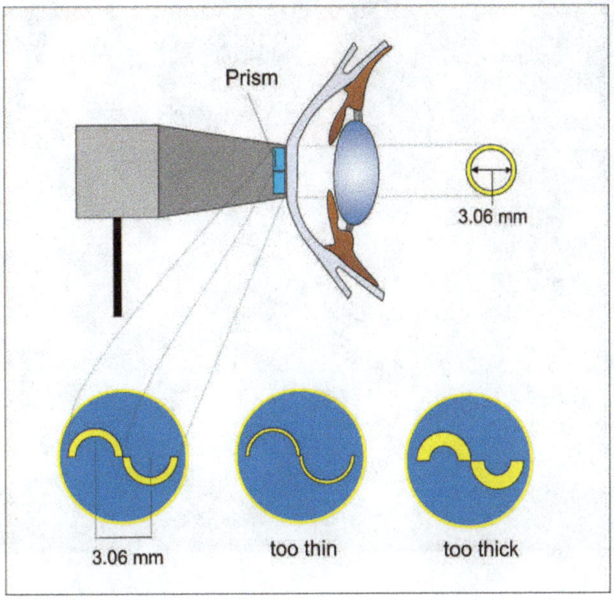

Figure 2. A schematic representation of IOP measurement with Goldman applanation tonometer.

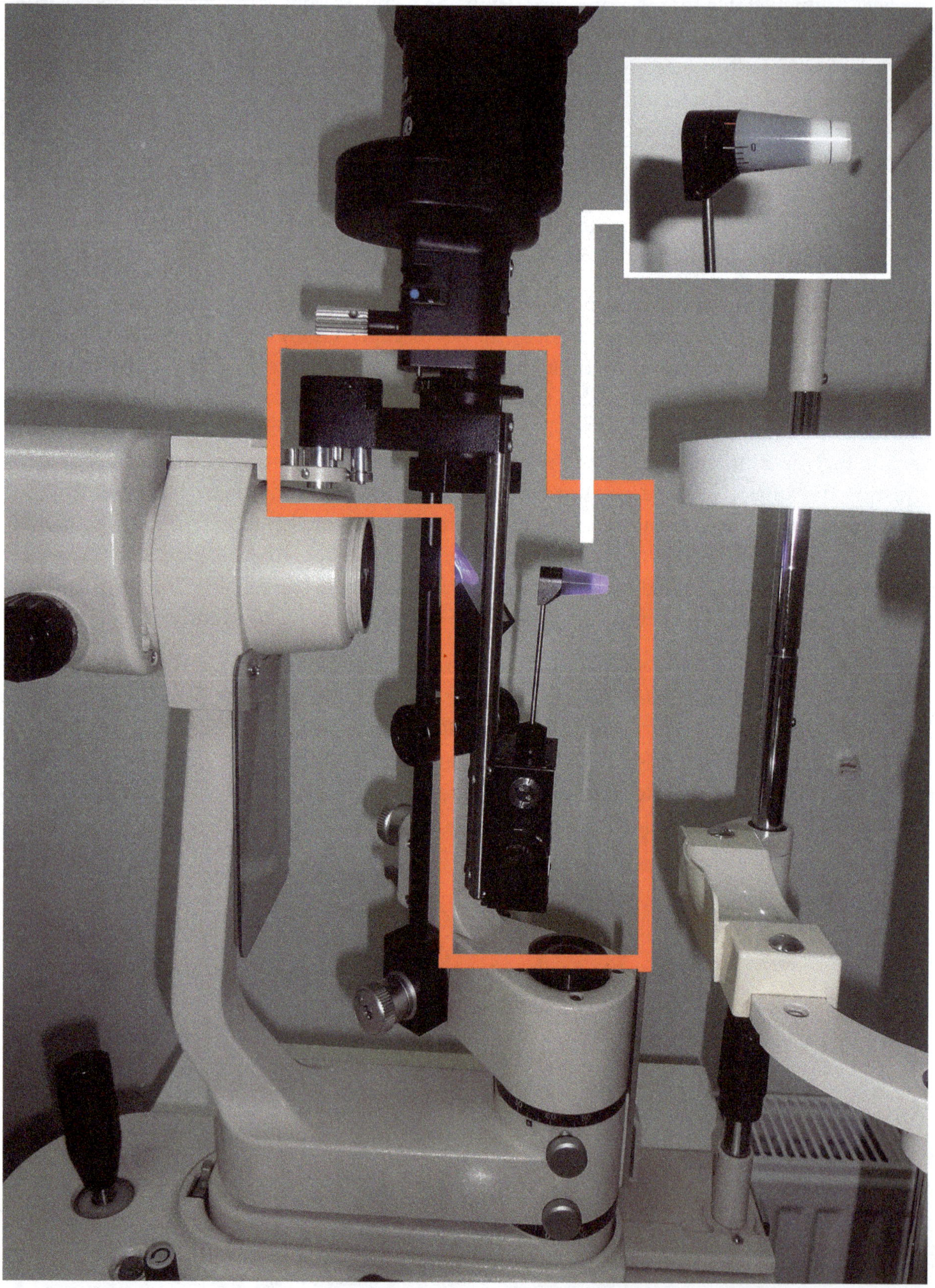

Figure 3. Goldman applanation tonometer, red line outlines tonometer mounted on a slit lamp, and white line magnifies tip of the tonometer.

can cause underestimation of IOP with GAT. Central corneal thickness greatly varies among the general population, and it should be corrected according to the thickness of the cornea [9]. Measurement of GAT may be affected by using excessive or insufficient amount of fluorescein, Valsalva's maneuver, corneal curvature, astigmatism, corneal scarring, eyelid squeezing, prior refractive surgery and indirect pressure on the globe [10]. High corneal curvature can be compensated by rotating tip to the axis of astigmatism. GAT must be calibrated by the user on a regular basis to maintain its accuracy. Despite these limitations, it is still popular and widely used due to low cost, simplicity and lack of consumables.

Goldman tonometry is not portable, and the subject must be in upright position. Handheld, portable version of GAT is called as Perkins tonometer. It is battery powered, uses GAT tip, and requires fluorescein dye. It has an internal mechanism and allows using either in supine or in upright position. Disinfection of the tip for both tonometers must be done properly. Wiping with alcohol solution does not kill all pathogens, and tip should be soaked in hydrogen peroxide or bleach solution at least 10 min and then should be washed.

4. Noncontact tonometer

Noncontact tonometry (NCT) also known as air puff tonometer works in a similar fashion as applanation tonometry, but it uses compressed air to flatten the corneal apex. It does not require direct contact with the cornea or topical anesthesia and can be used in uncooperative patients and children (**Figure 4**). No disinfection procedure is also required.

During the procedure, the device emits a column of air with gradually increasing intensity to the subject's cornea. Highly sensitive electro-optical sensors scan and detect the exact time of the corneal flattening and shut off the air pulse. Thereafter, the device records the value of force information at the moment of corneal flatting and calculates the IOP in mmHg.

Similar with GAT, NCT is also affected by corneal biomechanical factors such as ocular rigidity and central corneal thickness [11]. NCT measures IOP in a few milliseconds, and therefore, it may be affected by ocular pulse amplitude. A minimum of three measurements should be averaged to estimate the mean IOP. Modern NCT devices are advanced greatly than previous models and are well correlated with GAT measurements [12].

5. Pneumotonometer

The pneumotonometer was first invented by Durham et al. and modified by Langham and McCarthy [13]. It basically works like applanation tonometer; however, sensor of the device is air pressure. A slightly convex plunger with a 5-mm tip moves on a cushion of an air stream. The anesthetized cornea is intended by the tip and air pressure. When the tip and cornea are flat, pushing pressure equals the pressure in the eye. After measurement of IOP, the tip keeps indentation for 5–10 s more and provides real-time pressure monitoring of the eye during this period. The device measures the pressure in the system and displays or writes on graph paper for about 5 or 10 s.

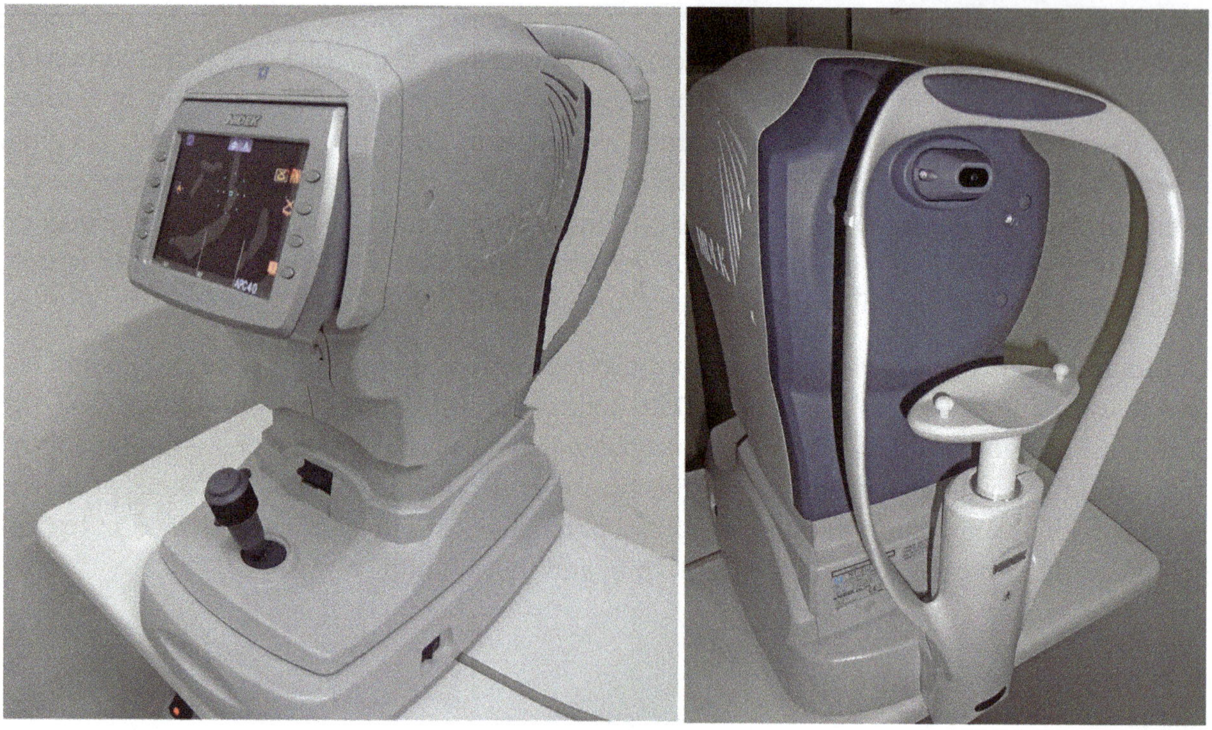

Figure 4. External view of a noncontact tonometer.

Unit of the pneumotonometer is portable and does not need to be mounted on a slit lamp. Measurement procedure is easy to learn and requires less skill than GAT. On the other hand, the tip must be sanitized for each patient. Tip can be cleaned in 70% isopropyl alcohol for 5 min and disinfected in 3% hydrogen peroxide solution.

The pneumotonometer gives 1–3 mmHg higher reading in normal IOP range than GAT, but readings tend to be similar in glaucomatous eyes [14]. A manometry study showed that pneumotonometer overestimates IOP at 10, 20, and 30 mmHg set points [15]. However, another study showed that pneumotonometer consistently underestimated IOP in the range of 5–58 mmHg. Like other applanation tonometers, pneumotonometer is susceptible to corneal thickness changes and measurements are positively correlated with increasing thickness [16, 17].

6. Mackay-Marg tonometer and Tono-Pen tonometry

Mackay-Marg tonometer was first described in the 1950s by Mackay et al., which is an electronic applanation tonometry working with Imbert-Fick principle. It uses a free plunger and a strain gauge for measuring the force necessary to flatten the cornea. A newer version of the Mackay-Marg tonometer is Tono-Pen, which was introduced in the 1980s as a small handheld device. The device is portable, easy to use, and powered by a battery. Tip of the tonometer has an applanating surface and a microscopically small plunger protruding from the center of the applanating surface. When applanating surface contacted with the cornea, plunger takes the corneal resistance and IOP shows an increasing record. Strain gauge linked to the plunger measures the force change and converts to mmHg electronically (**Figure 5**).

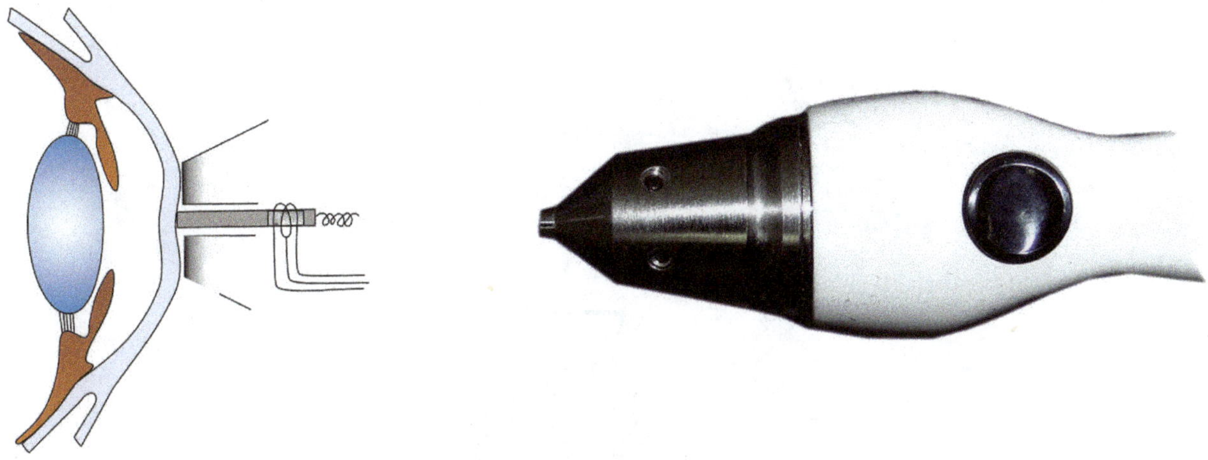

Figure 5. A schematic representation describing the working principle of Tono-Pen.

Tono-Pen tonometry uses a very small area of the cornea, and IOP measurement can be achieved from any normal portion of the cornea. Therefore, it is especially handy in the presence of corneal scarring, corneal grafts, band keratopathy, or similar cases. As Tono-Pen is designed to estimate IOP from especially center part of the cornea, it is affected by changes in corneal thickness and tends to overestimate IOP compared to GAT [18]. Moreover, in case of measurement from the peripheral portion of the cornea, the device may estimate IOP higher than normal [19]. Excessive pressure application on the globe during the measurement procedure may cause higher IOP estimation than normal. In optimal conditions, Tono-Pen readings are well correlated with GAT measurements within normal IOP ranges [20]. Single-use disposable covers are available for the tip of the Tono-Pen. Tip should not be disinfected with solvent and cleaning solutions.

7. Transpalpebral tonometry

Several centuries ago, IOP was first evaluated by eye palpation through the eyelids. However, this method is subjective and uncertain. This device aims to perform this evaluation method (ballistic) by sensors in an automated fashion. It applies pressure on an area of 1.5 mm in diameter by a rod through the eyelid, and the eyelid acts as a transmissive part. The device can be used in supine or upward position and does not require corneal anesthesia. In supine position, patient is instructed to look up 45° superiorly and the device is placed appropriately on the cartilaginous part of the lid while keeping the tonometer vertically. Rod of the device falls automatically with gravity and after analyzing the momentary change of the rebound; IOP is estimated and displayed in mmHg. Sterilization is not required. The device does not have a guiding feature for proper placement, stabilization, and orientation. It has been reported that results seem to be affected by corneal thickness, especially thinner corneas [21]. Results of Diaton were showed high variability and poor agreement with GAT results. Hereby, the authors recommend this device only for screening purposes (**Figure 6** and **Table 1**) [22, 23].

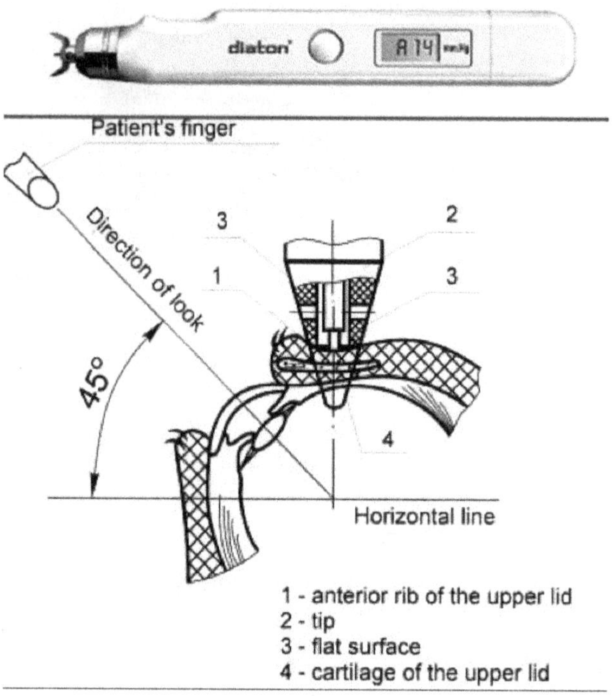

Figure 6. Diaton transpalpebral tonometer.

	Working principle	Brand name	Contact/noncontact
Conventional tonometers			
Goldmann applanation tonometer	Fixed area applanation	Goldman tonometer/perkins tonometer in various brands	Contact
Electronic applanation tonometer	Mackay-Marg applanation	Tono-Pen, Accupen	Contact
Noncontact tonometry	Air puff applanation	Various brands	Noncontact
Pneumatic tonometer	Fixed area applanation with air pressure	Reichert Model 30	Contact
Newer tonometers			
Ocular response analyzer	Bidirectional air puff	Reichert ocular response analyzer	Noncontact
Scheimpflug noncontact tonometer	Air puff; corneal analysis with Scheimpflug imaging	Oculus Corvis ST	Noncontact
Dynamic contour tonometer	Contour-matched piezoresistive sensor	Pascal DCT	Contact
Rebound tonometer	Ballistic probe	iCare Rebound tonometer	Contact
Transpalpebral tonometer	Ballistic probe through eyelid	Diaton	Contact (eyelid)

Table 1. Currently available tonometers in the market.

8. Manometry

Manometry is an invasive technique that precisely measures the real pressure inside the eye. Results of the manometry are the reference pressure for all other tonometers. It is especially used in laboratory conditions for continuous IOP measurement. It evaluates the effects of pharmacologic of physiologic manipulators and useful in exploring the aqueous humor dynamics. It is also used for calibrating and validating the results of various types of tonometers on postmortem human eyes.

The ideal tonometer would be easy to use, portable, reliable, and comfortable for both the patient and physician. It should have low inter- and intraoperator variability and provide an IOP reading that is close to the manometric IOP of the individual. To date, no such tonometer exists. Till date, the gold standard for IOP measurements is Goldmann applanation tonometer.

Author details

Umit Yolcu*, Abdullah Ilhan and Ahmet Tas

*Address all correspondence to: umit_yolcu@hotmail.com

Mevki Military Hospital, Ophthalmology Service, Ankara, Turkey

References

[1] Leske MC, Heijl A, Hyman L, Bengtsson B, Dong L, Yang Z, et al. Predictors of long-term progression in the early manifest glaucoma trial. Ophthalmology. 2007;114:1965–72. doi:10.1016/j.ophtha.2007.03.016

[2] Shiose Y. Intraocular pressure: new perspectives. Surv Ophthalmol. 1990;34:413–35

[3] Kass MA, Heuer DK, Higginbotham EJ, Johnson CA, Keltner JL, Miller JP, et al. The Ocular Hypertension Treatment Study: a randomized trial determines that topical ocular hypotensive medication delays or prevents the onset of primary open-angle glaucoma. Arch Ophthalmol. 2002;120:701–13; discussion 829–30

[4] Goel M, Picciani RG, Lee RK, Bhattacharya SK. Aqueous humor dynamics: a review. Open Ophthalmol J. 2010;4:52–9. doi:10.2174/1874364101004010052

[5] Glaucoma. 2007–2008 ed. San Francisco, CA: American Academy of Ophthalmology; 2007.

[6] Goldmann H, Schmidt T. Applanation tonometry. Ophthalmologica. 1957;134:221–42

[7] Whitacre MM, Stein RA, Hassanein K. The effect of corneal thickness on applanation tonometry. Am J Ophthalmol. 1993;115:592–6

[8] Herndon LW, Choudhri SA, Cox T, Damji KF, Shields MB, Allingham RR. Central corneal thickness in normal, glaucomatous, and ocular hypertensive eyes. Arch Ophthalmol. 1997;115:1137–41

[9] Gunvant P, O'Leary DJ, Baskaran M, Broadway DC, Watkins RJ, Vijaya L. Evaluation of tonometric correction factors. J Glaucoma. 2005;14:337–43

[10] Whitacre MM, Stein R. Sources of error with use of Goldmann-type tonometers. Surv Ophthalmol. 1993;38:1–30

[11] Tonnu PA, Ho T, Newson T, El Sheikh A, Sharma K, White E, et al. The influence of central corneal thickness and age on intraocular pressure measured by pneumotonometry, non-contact tonometry, the Tono-Pen XL, and Goldmann applanation tonometry. Br J Ophthalmol. 2005;89:851–4. doi:10.1136/bjo.2004.056622

[12] Vincent SJ, Vincent RA, Shields D, Lee GA. Comparison of intraocular pressure measurement between rebound, non-contact and Goldmann applanation tonometry in treated glaucoma patients. Clin Exp Ophthalmol. 2012;40:e163–70. doi:10.1111/j.1442-9071.2011.02670.x.

[13] Langham ME, McCarthy E. A rapid pneumatic applanation tonometer. Comparative findings and evaluation. Arch Ophthalmol. 1968;79:389–99

[14] Condon PI, Ryan JL. Comparative evaluation of two new applanation tonometers-preliminary study. Doc Ophthalmol. 1977;44:127–35.

[15] Currie BD, Bagga H, Rademaker AW, Tanna AP. Effect of instrument orientation on the accuracy of intraocular pressure measurements in human cadaveric eyes: manometric evaluation of the model 30 classic Pneumatonometer and Tono-Pen XL. J Glaucoma. 2011;20:465–9. doi:10.1097/IJG.0b013e3181f46324

[16] Morgan AJ, Harper J, Hosking SL, Gilmartin B. The effect of corneal thickness and corneal curvature on pneumatonometer measurements. Curr Eye Res. 2002;25:107–12

[17] Saleh TA, Adams M, McDermott B, Claridge KG, Ewings P. Effects of central corneal thickness and corneal curvature on the intraocular pressure measurement by Goldmann applanation tonometer and ocular blood flow pneumatonometer. Clin Experiment Ophthalmol. 2006;34:516–20. doi:10.1111/j.1442-9071.2006.01266.x

[18] Kim NR, Kim CY, Kim H, Seong GJ, Lee ES. Comparison of Goldmann applanation tonometer, noncontact tonometer, and TonoPen XL for intraocular pressure measurement in different types of glaucomatous, ocular hypertensive, and normal eyes. Curr Eye Res. 2011;36:295–300. doi:10.3109/02713683.2010.542865

[19] Amaral WO, Teixeira RM, Alencar LM, Cronemberger S, Calixto N. Central and peripheral corneal thickness: influence on the iop measurement by Tonopen. Arq Bras Oftalmol. 2006;69:41–5. doi:S0004–27492006000100009

[20] Iester M, Mermoud A, Achache F, Roy S. New Tonopen XL: comparison with the Goldmann tonometer. Eye (Lond). 2001;15:52–8. doi:10.1038/eye.2001.13

[21] Toker MI, Vural A, Erdogan H, Topalkara A, Arici MK. Central corneal thickness and Diaton transpalpebral tonometry. Graefes Arch Clin Exp Ophthalmol. 2008;246:881–9.

[22] Li Y, Shi J, Duan X, Fan F. Transpalpebral measurement of intraocular pressure using the Diaton tonometer versus standard Goldmann applanation tonometry. Graefes Arch Clin Exp Ophthalmol. 2010;248:1765–70.

[23] Doherty MD, Carrim ZI, O'Neill DP. Diaton tonometry: an assessment of validity and preference against Goldmann tonometry. Clin Exp Ophthalmol. 2012;40:e171–5.

4

Strategies for Managing Difficult Cases

Baris Komur

Abstract

Standard cataract surgery is considered as low-risk surgery for both patients and the surgeon, but some eyes have higher risk of complication due to some reasons that are generally known or can be predicted preoperatively. Knowing risky eyes and management of possible complications is important point for achieving good visual outcome after cataract surgery. We issued most encountered problems during surgery and some solutions to manage these difficult cases.

Keywords: small pupil, brunescent, hard, white, cataract, weak zonules, zonulopathy, postural problems, shallow anterior chamber, posterior polar, reverse pupillary block

1. Introduction

In ophthalmology, the clinical management of patients is constantly evolving and complication rate is getting low. On the other hand, patient expectations are increasing. Currently, the patient now expects excellent uncorrected visual acuity following cataract surgery [1]. Although routine cataract surgery considered as low-risk surgery for both patients and the surgeon, some eyes have higher risk of complication during cataract surgery. Operations on such difficult cases are also more likely to yield a poor visual outcome which is defined as best corrected vision less than 6/60 after surgery [2].

It is extremely important to recognize when eyes are at greater risk, and act accordingly, to reduce complications. Also, before the operation takes place, it is better to spare extra time on these difficult cases, explaining that surgery is somewhat different and difficult than "routine cataract surgery" and poor outcome is a possibility. Some patients may want to take a second opinion from another clinic, letting or even encouraging them to do so will be a better option than trying to explain complication may occur at every clinic after an undesired result occured. The patients should have realistic expectations, and understand possible complications and their other ocular problems [3]. This approach makes patients expectations much more realistic and improves postoperative compliance and follow-up. In rare cases, patients with complicated cataract will be happy if they achieve some improvement in their vision.

It is also important to prepare for difficult case both mentally and physically. Mentally, the surgeon must know what to do if any complication occurs, physically, the surgeon must prepare all the equipment to manage a possible complication, like pupil devices for small pupils, capsule tension rings (CTR) for weak zonules, sutures for scleral fixation or Cionni ring fixation and vitrectomy devices in the case of capsular rupture and vitreous loss.

In this chapter, we discuss some frequently encountered difficult situations and their solutions.

2. Small pupil

It is very important to obtain sufficient pupillary dilation that lasts for the duration of the cataract surgery. A small pupil is defined as having a diameter equal to or less than 4 mm; in these cases, although experienced surgeon can continue to surgery without any manipulation; beginner surgeon must enlarge the pupil. The surgeon must plan the operation very carefully, taking into consideration all possible situations. Methods used to deal with small pupil, must aim good return of pupil function, not causing esthetically bad results or functional problems such as photophobia and diplopia. The postoperative esthetic results of this type of surgery are potentially disturbing for the patient; any surgical alteration of the pupil may have a significant effect on its function with side effects such as iatrogenic glare that can be debilitating [4].

Preoperatively using a nonsteroidal anti-inflammatory drug (NSAID) in addition to cycloplegics and mydriatics may reduce probability of pupil contraction during the operation [5–7]. There are preparations, containing NSAID for intraoperative usage, approved by the US Food and Drug Administration, also there are some preparations combining both mydriatics and NSAIDs which can be used intraoperatively, but these preparations may not be available worldwide or may be very expensive [8–10]. Another (cheaper) option is 0.5 mL of 1:1000 preservative free adrenaline diluted in 10 mL of balanced salt solution (BSS); this is injected at the beginning of surgery, through the side-port incision or added to the infusion bottle (4 IU of 1:1000 adrenaline in 500 cc) [11, 12].

Even with pharmacological dilation, pupil may still not be large enough to allow safe surgery. Although there is no absolutely safe pupil size, generally if pupil allows creation of an adequate capsulorrhexis, it also may be sufficient for the remaining steps of the surgical procedure. Safe pupil size may depend on surgical expertise, cataract hardness, patient compliance and other anatomical restrictions.

First thing to try after failed pharmacological dilation may be viscomydriasis, which is injecting viscoelastic substance (VES) toward the iris, hoping a peripheral displacement of the central portion of the iris, resulting in expansion of the pupil. Keep in mind that, VES will enlarge the pupil only when it is anterior chamber (AC); the effect of VES is less when phacoemulsification and aspiration begins. High molecular weight cohesive products will be more effective for this purpose.

Synechiolysis can be utilized, when pupil is fixed by adhesions between the iris and the underlying lens capsule (posterior synechiae). Synechiae is broken with a blunt spatula or VES cannula that is inserted through a paracentesis, while AC filled with VES. Excessive traction may cause bleeding. Fibrous pupillary band also must be removed with a forceps for capsulorrhexis or vitreoretinal surgery [13].

Pupil stretching is more invasive procedure that induces numerous, very fine partial ruptures of the sphincter that induce mydriasis. Pupil stretching must be performed under VES protection to maintain AC depth. Two hooks are introduced into the AC; the pupil is engaged at two opposite points; and the surgeon applies peripheral pressure, sufficient to ensure moderate and controlled relaxation of the pupil edge to increase mydriasis. Repetitive gentle and progressive "push-pull" movements of the instruments are recommended. With this, rupture of the sphincter is minimized. Rapid movements may cause serious damage to the sphincter. The hook is inserted through the side-port incision and through the main incision; it is used to stretch the pupil in several different and opposite directions (initially at the 12 and 6 o'clock positions and then at the 3 and 9 o'clock positions). Then, oblique positions can be used if needed (**Figure 1**).

There are also one-handed dilators are available; inserted through the main incision, these devices stretch the pupil with a single maneuver. These instruments have been designed as a handpiece with a narrow cannula containing several hooks (between 2 and 4), with a fixed hook on its outside edge. There are fewer possibilities for adjustment with this technique and the dilator instrument itself can be expensive [14].

Sphincterotomy is an invasive procedure but useful in cases in which the sclerosis of the iris tissue is restricted to the central zone, typical of the senile pupil, capsular pseudoexfoliation, postinflammatory miosis, or iatrogenic inflammation resulting from the prolonged use of miotics. The microincisions (mini-sphincterotomies), usually 6–8, are created using fine microscissors. The incisions continue radially for approximately two-thirds of the length of the iris sphincter (**Figure 2**). The length of the corneal incision through which the scissors are inserted determines the degree of circumferential extension of the incisions [15].

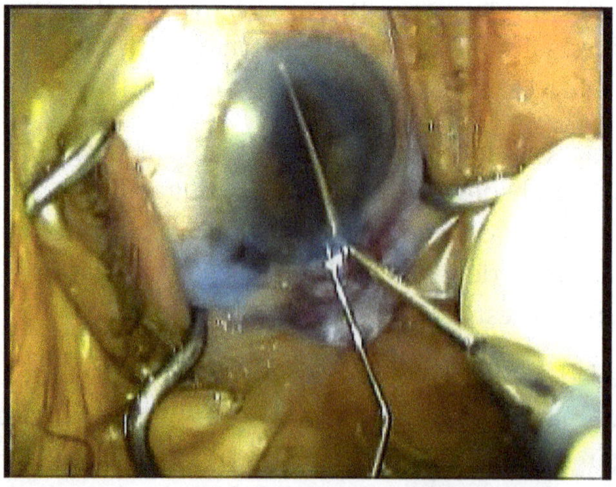

Figure 1. Pupil streching with two instruments.

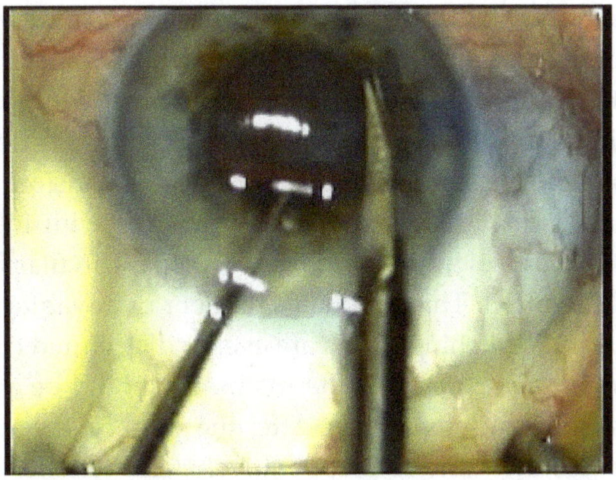

Figure 2. Mini-sphincterotomies with fine scissors.

In some cases, even after pupil stretching; size may still not be sufficient or iris laxity may cause repeated aspiration of the iris tissue itself by phaco tip. In these cases, mechanical hook retractors (dilator hooks) or iris rings can be used. Iris tissue must be sufficiently elastic to allow distention without causing lacerations. Technique for positioning iris hooks involves the creation of limbal paracenteses for the insertion of the hooks under VES. Iris hooks engage pupil margin and pull it centrifugally with silicone fragment that is engaged at the limbus. Generally, four hooks are positioned, producing a square-shaped iris. Positions of limbal paracenteses are important. For correct stretching, hooks should pull in a direction parallel to iris plane and iris must not be elevated. For this reason, incisions made close as possible to the limbus with an appropriate orientation (**Figure 3**). Once hooks positioned, the surgeon can cut the excess to avoid displacement of the hooks if the patient moves his or her eye, if topical anesthesia chosen. Iris hooks can be removed quite easily through the insertion incisions. Hooks create mydriasis that is adequate for surgery but not excessively large that can cause lax pupil postoperatively.

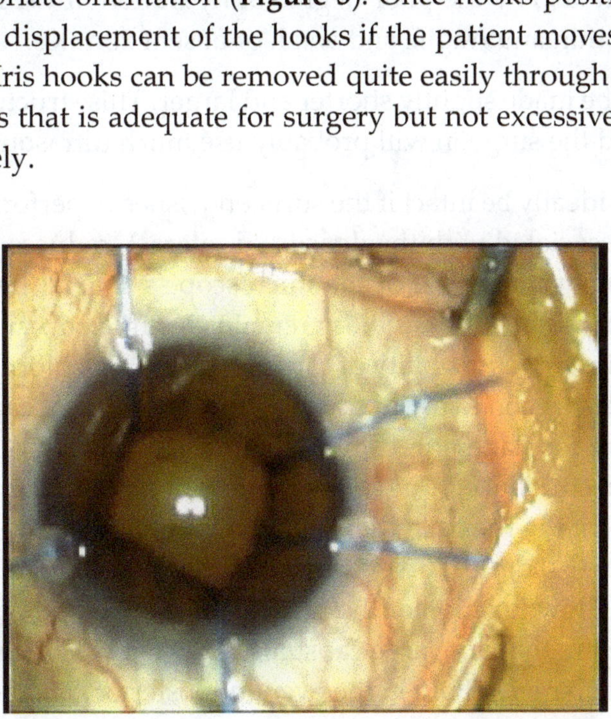

Figure 3. Iris hooks direction are better when parallel to iris plane and iris is not elevated.

Pupil expansion rings are another set of instruments designed to enlarge pupil without damaging the sphincter. These can be complete or incomplete rings; some are manufactured in polymethylmethacrylate (PMMA), others are silicone or expandable hydrogel [16]. Recently, Malyugin presented a new pupil expander [17, 18]. The use of this device also appears to be easier and faster compared to iris hooks and other pupil expansion rings. This device may be safer for dealing with a small pupil, particularly in eyes with intraoperative floppy iris syndrome. This device is a one-piece device of 5-0 Prolene. Circular buttonholes engage the pupil edge and expand the pupil. This ring has a number of advantages: it is easy to implant and induces less trauma and stretching forces are evenly distributed over the pupil edge. This may be useful in patients in which cutting the iris tissue should be avoided (e.g., iris rubeosis, chronic iritis, or systemic coagulopathies). After the surgery, the appearance of the majority of pupils is more or less the same as preoperatively, and functional activity is preserved. Additional corneal incisions are not necessary, and device is inserted through the main incision using an injector. Only negative point may be the cost of Malyugin ring.

Regardless of the method used to expand the pupil, at the end of surgery, the pupil must be constricted to avoid it being captured by part of the optic, adhering to the capsule, or other deformities.

3. Hard nucleus

Dense cataracts have always been considered challenging in phacoemulsification. The problems encountered in hard cataracts are determined not just by the hardness and the dimensions of the nucleus but also by the poor degree of hydration of the lens, absence of the red reflex, a capsule that is thin and fragile and weak or absent zonules.

Corneal tunnel should be made slightly shorter and larger. This structure will reduce the danger of wound burn, and the surgeon will probably use much ultrasound energy.

Capsulorrhexis should ideally be intact if the surgeon wishes to perform phacoemulsification. A reduced red reflex associated with the density of cataract, reduces the visualization of the anterior capsule. Changing the angle of the microscope's coaxial light beam may produce better visibility of the capsule. If the visibility remains insufficient, vital dyes (such as trypan blue) may be useful. It improves visibility of capsule during capsulorrhexis and phacoemulsification, which help the surgeon to avoid traumatizing the edge of capsulorrhexis. Adequate use of VES is important for flattening convex shape of the anterior lens surface, increasing AC depth (which has been reduced due to the large volume of the crystalline lens) to reduce zonular stretch and orient the rhexis in the desired direction [19]. Capsulorrhexis should ideally be a large rhexis (5.5–6.0 mm) to ease manipulations in the bag. In the event of difficulties, a large rhexis can also allow luxation of the nucleus in the AC and converting extracapsular cataract extraction. Beware that, too large capsulorrhexis may also make them unable to capture the optic of intraocular lens (IOL) in the event of posterior capsule rupture. In extremely mature cataracts, the anterior capsule may contain deposits of calcium or dense focal plaques, in these areas, the surgeon can cut through these dense areas with scissors.

Hydrodissection must be performed delicately. After half of the hydrodissection completed, center of raised nucleus should be pressed with cannula to depress the nucleus posteriorly; a further hydrodissection is performed on the opposite side (if needed, the surgeon can combine viscodissection procedure to rotate the nucleus). This pressing is important as the anterior shift of the large brunescent nucleus during hydrodissection may cause a capsule-lenticular blockage. In this case, if the surgeon proceeds with further and aggressive injections of liquid below the nucleus, the posterior capsule may be distended and ruptured. There may be strong corticocapsular adhesions that interfere with rotation of the nucleus; this procedure must be performed delicately without excessive force being applied. Before the surgeon begins ultrasound, it is essential that the nucleus rotate freely inside the capsular bag.

Weak zonules may be associated with the advanced age of these patients, with previous traumatic episodes that may have gone unnoticed, or with various reasons. The posterior capsule will have a greater tendency to shift toward the phaco tip even with a minimal degree of postocclusion surge. If the surgeon suspects clinically significant zonular weakness then he or she should not hesitate to use a capsular tension ring (CTR). There is a debate regarding the most suitable timing for this particular maneuver; some surgeons believe that the tension ring should be inserted as soon as any degree of weakness is observed, usually prior to the phacoemulsification procedure, while others feel that it should be inserted prior to irrigation/aspiration or before IOL is implanted.

These cataracts must be operated by expert surgeons who know modification of parameters and techniques to manage hard cataracts. When removing these nuclei, many surgeons proceed with sculpting procedures, but using techniques like "phaco chop" and the "stop and chop" technique that reduce the capsular and zonular stress, may reduce complications in these eyes [20, 21]. The "quick chop" technique is a variation of the "phaco chop" with a reduction in the amount of ultrasound used and manual fragmentation required. This allows reduction of energy with a reduction in the risk of wound burn, shortened operating times, and a reduction in the amount of stress to the zonules. Technique involves use of high vacuum and a chopper; the phaco tip is used as a pivot point to fracture the nucleus into pieces, moving them toward the chopper, which has been pushed from top down in front of the phaco tip. Regardless of the technique preferred by the modern surgeon (divide and conquer, stop and chop, chop), the basic principle is the same, to create multiple, small-size fragments. These fragments are larger and much denser than those of other types of nucleus. Comparing a standard cataract, the vacuum is much higher and occasional short bursts of ultrasound (20–40%) will be required. During this step, non-dominant hand movements are essential.

In the past, blockage of the tubing by rigid nuclear fragments was a frequent problem, as these pieces may occlude the phaco tip resulting in poor followability and in excessive turbulence which causes trauma to the endothelium. Thanks to modern phacoemulsification machines that considerably reduce the amount of energy and heat produced with increased followability associated with reduced vibration of the fragments inside the phaco tip. This technology is implemented by various companies [22, 23]. Despite this technology, signs that the surgeon must recognize when the phaco tip is partially or completely occluded are sudden appearance of emulsified milky material in front of the ultrasound tip and suddenly decreased followability. Posterior capsule is frequently thinner and stretched by the large volume of the lens; it will be weak and flaccid and will tend to be aspirated into the phaco tip with a major risk of rupture. Also, these cases generally have an absence or reduced amount of an epinucleus to protect the posterior capsule, forcing the surgeon to work closer to the posterior capsule and the equatorial periphery. Therefore, it is advisable for several small injections of a dispersive VES, behind the nucleus during phacoemulsification, injecting it into various areas to create a thin yet uniform layer of VES between the nucleus and the posterior capsule, creating an artificial epinucleus that separates the posterior capsule from the operating plane. Because of its intrinsic properties, it is not easily aspirated by the phaco tip, and this facilitates the safe emulsification of the fragments.

Once the nucleus has been completely removed, the remaining portion of the surgery is like a standard cataract. However, at the end of the procedure, if the capsular bag appears to be too compromised as it will not support the IOL, the surgeon may consider to implant a posterior chamber IOL with transscleral or iris fixation or an anterior chamber IOL.

4. Posterior polar cataracts

Posterior polar cataract is a type of congenital cataract that occurs in the central cortex adjacent to the posterior capsule. There is an increased risk of a posterior capsular tear during cataract surgery because a capsular defect is often present. Even if a discrete capsular defect is not detected (usually visible as small vacuole), there is an increased risk of a capsular complication. Hydrodissection increases the risk of blowing out the posterior capsule. While some authors did hydrodissection in multiple quadrants with tiny amount of fluid without allowing the wave to transmit across the posterior capsule, cortical cleaving hydrodissection is considered a contraindication in eyes with posterior polar cataract [24]. A weak point can produce hydraulic posterior capsule rupture during hydrodissection. Meanwhile, hydrodelineation, which is the separation between the nucleus and the epinucleus, is mandatory. It is worth mentioning that the surgeon should avoid vigorous decompression of the capsular bag after the delineation. In addition, nuclear rotation is contraindicated as it can act as a trephine to the posterior capsule. Some authors described a technique that was described for dense and posterior polar cataract called inside-out delineation [25]. In this technique, a trench is first sculpted and a right-angled cannula is used to subsequently direct the fluid perpendicularly to the lens fibers in the desired plane through one wall of the trench. This would avoid the possibility of inadvertent subcapsular injection and overcome the difficulty of introducing cannula to a significant depth in a dense cataract.

Capsular stress must be minimized by lowering the irrigation bottle height, reducing flow and vacuum settings which is named as slow-motion phaco, maintaining a stable anterior chamber (avoid surge and chamber bounce), and minimizing manipulations of the lens [26]. Attempting to polish any residual posterior capsular plaque in the area where the posterior polar cataract was located can easily create a tear in the weakened/defective posterior capsule. Leaving a small plaque may affect the patient's vision postoperatively, but it is much better to just perform a laser posterior capsulotomy when necessary.

5. Traumatic cataract

Cataract surgery in traumatized eyes is one of the most difficult clinical situations an anterior segment surgeon is likely to encounter. Preoperative good examination is essential. Presence and extent of phacodonesis and decentration of the lens zonular disinsertion must be recorded. A wrinkled anterior capsular surface may indicate discontinuity of the capsule itself or the zonules. It should be remembered that the integrity of the capsule may be compromised even with contusive (not penetrating) trauma [27].

Sometimes it is possible to examine the fundus depending on the opacity of the media, and its examination should include identification of holes, retinal lacerations, or retinal edema. The presence of subretinal or suprachoroidal hemorrhage should lead to greater prognostic caution, as any degree of suprachoroidal hemorrhage would cause posterior pressure during surgery.

If fundus examination is not possible, only B-scan may modify the surgeon's approach to the cataract surgery itself. When a suprachoroidal hemorrhage is detected, the surgeon should consider a pars plana vitrectomy. A computed tomography (CT) scan of the orbit is indicated if the surgeon suspects the presence of an intraocular or intraorbital foreign body. With an open corneal and/or scleral laceration, generally good slit-lamp examination will be impossible, making surgical planning more critical. If a penetration of anterior capsule present, cornea is sutured without removing the cataract; capsule may heal by itself with a little opacity [28].

A foreign body of a ferrous nature must be removed, as it could lead to ocular siderosis, while inert foreign bodies (such as glass) are well tolerated even when left in eye [29, 30]. Choice of local or general anesthesia depends on the surgeon expertise and clinical situation. Conjunctival peritomy must leave a room for pars plana sclerotomy, suturing of an IOL with scleral fixation or insertion of a Cionni ring. Conjuntiva should be spared for possible glaucoma surgery in the future. If anterior hyaloid is partly exposed, a dispersive VES can tamponade the vitreous. Dispersive VES may also provide protection for the endothelium, as endothelial cell density has been already reduced by the trauma [31].

Using vital dyes such as trypan blue has advantages: useful for finding thorn point of a capsule if needed.

With significant zonular damage, CTR can also be used to stabilize the bag. If the zonular damage involves more than 4 h (90°), suturing a Cionni ring can strengthen the area of greater zonular weakness [32]. This will improve the stability of the lens during all of the successive steps of the operation.

If introduction of ring is impossible prior to phaco, the surgeon can enhance zonular support with flexible nylon iris retractors or special capsule hooks introduced through a limbal incision, these hooks support the edge of capsulorrhexis (**Figure 4**). After emulsification of nucleus, CTR or Cionni ring can be positioned much more easily.

In case of vitreous present in anterior chamber, the surgeon must always avoid aspirating vitreous. Any traction exerted on anterior vitreous can create retinal tears and eventually lead to retinal detachment. Once vitreous removed from anterior chamber, the surgeon should then concentrate on the lens material.

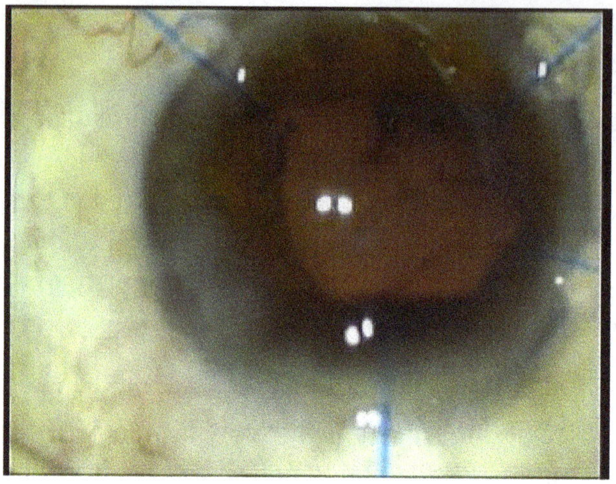

Figure 4. Iris hooks support the edge of capsulorrhexis vertically, acting like artifical zonules.

For soft nucleus, phacoaspiration of nucleus is generally safe and rapid. If there is a rupture of anterior or posterior capsule, manual aspiration with a Simcoe cannula and/or automated bimanual or coaxial irrigation and aspiration can be utilized. For harder nucleus, main principle is to reduce traction forces on remaining zonules. Many variations of delicate divide and conquer and particularly, phaco chop techniques can be chosen with low parameters of slow-motion phaco as described previously. If there is a significant zonular weakness and/or posterior capsular defect with a large lateral or inferior movement of the nucleus, then converting to manual extracapsular or intracapsular extraction techniques may be the only option.

It may be difficult for the surgeon to aspirate cortical material due to a lack of resistance of zonular fibers and manipulation may increase zonular dialysis. Using tangential movement as opposes to radial may be beneficial. If there is a capsular rupture, intact anterior hyaloid may covered with VES, after the surgeon can complete the removal of the cortex using manual dry aspiration. This technique utilizes a 25- or 27-gauge cannula attached to a 3-mL syringe, chamber filled with VES without allowing vitreous escape.

If there is an inadequate capsular support, the surgeon may try to suture one or both haptics of IOL to the sclera or the iris. With inadequate capsular support, the surgeon has several types of IOL such as scleral fixation, iris suture fixation, angle-supported anterior chamber IOL, or iris enclavation IOL. IOL Choice depends on the surgeon expertise and clinical situation.

After IOL has been inserted and appears to be well-centered, fixation can be confirmed using "Bounce test." This test is decentering the optic toward each one of two haptics and then releasing it. IOL should recenter spontaneously.

6. Femtosecond laser assistance in difficult cases

For white intumescent cataracts, using femtosecond laser to make capsulorrhexis without decompressing the anterior chamber allows round capsulorrhexis without any radial tears.

The surgeon may want to use additional vital dye to ensure the integrity of capsulorrhexis [33]. In traumatic cases and weak zonules even there is vitreous in the anterior chamber, femtosecond laser can make round capsulorrhexis.

Femtosecond laser assistance cataract surgery (FLACS) does not provide superior outcomes in all cases. In a recent study, two patients with bilateral posterior polar cataracts underwent traditional phacoemulsification in one eye and FLACS in the other eye. In both cases, the eye treated with FLACS developed a posterior capsule rupture during lens removal [34]. Caution may also be needed in the use of FLACS in glaucoma as docking procedure may raise intraocular pressure [35, 36]. In presence of silicone oil in AC, FLACS may result incomplete capsulotomy and lens fragmentation [37].

Use of femtosecond lasers in cataract surgery is continuing to evolve, together with its potential applications, but we think that its cost must be reduced to become popular among clinics.

7. Conclusions

Cataract surgery in difficult cases can be both enjoyable and troublesome. Knowing that every case has its own distinct features, the surgeon must treat each case in a unique way. We summarized some of the most encountered problems and solutions in this chapter. Each technique must be practiced preferably in animal's eyes or in simulation environments and then in easy standard cases. Before to try techniques for real difficult cases in real difficult situations, the surgeon must feel confident and relaxed about using mentioned techniques.

Author details

Baris Komur

Address all correspondence to: bkomur@gmail.com

Haseki Education and Research Hospital, Istanbul, Turkey

References

[1] Rana M, Shah S. Modern-day cataract surgery: Can we match growing expectations? The British Journal of Ophthalmology. 2014;**98**:1313-1314

[2] Limburg H. Monitoring cataract surgical outcomes: Methods and tools. Community Eye Health Journal. 2002;**15**:51-53

[3] Jackson H, Garway-Heath D, Rosen P, Bird AC, Tuft S. Outcome of cataract surgery in patients with retinitis pigmentosa. The British Journal of Ophthalmology. 2001;**85**:936-938

[4] Masket S. Relationship between postoperative pupil size and disability glare. Journal of Cataract and Refractive Surgery. 1992;**18**:506-507

[5] Solomon KD, Turkalj JW, Whiteside SB, Stewart JA, Apple DJ. Topical 0.5% ketorolac vs 0.03% flurbiprofen for inhibition of miosis during cataract surgery. Archives of Ophthalmology. 1997;**115**:1119-1122

[6] Stewart R, Grosserode R, Cheetham JK, Rosenthal A. Efficacy and safety profile of ketorolac 0.5% ophthalmic solution in the prevention of surgically induced miosis during cataract surgery. Clinical Therapeutics. 1999;**21**:721-732

[7] Donnenfeld ED, Perry HD, Wittpenn JR, Solomon R, Nattis A, Chou T. Preoperative ketorolac tromethamine 0.4% in phacoemulsification outcomes: Pharmacokinetic-response curve. Journal of Cataract and Refractive Surgery. 2006;**32**:1474-1482

[8] Morgado G, Barros P, Martins J, Lima A, Martins N. Comparative study of mydriasis in cataract surgery: Topical versus Mydriasert versus intracameral mydriasis in cataract surgery. European Journal of Ophthalmology. 2010;**20**:989-993

[9] Korobelnik JF, Tavera C, Renaud-Rougier MB, El Meski S, Colin J. The Mydriasert insert: An alternative to eye drops for preangiographic mydriasis. Journal Francais D'Ophtalmologie. 2004;**27**:897-902

[10] Levet L, Touzeau O, Scheer S, Borderie V, Laroche LA. Study of pupil dilation using the Mydriasert ophthalmic insert. Journal Français d'Ophtalmologie. 2004;**27**:1099-1108

[11] Liou SW, Chen CC. Maintenance of mydriasis with one bolus of epinephrine injection during phacoemulsification. Journal of Ocular Pharmacology and Therapeutics. 2001;**17**:249-253

[12] Lundberg B, Behndig A. Intracameral mydriatics in phacoemulsification cataract surgery. Journal of Cataract and Refractive Surgery. 2003;**29**:2366-2371

[13] Osher RH. Pupillary membranectomy. Video. Journal of Cataract and Refractive Surgery. 1991;**7**:7

[14] Barboni P, Zanini M, Rossi A, Savini G. Monomanual stretcher. Ophthalmic Surgery and Lasers. 1998;**29**:772-773

[15] Shingleton BJ, Campbell CA, O'Donoghue MW. Effects of pupil stretch technique during phacoemulsification on postoperative vision, intraocular pressure, and inflammation. Journal of Cataract and Refractive Surgery. 2006;**32**:1142-1145

[16] Goldman JM, Karp CL. Adjunct devices for managing challenging cases in cataract surgery: Capsular staining and ophthalmic viscosurgical devices. Current Opinion in Ophthalmology. 2007;**38**:32-57

[17] Chang DF. Use of Malyugin pupil expansion device for intraoperative floppy-iris syndrome: Results in 30 consecutive cases. Journal of Cataract and Refractive Surgery. 2008;**34**:832-841

[18] Agarwal A, Malyugin B, Kumar DA, Jacob S, Agarwal A, Laks L. Modified Malyugin ring iris expansion technique in small-pupil cataract surgery with posterior capsule defect. Journal of Cataract and Refractive Surgery. 2008;**34**:324-326

[19] Miyata K, Nagamoto T, Maruoka S, Tanabe T, Nakahara M, Amano S. Efficacy and safety of the soft-shell technique in cases with a hard lens nucleus. Journal of Cataract and Refractive Surgery. 2002;**38**:1546-1550

[20] Nagahara K. Video presentation. Seattle, WA: ASCRS; 1993

[21] Koch PS, Katzen LE. Stop and chop phacoemulsification. Journal of Cataract and Refractive Surgery. 1994;**20**:566-570

[22] Zeng M, Liu X, Liu Y, et al. Torsional ultrasound modality for hard nucleus phacoemulsification cataract extraction. The British Journal of Ophthalmology. 2008;**92**:1092-1096

[23] Fakhry MA, El Shazly MI. Torsional ultrasound mode versus combined torsional and conventional ultrasound mode phacoemulsification for eyes with hard cataract. Clinical Ophthalmology. 2011;**5**:973-978

[24] Fine IH, Packer M, Hoffman RS. Management of posterior polar cataract. Journal of Cataract and Refractive Surgery. 2003;**29**:16-19

[25] Vasavada AR, Raj SM. Inside-out delineation. Journal of Cataract and Refractive Surgery. 2004;**30**:1167-1169

[26] Osher RH, Yu BC, Koch DD. Posterior polar cataracts: a predisposition to intraoperative posterior capsular rupture. Journal of Cataract and Refractive Surgery. 1990;**16**:157-162

[27] Saika S, Kin K, Ohmi S, Ohnishi Y. Posterior capsule rupture by blunt ocular trauma. Journal of Cataract and Refractive Surgery. 1997;**23**:139-140

[28] Pieramici DJ, Capone A Jr, Rubsamen PE, Roseman RL. Lens preservation after intraocular foreign body injuries. Ophthalmology. 1996;**103**:1563-1567

[29] O'Duffy D, Salmon JF. Siderosis bulbi resulting from an intralenticular foreign body. American Journal of Ophthalmology. 1999;**127**:218-219

[30] Ozdemir O, Şengör T. Intraocular foreign body Detectedby Gonioscopy in the anterior chamber angle. Turkish Journal of Ophthalmology. 2013;**43**:278-281

[31] Fukagawa K, Tsubota K, Kimura C. Corneal endothelial cell loss induced by air bags. Ophthalmology. 1993;**100**:1819-1823

[32] Cionni RJ, Osher RH. Management of profound zonular dialysis or weakness with a new endocapsular ring designed for scleral fixation. Journal of Cataract and Refractive Surgery. 1998;**24**:1299-1306

[33] Asena BS, Erdur SK, Kaşkaloğlu M. Early experience in femtosecond laser assisted cataract surgery. Turkish Journal of Ophthalmology. 2015;**45**:97-101

[34] Alder BD, Donaldson KE. Comparison of 2 techniques for managing posterior polar cataracts: Traditional phacoemulsification versus femtosecond laser-assisted cataract surgery. Journal of Cataract and Refractive Surgery. 2014;**40**:2148-2151

[35] Darian-Smith E, Howie AR, Abell RG. Intraocular pressure during femtosecond laser pretreatment: Comparison of glaucomatous eyes and nonglaucomatous eyes. Journal of Cataract and Refractive Surgery. 2015;**41**:272-277

[36] Küçümen RB, Yenerel NM, Görgün E, Kohen MC, Başar D, Alimgil ML. Evaluation of changes in corneal biomechanical properties by ocular response Analyzer after femtosecond laser assisted LASIK. Turkish Journal of Ophthalmology. 2009;**39**:250-255

[37] Grewal DS, Singh Grewal SP, Basti S. Incomplete femtosecond laser-assisted capsulotomy and lens fragmentation due to emulsified silicone oil in the anterior chamber. Journal of Cataract and Refractive Surgery. 2014;**40**:2143-2147

5

Schlemm's Canal: The Outflow "Vessel"

Joanna Jabłońska, Katarzyna Lewczuk and

Marek Rękas

Abstract

The aim of this chapter is to review the knowledge about the aqueous outflow through Schlemm's canal. Morphology of this canal and aqueous humor pathways from the anterior chamber through the trabeculum into suprascleral and conjunctival veins via connector channels are described. Additionally, the role of Schlemm's canal in the development of glaucoma and outflow resistance is discussed. Canalography as a more precise method of assessing the conventional drainage pathway and facilitating localization of an uncollapsed collector and aqueous veins is shown. Attention is also drawn to the relationship between aqueous and suprascleral veins and heartbeat.

Keywords: Schlemm's canal, aqueous humor, conventional drainage pathway, outflow resistance, canalography, glaucoma

1. Introduction

Aqueous humor (AH) is drained from the eye via two physiological pathways. The conventional path begins at the level of the irido-corneal trabecular meshwork (TM) and is responsible for approximately 83–96% of drainage. From the anterior chamber, the aqueous humor moves through the trabecular meshwork to Schlemm's canal (SC) and then to intrascleral collector channels (CCs), which lead to the intrascleral venous plexus, aqueous vessels, and venous vessels of the suprascleral space. Aqueous vessels begin as collector channels in the exterior wall of Schlemm's canal and can be seen on the surface of the eye in the corneal limbus.

Aqueous humor flows out of the anterior chamber as a mass stream regulated by a pressure gradient. In healthy human eyes, outflow facility has a value of 0.40 at 10 mmHg and is reduced with age. From a physiological perspective, the trabeculum, particularly the interior wall of

Schlemm's canal, and the trabecular meshwork near collector channels are the main sources of resistance to aqueous outflow, and the remaining part of resistance is located in the exterior wall and surrounding tissues. Elevated IOP in glaucoma is caused by an increase in aqueous outflow resistance on its drainage pathways, not by an increase in aqueous production. Many authors believe that the source of outflow resistance in correct eyes is found close to or in the area of the interior wall of Schlemm's canal. Outflow resistance is not constant but a function of IOP and rises as IOP rises.

The aqueous humor flows out of Schlemm's canal through one of 30 collector channels and aqueous veins (AVs) and then to the system of suprascleral veins, ophthalmic veins, and general circulation. According to Poiseuille's law, the resistance of aqueous veins should be insignificant if they are not collapsed or compressed. Provocative gonioscopy, during which blood reflux into Schlemm's canal is observed, is the simplest method of assessing the conventional drainage pathway and facilitating localization of an uncollapsed collector and aqueous vein. Assessment of the distribution of aqueous veins in canalography is a more precise method. Studies by Grieschaber et al. showed a relationship between postoperative intraocular pressure (IOP) level and the presence of reflux in Schlemm's canal before surgery and between the degree to which water veins were filled. Zou introduced the trabeculum bypass theory, which reduces resistance in this part of the drainage route. He observed increased flow through Schlemm's canal only in the quadrant where the implant was applied, and intraocular pressure reduction was dependent on initial pressure.

Aqueous and suprascleral veins oscillate according to heartbeat. These oscillations enable continuous lamellar flow. Pressure in aqueous veins is sufficiently high and enables reverse lamellar flow from suprascleral veins at cardiac diastole. At cardiac systole, pressure in aqueous veins increases and reverses the direction of aqueous flow with simultaneous blood reflux.

2. Schlemm's canal

Schlemm's canal (SC) was named in honor of the German anatomist, Friedrich Schlemm, who, in 1830, discovered the canal in the anterior chamber angle, draining aqueous humor (AH) into the bloodstream [1, 2]. It is a ring-like canal with a length of 36–40 mm encircling the cornea [3, 4] and directly adjacent to the juxtacanalicular trabecular meshwork (JCT) [5], and together with the trabecular meshwork (TM), it forms the conventional outflow pathway, which accounts for 50–90% of AH flow [6, 7]. Its cross-section has the shape of an elongated ellipse, with its longer axis measuring 150–350 μm. Three-dimensional visualizations have made it possible to take precise measurements of the canal, the cross-sectional area of which ranges from 4064 to 7164 μm^2 [8–12]. Rarely, the canal may be bi- or tripartite [13], and it may sometimes contain septa [14]. One of the primary functions of SC is to drain aqueous humor from the trabeculum to collector channels (CCs).

Due to its direct adjacency to the trabeculum, not all SC cells are identical [5, 15]. Owing to the canal's microanatomy, we can distinguish between the inner and outer wall, each built of a continuous, single-cell layer of endothelium. The cells of both walls differ in terms of morphology [16], the presence of different marker expressions, cell organelles, and function [17]. The inner wall is more frequently analyzed because it presents the greatest resistance to drainage of AH [18–20]. Endothelial cells of the inner wall are shaped like paver stones, while the cells of the outer wall are smooth and flat [15]. Tight junctions of VE-cadherin as well as characteristic giant vacuoles and pores are the markers for cells of the inner wall. Desmin, reactivity to Factor VIII-related antigen, and the presence of Weibel-Palade bodies are the markers for cells of the outer wall [6, 21–26].

2.1. Embryogenesis

Schlemm's canal is a highly specialized vessel. Despite many similarities to vascular endothelium, the canal's embryonic origin and progression of its development have still not been precisely determined [5]. Earlier research suggested a vascular origin of cells [24, 27–29], but recent publications have classified them as unique endothelial cells with phenotypical traits of the endothelial cells of both blood and lymphatic vessels [30–33]. In humans, the prenatal development of SC begins with development of the trabeculum in the 17th week [15]; in the 24th week, the canal is already defined and encircles the limbus over 360°; and in the 36th week, the canal and collector channels are fully developed [34].

The organogenesis of SC was described by Kizhatil as a combination of the vascular developmental factors of angiogenesis and lymphangiogenesis. He termed this process "*canalogenesis,*" which begins from the limbal vascular plexus [30]. The development of SC can be divided into four stages, starting from differentiation of the canal's precursor cells, proliferation and migration of frontal cells, formation of the canal's lumen, and separation from the venous vascular system [5]. PROX1 and VEGFR-3 expression is required for division of frontal cells and shaping them into the canal.

2.2. Genetics

PROX1 (*prospero homeobox protein 1*) is the main regulator of lymphangiogenesis, and its expression is critical in transforming cells of the vascular endothelium into cells of the lymphatic endothelium [5, 30, 32]. Truong was the first to demonstrate a high level of expression of the PROX1 lymphatic transcription factor in the canal's endothelial cells, thus showing the similarity to lymphatic endothelial cells [7]. VEGFR-3 (*vascular endothelial growth factor receptor 3*), or FLT4, is a receptor belonging to the RTKs-KDR (*kinase insert domain-containing receptor*) family; it binds the VEGF-C and VEGF-D vascular endothelial growth factors, and its expression is typical of endothelium in lymphatic vessels [35]. Aspelund et al. [31] and Park et al. [32] presented the properties of the precursor cells of Schlemm's canal as well as key molecular mechanisms required for differentiation of these cells into the mature cells of the canal [31, 32]. Aspelund demonstrated that the VEGF-C vascular endothelial growth factor is necessary for activating migration of vascular endothelial cells and their further formation from transscleral venous vessels. He also demonstrated that precursor cells are, in essence, vascular endothelial cells with VEGFR-2 and TIE-2 (*tunica interna endothelial cell kinase*) expression. Precursor cells then gain PROX1 expression in order to create and form the canal's lumen and also VEGFR-3 for later maturing of the canal's cells [31, 32]. Both aqueous humor and VEGF-C are required for proper SC development. A reduction in AH in mice resulted in the loss of elements of canal cells' lymphatic identity [32]. The direct relationship of the SC endothelium with JCT and the fact that the development of TM precedes the development of SC allow for the hypothesis that soluble factors from JCT cells may be of critical significance for obtaining phenotypical traits of SC cells. Because the inner wall of SC is in direct contact with the TM over a 360° circumference, modern canal surgery provides access to the entire inner wall of SC and the juxtacanalicular region without affecting the cornea, iris, and ciliary body. Canaloplasty may be used to deliver transgenic SC/TM vectors in glaucoma gene therapy [36].

2.3. Role of NO

Several studies have also documented the influence of cytokines (tumor necrosis factor (TNF)-α, interleukin (IL)1-α, IL-β, IL-8) released by TM cells on SC cells, as well as their influence on regulation of aqueous drainage [37, 38]. Nitrogen oxide (NO) was widely studied from the perspective of its role in modulating the behavior of SC cells and regulating aqueous flow [39, 40]. Stresses in the SC endothelium trigger no production in SC cells, similarly as in other vascular endothelial cells [39]. Nitrogen oxide also mediates volume reduction in SC cells, which is linked to facilitation of AH drainage [40].

2.4. Biomechanics

The hydraulic conductivity of the conventional aqueous drainage pathway amounts to approximately 10^{-7} $cm^2\,s^{-1}g^{-1}$, and this value also sets the lower limit for hydraulic conductivity of the SC endothelium, which is 2–5 times greater than the hydraulic conductivity of brain endothelium and the greatest in the entire human body [41]. In SC, the biomechanical conditions acting on endothelial cells resemble the microenvironment in a lymphatic vessel [30]. In SC endothelial cells, the pressure gradient is distributed from the base to the apex of a cell similarly as in lymphatic vessels, but inversely to the distribution in the case of vascular endothelium [42]. In a typical blood vessel, the basement membrane and surrounding tissue provide additional support for endothelial cells, reducing circumferential, and radial stresses acting on cells. In the case of SC cells, the inverted pressure gradient caused by AH flowing into the canal's lumen generates a force that pushes cells away from the basement membrane [43]. However, in contrast to a lymphatic vessel, SC cells are bound by tight junctions, so they maintain the pressure difference between the eyeball and episcleral veins (EPV). Forces related to the pressure drop from the base to the apex of a cell result in cell deformation and the formation of large, dome-shaped diverticula into the canal's lumen, called giant vacuoles [41, 42, 44–47]. Besides tight junctions between endothelial cells, there are extensive links between endothelial cells and cells in the JCM area. These junctions are present when SC cells form protrusions to join with JCM cells, forming parachute-like structures. These junctions, described by Johnstone, play an important role in anchoring the canal's endothelial cells in response to increases in pressure [15, 48]. The size of SC's lumen changes in response to IOP fluctuations [48]. When IOP increases, the TM widens while the canal narrows, and this is caused by an increase in the number of vacuoles and of the area of the extracellular matrix (ECM), as well as by the fact that both walls of the canal are closer to one another. At high IOP, the probability that the canal's walls will collapse and resistance on drainage outflow pathways will grow increases significantly [48]. When IOP increases to approximately 40 mmHg, the canal collapses, with the exception of segments containing septa [20, 49], which support the walls of SC and prevent occlusion of CCs [20, 48, 49]. In eyes with glaucoma, the lumen of SC is smaller than in healthy eyes [50].

2.5. Microanatomy-giant vacuoles and pores

Giant vacuoles are potential spaces between extracellular matrix (ECM) and the SC's inner wall cells [15]. Giant vacuoles form dynamically and respond to changes in intraocular pressure (IOP) instantaneously [5, 51]. Their quantity and size increase as IOP increases. After enucleation, the IOP drops to zero, and vacuoles disappear within a time of <3 min [52]. The majority of giant vacuoles are found near CCs outlets [52], which suggests that a greater pressure gradient is present at CCs outlets due to the greater aqueous flow [15]. Most probably due to the specific biomechanical microenvironment, endothelial cells are characterized by contractile properties and by an elastic modulus of 1–3 kPa [41], which is slightly greater than in the case of other endothelial cells [42, 47]. SC cells owe their capability of adapting to deformations to the cytoskeleton system fortified with actin microfilaments. Cells of the outer wall have star-shaped F-actin systems that pass through most cells, in contrast to the circumferential F-actin bands observed in endothelial cells of the inner wall [53]. The position of SC cells relative to ECM allows for reception of biomechanical signals from the ECM [37], which affect the expression of cells' genes and adapt them to changes in the rigidity. The rigidity and contractility of SC cells exhibited a strong response to pharmacological stimulation. Medications increasing resistance to drainage increased the rigidity of SC cells, and inversely, medications reducing resistance to drainage reduced the rigidity of these cells [41]. In eyes with glaucoma, endothelial cells are more sensitive and exhibit an amplified response to the increase in the substrate's rigidity that occurs in glaucoma [42]. Stress caused by a rise in IOP can increase cell surfaces by up to 50% and even cause them to thin out [22]. Tight junctions between endothelial cells of the inner wall are very sensitive to increases in IOP and become less complex when IOP is elevated [37]. Endothelial deformation may initiate the formation of pores mediating aqueous transport by loosening intercellular junctions [54–56].

Pores are structures in the inner wall with sizes ranging from 0.6 to 3 μm [25, 43, 57], and they are responsible for 10% of the resistance to aqueous drainage [37]. They may be found in the walls of giant vacuoles, but they may also be unrelated to them [21]. They form the main pathway of aqueous flow through the inner wall of SC. Two pore types have been identified and characterized: type I pores (transcellular) and type B pores (paracellular) [25]. They differ in their locations, filtration ability, and formation mechanisms [43]. B pores are larger, but they are outnumbered 3–4 to 1 by I pores. Type B pores form as a result of local loosening and widening of intercellular junctions [43]. Braakman et al. [26] presented a segmentation of the aqueous drainage stream, and type B pores account for the majority of aqueous flow. Type I pores may form as a result of a combination of deformations of the cellular membrane at the base and apex of an endothelial cell, which may occur under the influence of the aqueous filtration stream, and caveolae, vesicles, and minipores [43, 58]. Pores in Schlemm's canal are most frequently formed from minipores 60 nm in size, covered by a diaphragm containing PLVAP (plasmalemma vesicle-associated protein) [43, 58]. Molecular pore formation processes are not well known, but PLVAP is most probably involved in them, considering that pore formation is significantly impaired in mice with PLVAP deficiency [58, 59]. Pore density in the interior wall fluctuates between 1000 and 2000/mm^2 [55, 60]. When IOP is elevated, the number of pores in the inner wall increases [25, 51, 55]. Giant vacuoles and pores are unique features of the endothelium of SC's inner wall and of the endothelium of the arachnoid villi in the central nervous system [42, 61, 62]. Scanning electron micrograph of the inner wall of Schlemm's canal can visualize the giant vacuoles and pores at the base of a bulging structure (**Figure 1**) [56].

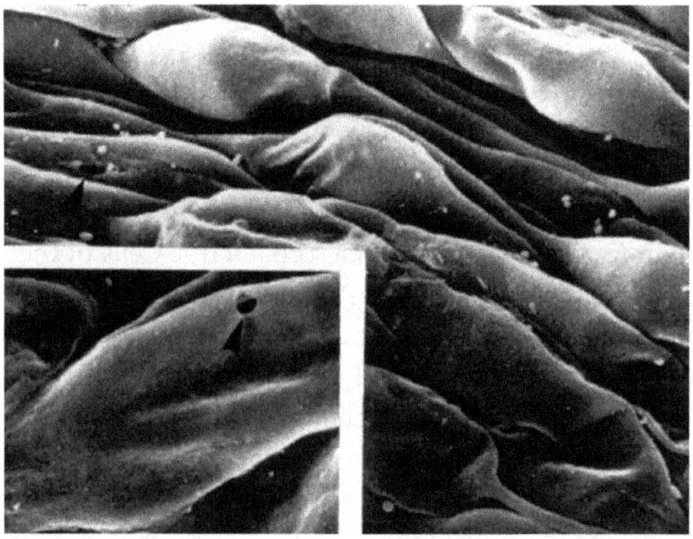

Figure 1. Scanning electron micrograph of the giant vacuoles and pores of the inner wall of Schlemm's canal. A pore (arrow) is observed at the base of a bulging structure (modified from Allingham et al. [56]).

The formation of giant vacuoles is directed in one direction, providing a preferential aqueous drainage pathway through the endothelium by means of a one-way valve mechanism. In the case of a pressure increase in episcleral veins and in SC that exceeds IOP, the number of vacuoles and pores decreases, preventing blood reflux from SC into the anterior chamber [42, 63, 64]. Certain medications, such as glycocorticosteroids or sphingosine-1-phosphate (S1P), which induce polymerization of the cytoskeleton's proteins [65, 66], may inhibit the formation and reduce the density of vacuoles, increasing resistance to drainage [67, 68]. Eyes with glaucoma exhibit reduced pore density, which emphasizes the critical role of the inner wall in maintaining homeostasis of AH. The aqueous flow resistance is considerably increased by the hydrodynamic interaction between pores and their basal substrate- subendothelial (basement membrane of SC cells and extracellular matrix of JCT) [69]. In particular, flow is concentrated near every pore, forming funnels that flow through the region of extracellular matrix closest to a given pore, which significantly reduces the effective area available for flow through these regions [42]. The goal of glaucoma therapy oriented toward SC may be to increase pore density, and thus drainage, leading to reduction in IOP [55].

2.6. Distribution of aqueous humor

AH in Schlemm's canal is not distributed uniformly through the canal's inner wall, but rather appears preferentially at certain locations. Drainage of AH most frequently occurs near CCs [70]. Twice as many giant vacuoles are present near collectors, which suggests that aqueous flow through the inner wall is dependent on the value of pressure [52]. Studies involving the application of fluorescent markers have also demonstrated an elevated level of markers in the pigmented part of TM adhering to CCs, suggesting that the preferred drainage outflow pathways are present near collectors [70]. Histological research on human eyes has proven that, between the 25th and 30th year of life, CCs are randomly distributed around the eye, with preferential dislocation in the inferior nasal quadrant [1, 71]. This has been confirmed by three-dimensional micro-CT tests [72]. There is high diversity in the size of CCs outlets, with values ranging between 5–50 μm and up to 70 μm depending on the type of test [1, 71, 72]. From the CCs, AH flows through a winding system of venous plexuses, from the deep scleral plexus, through the limbal plexus, to the intrascleral plexus, which ultimately leads to the episcleral veins [6].

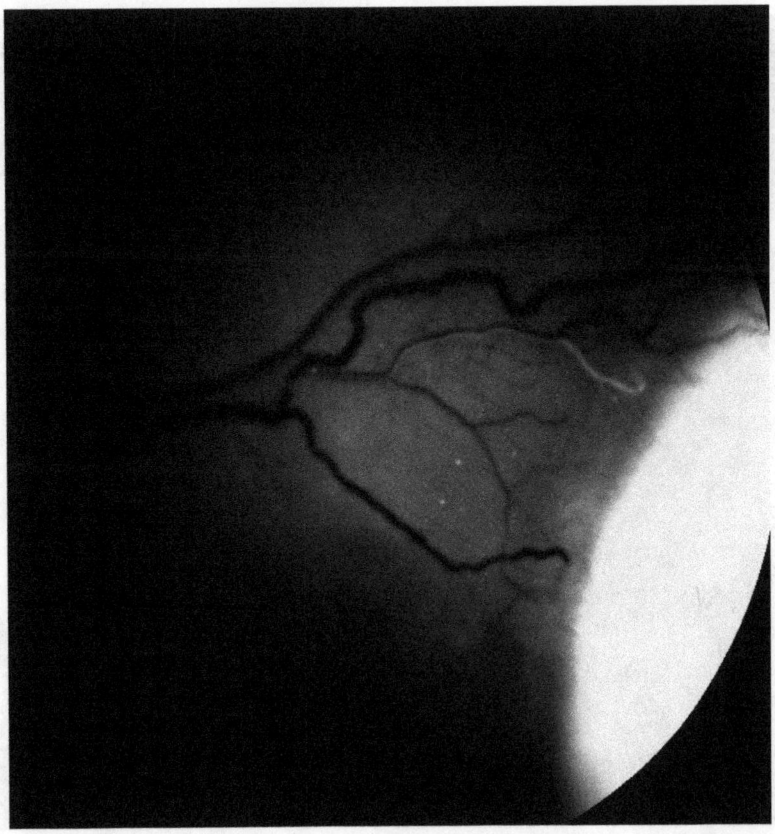

Figure 2. Aqueous veins.

2.7. Aqueous veins

Aqueous humor moves through the TM into SC, issuing forth from its lumen into CCs, aqueous veins (AVs) (**Figure 2**) and the system of episcleral veins (EPV) (**Figure 3**), ocular veins, and into the general circulation [21, 73]. AVs have lumens that are directly connected to CCs, and because of this, they are directly connected to the episcleral veins draining blood into the general circulation, bypassing the deep scleral and intrascleral venous plexuses [74, 75]. AVs containing initially clean AH are joined to episcleral veins filled with blood, which is why transition zones can be identified on the surface of the conjunctiva as large vessels with a transparent, central lumen bounded by dark blood from all sides. Linear stratification into AH and blood occurs due to the differences in these fluids' viscosity and density [76]. The composition of blood and aqueous in transition zones changes as IOP changes. Direct observation of these changes is a reliable indicator for assessment of the effectiveness of topical and surgical therapy oriented toward IOP reduction in glaucoma [77]. AVs differ in their position, size, and anatomical configuration. In a slit lamp test, 2–3 AVs are usually visible, and sporadically, up to 6 AVs may be seen [78, 79]. AVs are nonuniformly distributed and are present in the greatest number in the inferior nasal quadrants [78, 80]. Their size varies from 20 to 100 μm, 50 μm on average [78, 81, 82]. Histologically, AVs cannot be distinguished from conjunctival and EPV [80].

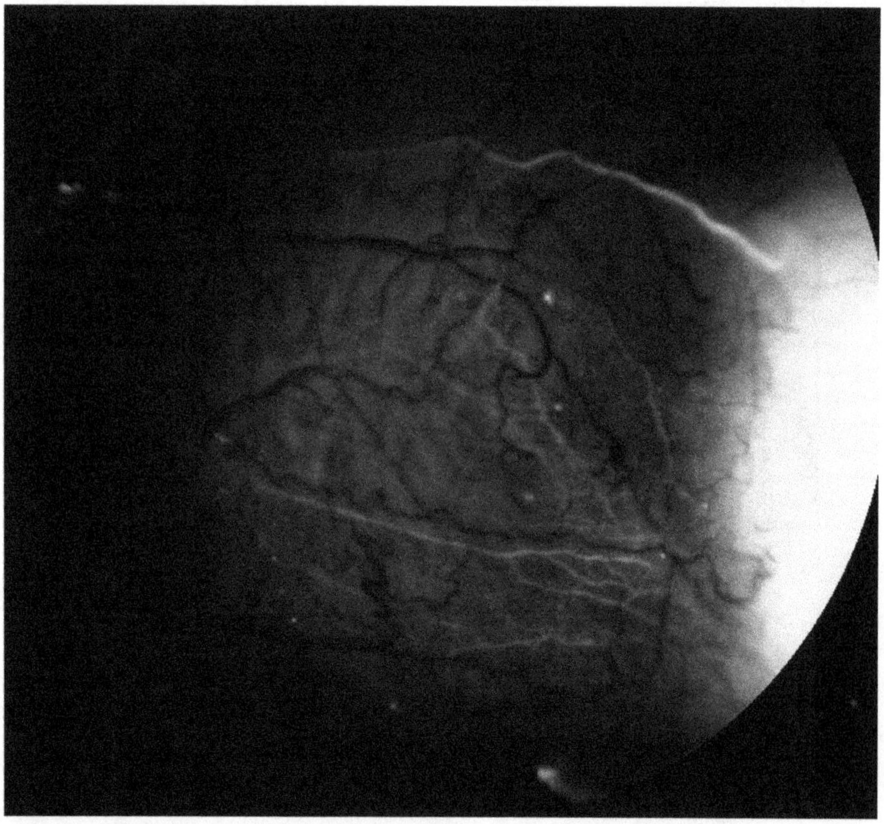

Figure 3. Episcleral veins.

2.8. Aqueous humor drainage

IOP is the primary factor affecting AH drainage. Drainage through the conventional outflow pathway is directly proportional to the IOP value within the range of physiological values [83, 84]. Drainage facility is the measure of how easily AH leaves the eye, and it is the inverse of resistance to drainage [20, 85]. In healthy human eyes, drainage facility has a value of 0.40 μl/min/mmHg at an IOP of 10 mmHg [86]. The main point of resistance to AH drainage is located at the JCM level in juxtacanalicular connective tissues, in the inner wall of SC, and its basement membrane [21, 69]. Elevated IOP in glaucoma is caused by an increase in aqueous outflow resistance on its drainage outflow pathways, not by an increase in aqueous production [87]. AH flow, defined as the movement of AH from the posterior chamber of the eye through the pupil into the anterior chamber, is lower than aqueous production because it does not include the AH that leaves the posterior chamber via other pathways [85]. The value of AH flow through the anterior chamber is not dependent on sex [88]. AH flow amounts to 2.4 ± 0.6 μl/min and decreases with age by 2% per decade [88], which may result in a reduction of up to 30% [89]. It has also been observed that flow is halved during the night (1.13–1.6 μl/min) as compared to the day (3.0–3.1 μl/min) [89, 90]. In studies with fluorescein, it was observed that flow value is also significantly lower in eyes with pseudoexfoliation syndrome than in physiologically correct eyes [88].

2.9. Effective filtration areas

Based on observations of the distribution of pigment and perfusion markers, it was determined that, circumferentially, drainage of AH in healthy eyes is nonuniform and segmented [91–94]. At any given time, only some AH drainage pathways are actively involved in aqueous percolation. These active areas are called effective filtration area (EFA) [50, 80, 95]. EFA is a valuable method for measuring resistance to flow and the effects of IOP changes. Segmented drainage has been described in mice [96], pigs [97], cows [91, 93], monkeys [94], and humans [70, 97, 98]. Higher marker concentration was present in the TM neighboring the outlets of CCs, and in humans, more pigment was also observed at this location, suggesting that EFA locations can be determined by using pigment distribution as a marker [80]. A sudden increase in IOP in cow eyes caused a significant reduction in EFA [91, 93]. When IOP increased suddenly, the marker was present in a greater concentration near CC outlets. When IOP was correct, the drainage patterns were more uniform, and when IOP was elevated, drainage became more segmented [91]. EFA reduction is linked to reduction in drainage facility and is reversed when pressure is reduced from high to normal level [99]. EFA reduction was also observed in an animal model, in eyes with glaucoma and chronic IOP elevation that had undergone laser therapy [100]. In this study, reduction in the marker level was determined in regions of the TM that had undergone laser therapy. It was stated that active drainage shifted from areas that had undergone laser therapy to areas not affected by therapy. In a study, where a marker was applied, significant EFA reduction was observed in eyes with glaucoma in comparison with healthy eyes [101]. In addition, the inversely proportional dependence between EFA and IOP has been documented on an animal model in the eyes of a mouse with ocular hypertension [96].

2.10. Pulsating flow

Drainage of AH is a complex process. Besides the traditional approach, according to which the AH moves passively in a combined stream through TM into SC, downward along the pressure gradient determined by the heart [102], a significant effect of the active process driven by means of a mechanical pump is also assumed [77]. Pulsating flow occurs as a result of oscillating compressive force caused by transitional IOP increases occurring during the cardiac cycle, blinking, and eye movements. These transitional IOP spikes cause microscopic deformations of the flexible structural elements of drainage outflow pathways. During contraction, the canal's endothelial cells move to the outside, forcing AH flow to the outlets of CCs and AVs. When the value of IOP drops, flexible elements move back to their original configuration, which leads to a relative reduction in pressure in SC inducing AH flow into the SC's lumen [11, 102, 103]. The theory that pulsating flow drives AH drainage is reflected in the dynamic equilibrium between AH and blood in AVs [104]. During contraction, the pulse wave causes flow of AH through AVs, resulting in visible widening of the aqueous layer in their lumens [78]. Eyes with glaucoma exhibit reduced pulsating flow in comparison with healthy eyes [105, 106]. In healthy eyes, the TM is susceptible to deformation under the influence of naturally occurring, dynamic changes in pressure and volume of AH flow from the anterior chamber to SC. Reduction in pulsating flow in glaucoma may be caused by changes in the TM's elasticity [75].

Author details

Joanna Jabłońska*, Katarzyna Lewczuk and Marek Rękas

*Address all correspondence to: joannajablonska.md@gmail.com

Department of Ophthalmology, Military Institute of Medicine, Warsaw, Poland

References

[1] Dvorak-Theobald G. Schlemm's canal: its anastomoses and anatomic relations. Trans Am Ophthalmol Soc. 1934;32:574–95. https://www.ncbi.nlm.nih.gov/pmc/articles/PMC1315493/

[2] Mansouri K, Shaarawy T. Update on Schlemm's canal based procedures. Middle East Afr J Ophthalmol. 2015;22:38–44. doi:10.4103/0974-9233.148347

[3] Freddo TF, Johnson M. The eye's aqueous humor. Aqueous humor outflow resistance. Curr Topics Membr. Elsevier; 2008;62:161–192 doi:org/10.1016/S1063-5823(08)00406-7

[4] Seiler T, Wollensak J. The resistance of the trabecular meshwork to aqueous humor outflow. Graefe's Arch Clin Exp Ophthalmol = Albr von Graefes Arch für Klin und Exp Ophthalmol. 1985;223:88–91. doi:10.1007/BF02150951

[5] Dautriche C, Tian Y, Xie Y, Sharfstein S. A closer look at Schlemm's canal cell physiology: implications for biomimetics. J Funct Biomater. 2015;6:963–85. doi:10.3390/jfb6030963

[6] Goel M, Picciani RG, Lee RK, Bhattacharya SK. Aqueous humor dynamics: a review. Open Ophthalmol J. 2010;4:52–9. doi:10.2174/1874364101004010052

[7] Truong TN, Li H, Hong Y, Chen L. Novel characterization and live imaging of Schlemm's canal expressing Prox-1. PLoS One. 2014;9:1–8. doi:10.1371/journal.pone.0098245

[8] Kagemann L, Wang B, Wollstein G, Ishikawa H, Nevins JE, Nadler Z, et al. IOP elevation reduces Schlemm's canal cross-sectional area. Invest Ophthalmol Vis Sci. 2014;55:1805–9. doi:10.1167/iovs.13-13264

[9] Kagemann L, Wollstein G, Ishikawa H, Bilonick R a, Brennen PM, Folio LS, et al. Identification and assessment of Schlemm's canal by spectral-domain optical coherence tomography. Invest Ophthalmol Vis Sci. 2010;51:4054–9. doi:10.1167/iovs.09-4559

[10] Kagemann L, Nevins JE, Jan N-J, Wollstein G, Ishikawa H, Kagemann J, et al. Characterisation of Schlemm's canal cross-sectional area. Br J Ophthalmol. 2014;98:10–4. doi:10.1136/bjophthalmol-2013-304629

[11] Kagemann L,Wollstein G, Ishikawa H, et al. 3D visualization of aqueous humor outflow structures in-situ in humans. Exp Eye Res. 2011;141(4):520–9. doi:10.1016/*j*.exer.2011.03.019

[12] Sambasivarao S V. Visualization of the conventional outflow pathway in the living human eye. Ophthalmology. 2013;18(9):1199–216. doi:10.1016/j.ophtha.2012.02.032

[13] Ten Hulzen RD, Johnson DH. Effect of fixation pressure on juxtacanalicular tissue and Schlemm's canal. Investig Ophthalmol Vis Sci. 1996;37:114–24. http://iovs.arvojournals.org/article.aspx?articleid=2180115

[14] Dietlein TS, Jacobi PC, Lüke C, Krieglstein GK. Morphological variability of the trabecular meshwork in glaucoma patients: implications for non-perforating glaucoma surgery. Br J Ophthalmol. 2000;84:1354–9. doi:10.1136/bjo.84.12.1354

[15] Ethier CR. The inner wall of Schlemm's canal. Exp Eye Res. 2002;74:161–72. doi:10.1006/exer.2002.1144

[16] Lütjen-Drecoll E, Rohen JW. Endothelial studies of the Schlemm's canal using silver-impregnation technic. Albr von Graefe's Arch Clin Exp Ophthalmol. 1970;180:249–66. http://www.ncbi.nlm.nih.gov/pubmed/4938983

[17] Karl MO, Fleischhauer JC, Stamer WD, Peterson-Yantorno K, Mitchell CH, Stone RA, et al. Differential P1-purinergic modulation of human Schlemm's canal inner-wall cells. Am J Physiol Cell Physiol. 2005;288:784–94. doi:10.1152/ajpcell.00333.2004

[18] Vranka JA, Kelley MJ, Acott TS, Keller KE. Extracellular matrix in the trabecular meshwork: intraocular pressure regulation and dysregulation in glaucoma. Exp Eye Res. 2015;133:112–25. doi:10.1016/j.exer.2014.07.014

[19] Acott TS, Kelley MJ. Extracellular matrix in the trabecular meshwork. Exp Eye Res. 2008;86:543–61. doi:10.1016/j.exer.2008.01.013

[20] Johnson MC, Kamm RD. The role of Schlemm's canal in aqueous outflow from the human eye. Investig Ophthalmol Vis Sci. 1983;24:320–5. http://www.ncbi.nlm.nih.gov/pubmed/6832907

[21] Tamm ER. The trabecular meshwork outflow pathways: structural and functional aspects. Exp Eye Res. 2009;88:648–55. doi:10.1016/j.exer.2009.02.007

[22] Hamanaka T, Bill A, Ichinohasama R, Ishida T. Aspects of the development of Schlemm's canal. Exp Eye Res. 1992;55:479–88. doi:10.1016/0014-4835(92)90121-8

[23] Heimark RL, Kaochar S, Stamer WD. Human Schlemm's canal cells express the endothelial adherens proteins, VE-cadherin and PECAM-1. Curr Eye Res. 2002;25:299–308. http://www.ncbi.nlm.nih.gov/pubmed/12658549

[24] Hamanaka T, Bill A. Platelet aggregation on the endothelium of Schlemm's canal. Exp Eye Res. 1994;59:249–56. doi:10.1006/exer.1994.1106

[25] Ethier CR, Coloma FM, Sit AJ, Johnson M. Two pore types in the inner-wall endothelium of Schlemm's canal. Invest Ophthalmol Vis Sci. 1998;39:2041–8. http://www.ncbi.nlm.nih.gov/pubmed/9761282

[26] Braakman ST, Read AT, Chan DW-H, Ethier CR OD. Colocalization of outflow segmentation and pores along the inner wall of Schlemm's canal. Exp Eye Res. 2015;130:87–96. doi:10.1016/j.exer.2014.11.008

[27] Smelser GK, Ozanics V. The development of the trabecular meshwork in primate eyes. Am J Ophthalmol. 1971;71:366–85. http://www.ncbi.nlm.nih.gov/pubmed/5542135

[28] Wulle KG. Electron microscopic observations of the development of Schlemm's canal in the human eye. Trans Am Acad Ophthalmol Otolaryngol. 1968;72:765–73. http://www.ncbi.nlm.nih.gov/pubmed/5692862

[29] Foets B, van den Oord J, Engelmann K, Missotten L. A comparative immunohistochemical study of human corneotrabecular tissue. Graefe's Arch Clin Exp Ophthalmol = Albr von Graefes Arch für Klin und Exp Ophthalmol. 1992;230:269–74. doi:10.1007/BF00176303

[30] Kizhatil K, Ryan M, Marchant JK, Henrich S, John SWM. Schlemm's canal is a unique vessel with a combination of blood vascular and lymphatic phenotypes that forms by a novel developmental process. PLoS Biol. 2014;12:e1001912. doi:org/10.1371/journal.pbio.1001912

[31] Aspelund A, Tammela T, Antila S, Nurmi H, Leppänen V-M, Zarkada G, et al. The Schlemm's canal is a VEGF-C/VEGFR-3-responsive lymphatic-like vessel. J Clin Invest. 2014;124:3975–86. doi:10.1172/JCI75395

[32] Park D-Y, Lee J, Park I, Choi D, Lee S, Song S, et al. Lymphatic regulator PROX1 determines Schlemm's canal integrity and identity. J Clin Invest. 2014;124:3960–74. doi: 10.1172/JCI75392

[33] Karpinich NO, Caron KM. Schlemm's canal: More than meets the eye, lymphatics in disguise. J Clin Invest. 2014;124:3701–3. doi:10.1172/JCI77507

[34] Ramírez JM, Ramírez AI, Salazar JJ, Rojas B, De Hoz R, Triviño A. Schlemm's canal and the collector channels at different developmental stages in the human eye. Cells Tissues Organs. 2004;178:180–5. doi:10.1159/000082248

[35] Neufeld G, Cohen T, Gengrinovitch S, Poltorak Z. Vascular endothelial growth factor (VEGF) and its receptors. FASEB J. 1999;13:9–22. http://www.ncbi.nlm.nih.gov/pubmed/9872925

[36] Tian B, Kaufman PL. A potential application of canaloplasty in glaucoma gene therapy. Transl Vis Sci Technol. 2013;2(1):2. doi:10.1167/tvst.2.1.2

[37] Alvarado JA, Yeh R-F, Franse-Carman L, Marcellino G, Brownstein MJ. Interactions between endothelia of the trabecular meshwork and of Schlemm's canal: a new insight into the regulation of aqueous outflow in the eye. Trans Am Ophthalmol Soc. 2005;103:148–63. http://www.ncbi.nlm.nih.gov/pmc/articles/PMC1447570/

[38] Alexander JP, Acott TS. Involvement of the Erk-MAP kinase pathway in TNFalpha regulation of trabecular matrix metalloproteinases and TIMPs. Invest Ophthalmol Vis Sci. 2003;44:164–9. http://www.ncbi.nlm.nih.gov/pubmed/12506070

[39] Ashpole NE, Overby DR, Ethier CR, Stamer WD. Shear stress-triggered nitric oxide release from Schlemm's canal cells. Invest Ophthalmol Vis Sci. 2014;55:8067–76. doi: 10.1167/iovs.14-14722

[40] Ellis DZ, Sharif NA, Dismuke WM. Endogenous regulation of human Schlemm's canal cell volume by nitric oxide signaling. Invest Ophthalmol Vis Sci. 2010;51:5817–24. doi: 10.1167/iovs.09-5072

[41] Zhou EH, Krishnan R, Stamer WD, Perkumas KM, Rajendran K, Nabhan JF, et al. Mechanical responsiveness of the endothelial cell of Schlemm's canal: scope, variability

and its potential role in controlling aqueous humour outflow. J R Soc Interface. 2012;9:1144–55. doi:10.1098/rsif.2011.0733

[42] Stamer WD, Braakman ST, Zhou EH, Ethier CR, Fredberg JJ, Overby DR, et al. Biomechanics of Schlemm's canal endothelium and intraocular pressure reduction. Prog Retin Eye Res. 2014;44:1–13. doi:10.1016/j.preteyeres.2014.08.002

[43] Braakman ST, Pedrigi RM, Read AT, Smith JAE, Stamer WD, Ethier CR, et al. Biomechanical strain as a trigger for pore formation in Schlemm's canal endothelial cells. Exp Eye Res. 2014;127:224–35. doi:10.1016/j.exer.2014.08.003

[44] Miteva DO, Rutkowski JM, Dixon JB, Kilarski W, Shields JD, Swartz MA. Transmural flow modulates cell and fluid transport functions of lymphatic endothelium. Circ Res. 2010;106:920–31. doi:10.1161/CIRCRESAHA.109.207274

[45] Raviola G, Raviola E. Paracellular route of aqueous outflow in the trabecular meshwork and canal of Schlemm. A freeze-fracture study of the endothelial junctions in the sclerocorneal angle of the macaque monkey eye. Investig Ophthalmol Vis Sci. 1981;21(1 II):52–72.http://www.ncbi.nlm.nih.gov/pubmed/7251302

[46] Overby DR, Zhou EH, Vargas-Pinto R, Pedrigi RM, Fuchshofer R, Braakman ST, et al. Altered mechanobiology of Schlemm's canal endothelial cells in glaucoma. Proc Natl Acad Sci USA. 2014;111:13876–81. doi:10.1073/pnas.1410602111

[47] Zeng D, Juzkiw T, Read AT, Chan DWH, Glucksberg MR, Ethier CR, et al. Young's modulus of elasticity of Schlemm's canal endothelial cells. Biomech Model Mechanobiol. 2010;9:19–33. doi:10.1007/s10237-009-0156-3

[48] Johnstone MA. Pressure-dependent changes in nuclei and the process origins of the endothelial cells lining Schlemm's canal. Invest Ophthalmol Vis Sci. 1979;18:44–51. http://www.ncbi.nlm.nih.gov/pubmed/103860

[49] Van Buskirk EM. Anatomic correlates of changing aqueous outflow facility in excised human eyes. Invest Ophthalmol Vis Sci. 1982;22:625–32. http://www.ncbi.nlm.nih.gov/pubmed/7076408

[50] Allingham RR, de Kater AW, Ethier RC. Schlemm's canal and primary open angle glaucoma: correlation between Schlemm's canal dimensions and outflow facility. Exp Eye Res. 1996;62:101–10. doi:10.1006/exer.1996.0012

[51] Epstein DL, Rohen JW. Morphology of the trabecular meshwork and inner-wall endothelium after cationized ferritin perfusion in the monkey eye. Investig Ophthalmol Vis Sci. 1991;32:160–71. http://www.ncbi.nlm.nih.gov/pubmed/1987099

[52] Parc CE, Johnson DH, Brilakis HS. Giant vacuoles are found preferentially near collector channels. Invest Ophthalmol Vis Sci. 2000;41:2984–90. http://www.ncbi.nlm.nih.gov/pubmed/10967055

[53] Ethier CR, Read AT, Chan D. Biomechanics of Schlemm's canal endothelial cells: influence on F-actin architecture. Biophys J. 2004;87(4):2828–37. doi:10.1529/biophysj.103.038133 [cited 2016 Mar 12]

[54] Johnson M, Shapiro A, Ethier CR, Kamm RD. Modulation of outflow resistance by the pores of the inner wall endothelium. Investig Ophthalmol Vis Sci. 1992;33(5):1670–5. http://www.ncbi.nlm.nih.gov/pubmed/1559767

[55] Johnson M, Chan D, Read AT, Christensen C, Sit A, Ethier CR. The pore density in the inner wall endothelium of Schlemm's canal of glaucomatous eyes. Investig Ophthalmol Vis Sci. 2002;43(9):2950–5. http://www.ncbi.nlm.nih.gov/pubmed/12202514

[56] Allingham RR, De Kater AW, Ethier CR, Anderson PJ, Hertzmark E, Epstein DL. The relationship between pore density and outflow facility in human eyes. Investig Ophthalmol Vis Sci. 1992;33(5):1661–9. http://www.ncbi.nlm.nih.gov/pubmed/1559766

[57] Grierson I, Lee WR. Pressure-induced changes in the ultrastructure of the endothelium lining Schlemm's canal. Am J Ophthalmol. 1975;80:863–84. http://www.ncbi.nlm.nih.gov/pubmed/811121

[58] Herrnberger L, Ebner K, Junglas B, Tamm ER. The role of plasmalemma vesicle-associated protein (PLVAP) in endothelial cells of Schlemm's canal and ocular capillaries. Exp Eye Res. 2012;105:27–33. doi:10.1016/j.exer.2012.09.011

[59] Herrnberger L, Hennig R, Kremer W, Hellerbrand C, Goepferich A, Kalbitzer HR, et al. Formation of fenestrae in murine liver sinusoids depends on plasmalemma vesicle-associated protein and is required for lipoprotein passage. PLoS One. 2014;9(12):e115005. doi:10.1371/journal.pone.0115005 [cited 2016 Mar 26]

[60] Sit AJ, Coloma FM, Ethier CR, Johnson M. Factors affecting the pores of the inner wall endothelium of Schlemm's canal. Invest Ophthalmol Vis Sci. 1997;38:1517–25. http://www.ncbi.nlm.nih.gov/pubmed/9224279

[61] Bill A, Svedbergh B. Scanning electron microscopic studies of the trabecular meshwork and the canal of Schlemm–an attempt to localize the main resistance to outflow of aqueous humor in man. Acta Ophthalmol. 1972;50:295–320. doi:10.1111/j.1755-3768.1972.tb05954.x

[62] Tripathi BJ, Tripathi RC. Vacuolar transcellular channels as a drainage pathway for cerebrospinal fluid. J Physiol. 1974;239:195–206. http://www.ncbi.nlm.nih.gov/pubmed/4369428

[63] Pedrigi RM, Simon D, Reed A, Stamer WD, Overby DR. A model of giant vacuole dynamics in human Schlemm's canal endothelial cells. Exp Eye Res. 2011;92:57–66. doi:10.1016/j.exer.2010.11.003

[64] Alvarado JA, Betanzos A, Franse-Carman L, Chen J, González-Mariscal L. Endothelia of Schlemm's canal and trabecular meshwork: distinct molecular, functional, and

anatomic features. Am J Physiol Cell Physiol. 2004;286:621–34. doi:10.1152/ajpcell.00108.2003

[65] Filla MS, Schwinn MK, Nosie AK, Clark RW, Peters DM. Dexamethasone-associated cross-linked actin network formation in human trabecular meshwork cells involves β3 integrin signaling. Investig Opthalmol Vis Sci. 2011;52:2952. doi:10.1167/iovs.10-6618

[66] Clark AF, Wilson K, McCartney MD, Miggans ST, Kunkle M, Howe W. Glucocorticoid-induced formation of cross-linked actin networks in cultured human trabecular meshwork cells. Invest Ophthalmol Vis Sci. 1994;35:281–94. http://www.ncbi.nlm.nih.gov/pubmed/8300356

[67] Underwood JL, Murphy CG, Chen J, Franse-Carman L, Wood I, Epstein DL, et al. Glucocorticoids regulate transendothelial fluid flow resistance and formation of intercellular junctions. Am J Physiol. 1999;277:330–42. http://www.ncbi.nlm.nih.gov/pubmed/10444410

[68] Sumida GM, Stamer WD. Sphingosine-1-phosphate enhancement of cortical actomyosin organization in cultured human Schlemm's canal endothelial cell monolayers. Invest Ophthalmol Vis Sci. 2010;51:6633–8. doi:10.1167/iovs.10-5391

[69] Johnson M. What controls aqueous humour outflow resistance? Exp Eye Res. 2006;82:545–57. doi:10.1016/j.exer.2005.10.011

[70] Hann CR, Fautsch MP. Preferential fluid flow in the human trabecular meshwork near collector channels. Invest Ophthalmol Vis Sci. 2009;50:1692–7. doi:10.1167/iovs.08-2375

[71] Rohen JW, Rentsch FJ. Morphology of Schlemm's canal and related vessels in the human eye. Albr von Graefes Arch für Klin und Exp Ophthalmol Albr von Graefe's Arch Clin Exp Ophthalmol. 1968;176:309–29. http://www.ncbi.nlm.nih.gov/pubmed/5305008

[72] Hann CR, Bentley MD, Vercnocke A, Ritman EL, Fautsch MP. Imaging the aqueous humor outflow pathway in human eyes by three-dimensional micro-computed tomography (3D micro-CT). Exp Eye Res. 2011;92:104–11. doi:10.1016/j.exer.2010.12.010

[73] Toris CB. Aqueous humor dynamics and intraocular pressure elevation. Second Ed. Glaucoma. Elsevier Ltd; 2015. 47–56. http://linkinghub.elsevier.com/retrieve/pii/B9780702051937000066

[74] Ascher KW. The aqueous veins: I. Physiologic importance of the visible elimination of intraocular fluid. Am J Ophthalmol. 1942;25:1174–209. doi:10.1016/S0002-9394(42)90325-8

[75] Schacknow PN SJ. The glaucoma book: a practical, evidence-based approach to patient care. 1st ed. Vol. 53, J Chem Inf Model. New York: Springer-Verlag; 2010. 1689–1699

[76] Meighan SS. Blood vessels of the bulbar conjunctiva in man. Br J Opthalmol. 1956;40:513–26. http://www.ncbi.nlm.nih.gov/pubmed/13364178

[77] Johnstone MA. The aqueous outflow system as a mechanical pump: evidence from examination of tissue and aqueous movement in human and non-human primates. J Glaucoma. 2004;13:421–38. http://www.ncbi.nlm.nih.gov/pubmed/15354083

[78] De Vries S. De zichtbare afvoer van het kamerwater. 1st ed. Drukkerij Kinsbergen. Amsterdam; 1947

[79] Johnstone M, Jamil A, Martin E. Aqueous veins and open angle glaucoma. In: The Glaucoma Book. New York, NY: Springer New York; 2010:65–78. DOI: 10.1007/978-0-387-76700-0_7

[80] Surgical Innovations in Glaucoma. Springer Science & Business Media; 2014;307. https://books.google.com/books?id=7uS5BAAAQBAJ&pgis=1 http://www.springer.com/us/book/9781461483472

[81] Stepanik J. Measuring velocity of flow in aqueous veins. Am J Ophthalmol. 1954;37:918–22. doi:10.1016/0002-9394(54)91933-9

[82] Goldmann H. Weitere Mitteilung über den Abfluss des Kammerwassers beim Menschen. Ophthalmologica. 1946;112:344–9. http://www.ncbi.nlm.nih.gov/pubmed/20293720

[83] Morrison JC, Pollack IP. Glaucoma: science and practice. Thieme; New York Stuttgart 2003. https://books.google.pl/books?isbn=1588905918

[84] Glaucoma Research and Clinical Advances 2016 to 2018. Kugler Publications; 2016:336. https://www.kuglerpublications.com/index.php?p=316&page=publication

[85] Morrison JC, Freddo TF TC. Anatomy and physiology of aqueous humor formation. Glaucoma Science and Practice. Stuttgart: Thieme New York; 2003:4–41. http://s2.bitdownload.ir/Ebook/Biology/Medicine/Glaucoma%20-%20Science%20and%20Practice%20-%20J.%20Morrison,%20I.%20Pollack%20(Thieme,%202003)%20WW.pdf

[86] Brubaker RF. The effect of intraocular pressure on conventional outflow resistance in the enucleated human eye. Invest Ophthalmol. 1975;14:286–92. http://www.ncbi.nlm.nih.gov/pubmed/1123284

[87] Grant WM. Clinical measurements of aqueous outflow. AMA Arch Ophthalmol. 1951;46:113–31. http://www.ncbi.nlm.nih.gov/pubmed/14856471

[88] Brubaker RF. The flow of aqueous humor in the human eye. Trans Am Ophthalmol Soc. 1982;80:391–474. http://www.ncbi.nlm.nih.gov/pubmed/1748546

[89] Reiss GR, Lee DA, Topper JE, Brubaker RF. Aqueous humor flow during sleep. Invest Ophthalmol Vis Sci. 1984;1:776–8. http://www.ncbi.nlm.nih.gov/pubmed/6724850

[90] Viggiano SR, Koskela TK, Klee GG, Samples JR, Arnce R, Brubaker RF. The effect of melatonin on aqueous humor flow in humans during the day. Ophthalmology. 1994;101:326–31. doi:10.1016/S0161-6420(94)31332-7

[91] Battista SA, Lu Z, Hofmann S, Freddo T, Overby DR, Gong H. Reduction of the available area for aqueous humor outflow and increase in meshwork herniations into collector channels following acute IOP elevation in bovine eyes. Investig Ophthalmol Vis Sci. 2008;49:5346–52. doi:10.1167/iovs.08-1707

[92] Camp JJ, Hann CR, Johnson DH, Tarara JE, Robb RA. Three-dimensional reconstruction of aqueous channels in human trabecular meshwork using light microscopy and confocal microscopy. Scanning. 2006;19:258–63. doi:10.1002/sca.4950190402

[93] Lu Z, Overby DR, Scott PA, Freddo TF, Gong H. The mechanism of increasing outflow facility by rho-kinase inhibition with Y-27632 in bovine eyes. Exp Eye Res. 2008;86:271–81. doi:10.1016/j.exer.2007.10.018

[94] Lu Z, Zhang Y, Freddo TF, Gong H. Similar hydrodynamic and morphological changes in the aqueous humor outflow pathway after washout and Y27632 treatment in monkey eyes. Exp Eye Res. 2011;93:397–404. doi:10.1016/j.exer.2011.05.012

[95] Cha EDK, Xu J, Gong L, Gong H. Variations in active outflow along the trabecular outflow pathway. Exp Eye Res. 2016;146:354–60; doi:10.1016/j.exer.2016.01.008

[96] Swaminathan SS, Oh D-J, Kang MH, Ren R, Jin R, Gong H, et al. Secreted protein acidic and rich in cysteine (SPARC)-null mice exhibit more uniform outflow. Invest Ophthalmol Vis Sci. 2013;54:2035–47. doi:10.1167/iovs.12-10950

[97] Keller KE, Bradley JM, Vranka JA, Acott TS. Segmental versican expression in the trabecular meshwork and involvement in outflow facility. Invest Ophthalmol Vis Sci. 2011;52:5049–57. doi:10.1167/iovs.10-6948

[98] Yang CYC, Liu Y, Lu Z, Ren R, Gong H. Effects of Y27632 on aqueous humor outflow facility with changes in hydrodynamic pattern and morphology in human eyes. Investig Ophthalmol Vis Sci. 2013;54:5859–70. doi:10.1167/iovs.12-10930

[99] Zhu JY, Ye W, Wang T, Gong HY. Reversible changes in aqueous outflow facility, hydrodynamics, and morphology following acute intraocular pressure variation in bovine eyes. Chin Med J (Engl). 2013;126:1451–7. http://www.ncbi.nlm.nih.gov/pmc/articles/PMC3771502/

[100] Zhang Y, Toris CB, Liu Y, Ye W, Gong H. Morphological and hydrodynamic correlates in monkey eyes with laser induced glaucoma. Exp Eye Res. 2009;89:748–56. doi:10.1016/j.exer.2009.06.015

[101] Cha E, Jin R, Gong H. The relationship between morphological changes and reduction of active areas of aqueous outflow in eyes with primary open angle glaucoma. Invest Ophthalmol Vis Sci. 2013;54:2291–2291. http://iovs.arvojournals.org/article.aspx?articleid=2146968

[102] Bill A. Blood circulation and fluid dynamics in the eye. Physiol Rev. 1975;55:383–417. http://www.ncbi.nlm.nih.gov/pubmed/1153528

[103] Johnstone M, Martin E, Jamil A. Pulsatile flow into the aqueous veins: manifestations in normal and glaucomatous eyes. Exp Eye Res. 2011;92:318–27. doi:10.1016/j.exer.2011.03.011

[104] Zamir M, Budwig R. Physics of pulsatile flow. Appl Mech Rev. 2002;55:35. doi:10.1007/978-1-4612-1282-9

[105] Kleinert H. The visible flow of aqueous humor in the epibulbar veins. II. The pulsating blood vessels of the aqueous humor. Albr von Graefe's Arch für Ophthalmol. 1952;152:587–608. http://www.ncbi.nlm.nih.gov/pubmed/12976314

[106] Kleinert HW, Ascher KW, Goldmann H, Duke-Elder WS, Goldmann H, Ascher KW, et al. The compensation maximum. AMA Arch Ophthalmol. 1951;46:618. http://www.ncbi.nlm.nih.gov/pubmed/14868091

6

Managing Intraocular Pressure: Innovation in Glaucoma Management

Anne-Marie Bleau, Beatriz Vargas,
Ana Isabel Jiménez and Covadonga Pañeda

Abstract

Primary open-angle glaucoma is a progressive ocular neuropathy that if left untreated may lead to blindness. The main risk factor for developing glaucoma is increased intraocular pressure. Intraocular pressure is regulated by the balance of aqueous humour synthesis and secretion into the eye and outflow from the eye; therefore, most therapies for glaucoma seek lowering intraocular pressure to avoid disease progression. There are several types of drugs in the market for the treatment of glaucoma, but there are still unmet needs to be overcome; therefore, significant effort has been put in the last few years to develop new medicines with innovative mechanisms of action as well as devices to improve quality of life in glaucoma patients. The present review offers a thorough revision of the latest advances in the glaucoma therapy field, focusing on innovative approaches, new targets and new mechanisms of action.

Keywords: glaucoma, innovation, therapy, oligonucleotides, devices, stem cells, gene therapy

1. Introduction

Primary open-angle glaucoma (POAG) is a multi-factorial optic neuropathy characterized by retinal ganglion cell degeneration and progressive visual field loss [1]. The underlying molecular changes leading to ocular tissue damage in glaucoma are largely unknown, but it has been shown that reduction in intraocular pressure (IOP) correlates with a decrease in disease progression. As such, treatment in glaucoma is mainly oriented towards reducing IOP to reach a target reduction of approximately 25–30% from the patient's baseline [2]. Pressure in the eye is maintained by balancing the amount of fluid contained within the anterior and posterior chambers; thus, reduction in IOP is achieved either by reducing the amount of aqueous humour (AH) secreted into the eye or by increasing its outflow [1]. AH is produced by the epithelial cells of the ciliary processes through a complex mechanism that involves ultrafiltration, active transport and diffusion; AH is thereafter secreted into the posterior chamber. AH circulates from the posterior chamber around the lens and through the pupil into the anterior chamber and exits the eye trough one of two pathways: the conventional pathway or the uveoscleral route. AH exiting the anterior chamber through the conventional route crosses the trabecular meshwork (TM) to reach the Schlemm's canal (SC) located at the limbus. Contraction of the ciliary muscle causes the TM to expand and SC to open resulting in increased outflow through this route. The main source of outflow resistance through this route is the extracellular matrix of the TM and the inner wall endothelium of the SC. Through the unconventional or uveoscleral route, AH flows from the iris angle through the anterior face of ciliary muscle into the connective tissue located between the muscle bundles to finally reach the suprachoroidal space. The fluid is thereafter drained through the sclera or the perivascular spaces into the episcleral tissue where it enters the venous circulation. In contrast to the conventional route, the main source of AH outflow resistance is the ciliary body [3].

The eye is a contained organ that is partially isolated from the rest of the body; this isolation provides a certain immune privilege and limits the amount of compound needed to perform proof-of concept studies. In addition, the eye has a sophisticated structure with many different cell types and specialized barriers making it an ideal organ for studying delivery of larger compounds. As such, the eye has often been used to study new mechanisms of action and to obtain initial data for new compounds in development. Therefore, it is not surprising that most innovative new classes of drugs have, at some point, been tested in the eye, among these new classes of drugs are aptamers, antisense oligonucleotides (ASO), short interfering RNAs (siRNA), antibodies, stem cells, gene therapy and different types of delivery approaches and devices.

Here, we will review innovative programs developing drugs for the treatment of glaucoma focusing on the latest advances oriented towards lowering IOP, paying particular attention to the mechanisms used by these drugs and devices.

2. Pharmacological innovation

Progressive and irreversible loss of vision is the most feared complication for glaucoma. While current treatments focus on lowering IOP, up to date no therapies have been approved to address the critical issue of visual field deterioration. For this reason, high unmet needs remain for the development of innovative approaches to treat such aspect of the disease. Fortunately, beyond classic eye drop medicines, various exciting therapies are emerging in the field. Overall, these techniques aim to provide either a novel alternative to reduce IOP or a protection and regeneration of retinal ganglion cells (RGCs) to ultimately reverse vision loss. In this section, we will describe novel techniques for the treatment of glaucoma. Interestingly, these complex strategies have been combined in order to achieve broader efficacy.

Traditionally, drug discovery has been based on screening large libraries of compounds to select products with specific activities. However, in the last decades, advances in the molecular biology field have allowed the search for active candidates to become more rational. As a result, new pharmaceuticals with innovative mechanisms of action, target specific design and improved pharmaceutical properties have emerged. Some of the advantages of these new compounds include increased specificity, reduced toxicity and the ability to address targets that cannot be engaged by traditional small molecules. Among these new pharmaceuticals are biologicals, stem cells, gene therapy and therapies based on oligonucleotides.

Developing innovative compounds for the treatment of glaucoma entails thus targeting the function of cells and tissues related to IOP control; these tissues include the ciliary muscle, the TM, the SC, collector channels and aqueous veins. The latest discoveries in molecular biology allow the identification of key molecules that control AH dynamics in these tissues, and these molecules can be used as starting point for new therapeutic strategies and discovery of new targets. In order to fully take advantage of these approaches, the characteristics of these specific tissues have to be taken into account when designing the therapeutic strategy. The following characteristics are particularly interesting when developing innovative glaucoma therapies:

1. The TM is composed of phagocytotically active cells; this facilitates the entrance of compounds that exert their action inside the cell. Phagocytosis may be enhanced by some surgical procedures.

2. Many of the cells of the TM are non-proliferative, terminally differentiated cells; this prolongs the action of certain therapies that can exert their action inside cells such as genetic therapies, antibodies and oligonucleotide-based therapies.

3. The TM and the SC are structures with the ability to present antigens and induce tolerance; this may work in favour of some therapies that usually induce an immune response.

4. Tissues responsible for IOP control are located in the anterior chamber and are more accessible than tissues of the back of the eye; therefore, invasive procedures are not usually required.

2.1. New drug targets

As mentioned above, current approaches to develop new drugs for the treatment of glaucoma are aimed towards decreasing IOP to avoid further damage to the glaucomatous eye. Five drug-types are currently approved to treat glaucoma: alpha agonists, beta-blockers, carbonic anhydrase inhibitors, prostaglandin analogues and cholinergic drugs. Given the information available from the field of genetics, it is surprising that no new targets have reached the clinic since prostaglandin analogues, but this may change in the near future. Here, we review the information and mechanistic data existing for three new targets against which several compounds are currently under clinical development.

2.1.1. Rho-associated protein kinase (ROCK) inhibitors

2.1.1.1. Description and biological function

The Rho family consists of three guanosine triphosphate (GTP)-binding proteins named RhoA, RhoB and RhoC, which belong to the Ras-superfamily of GTPases [4]. Rho proteins bound to guanosine diphosphate (GDP) remain inactive in the cytoplasm of the cell; upon binding of GTP, these proteins become active and translocate to the cellular membrane where they exert their function [5]. The Rho activation and inactivation cycle is regulated by GTP-ase activating proteins (GAP) and guanine nucleotide-exchange factors (GEFs) that catalyse GTP and GDP exchange [6]. Rho proteins are ubiquitously expressed and participate in the regulation of cytoskeletal dynamics, thus playing a central role in cell morphology, adhesion and migration, as well as in numerous signalling pathways [7]. Increased levels of RhoA expression have been detected in optic nerve head of glaucomatous eyes [8].

One of the most comprehensively studied effectors of Rho proteins is the Rho-associated coiled-coil containing protein kinases (ROCK), which are serine-threonine kinases composed of a catalytic domain, a coiled-coin Rho-binding site and an auto-inhibitory domain [9]. In humans, ROCKs exist as two isoforms, ROCK1 and ROCK2, expressed in a wide variety of tissues including the TM and the ciliary muscle cells [10]. Multiple studies indicate that ROCK regulate the contractile properties of the TM, synthesis of extra-cellular matrix (ECM) and outflow of AH through the TM; factors known to be involved in AH dynamics [11]. In addition, ROCK1 and ROCK2 knock-out mice exhibit lower values of IOP when compared to those of their wild-type littermates [12].

2.1.1.2. Mechanism of action

Upon activation, ROCK phosphorylates a large number of substrates inducing their activation or inhibition; many of these substrates, such as the myosin light chain (MLC), the myosin phosphatase (MLP) and actin-binding LIM kinase (LIMK), actively participate in cytoskeletal dynamics and cell motility of the TM, SC and ciliary muscle [13, 14]. The contraction/relaxation status of these structures influences the resistance to AH outflow and as a result modulate IOP homeostasis. In consequence, the results of multiple studies have proposed a role of ROCK inhibitors in enhancing AH drainage through the TM by altering the cytoskeleton [15]. NF-κβ is another downstream effector of the ROCK pathway; its activation controls the translation of pro-inflammatory mediators such as interleukins or TNF-α.

The anti-fibrotic activity of ROCK inhibitors seems also to be relevant to the therapeutic role of these agents in glaucoma. Post-operative scaring is one of the main causes of filtration surgery failure; scaring tissue formed at the TM leads to poor IOP control and allows silent disease progression. The differentiation of fibroblasts to myofibroblasts during wound healing and scar formation is mediated by TGF-β that facilitates the contractile response of fibroblasts. ROCK inhibitors such as Y-27632 and AMA0526 have demonstrated to improve surgical outcome in animal models of glaucoma filtration surgery [16, 17]. Additionally, ROCK inhibitors such as Y-39983 and fasudil have been found to improve blood flow to the optic nerve head, seemingly due to their action on MLC that regulates the contraction of smooth muscle cells in the blood vessels irrigating this area [18, 19]. Finally, it has been shown that ROCK may also have an effect on central nervous system (CNS) targets involved in neuronal survival and axonal regeneration thus giving ROCK inhibitors an added-on value to their role on AH dynamics [20].

2.1.1.3. *Drugs in development*

Y-27632 was the first identified ROCK specific inhibitor, and **SNJ-1656** (also known as Y-39983/ RKI983; Senju and Novartis Pharmaceuticals) was the first ROCK inhibitor to demonstrate an IOP-lowering effect in human subjects [21]. Despite its effect in humans, the clinical development of this compound was halted in Phase II due to insufficient efficacy and a poor tolerability profile [22]. ROCK inhibitors currently undergoing clinical trials in glaucoma include ripasudil (KowaCompany, Ltd; Japan), netarsudil (Aerie Pharmaceuticals, Inc; USA), PG324 (Aerie Pharmaceuticals, Inc; USA) and AMA0076 (Amakem; Belgium).

Ripasudil hydrochloride hydrate, formerly known as K-115 (Glanatec® ophthalmic solution 0.4%), was approved in Japan in September 2014 for the treatment of glaucoma and ocular hypertension when other therapeutic drugs are not effective or cannot be administered, at the dosage of one drop per eye, twice daily (b.i.d) [23, 24]. Compiled data from Phase II and III clinical trials indicated that this drug achieved a 15% IOP reduction (3.5 mmHg), being conjunctival hyperaemia the most frequently reported adverse event with incidence rates ranging from 55 to 74% [25, 26]. Non-clinical studies proved that ripasudil inhibited both ROCK1 and ROCK2 (IC50 0.051 and 0.019 μmol/L, respectively) and mechanistic studies performed in rabbits demonstrated that its ocular hypotensive effect is due to increased drainage of AH through the TM and SC [27]. Ripasudil induces cytoskeletal changes secondary to ROCK inhibition that lead to the retraction and rounding of the TM cells decreasing the compaction of the TM allowing aqueous outflow. Additionally, *in vitro* studies demonstrated that ripasudil reduced outflow resistance and increased SC endothelial cell permeability [28].

Netarsudil (Rhopressa™ ophthalmic solution, 0.02%), formerly known as AR-13324, is a ROCK and a norepinephrine transporter (NET) inhibitor currently in Phase III clinical trials [29]. In a Phase II study, this product achieved a 22% reduction in mean diurnal IOP after 28 treatment days when administered in eye drops once daily (*q.d*). However, non-inferiority versus latanoprost was not met [30]. IOP reduction is thought to be achieved by three different mechanisms of action: increasing AH outflow through the TM, reducing the pressure in the epliscleral vein and reducing AH synthesis. Real-time effect of netarsudil on AH dynamics was evaluated *in vivo* both in albino and pigmented mice using a custom-made optical coherence tomography system [31]. This technique confirmed that the IOP-lowering effect of netarsudil is related to its action both in proximal and distal steps of the outflow pathway. It was noted that the observed cytoskeletal changes induced by netarsudil caused the expansion of the conventional outflow tissues such as the TM and the SC avoiding its collapse at elevated IOP. As a NET inhibitor, netarsudil is thought to decrease AH secretion since elevated norepinephrine levels activate $\alpha 2$ adrenergic receptors responsible for AH production at the ciliary processes [32]. Finally, netarsudil is also thought to have vasodilator properties as it reduces episcleral venous pressure in rabbits facilitating AH drainage to the bloodstream [32]. Similarly to ripasudil, ocular hyperaemia was the most frequently reported AE during clinical development with incidence rates of 57% which improved during the course of the study decreasing to 24% after 28 treatment days.

Roclatan™, formerly known as PG323, is a fixed dose combination (FDC) of netarsudil 0.02% and latanoprost 0.005%, which combines the previously described mechanisms of action with the capacity of the prostaglandins of increasing AH outflow through the uveoscleral pathway [33, 34]. This fixed combination currently in Phase III clinical trials achieved clinically and statistically superiority in terms of ocular hypotensive efficacy when compared to its individual active components at the same concentrations. However, incidence rates of ocular hyperaemia were superior in the FDC than those observed in the latanoprost group (40 vs. 60%).

AMA0076 is a locally acting ROCK inhibitor currently in Phase II clinical trials specifically designed to reduce IOP while minimizing side effects such as hyperemia. *In vivo* studies conducted in an acute hypertensive rabbit model showed that AMA0076 prevented IOP elevation more efficiently than latanoprost and bimatoprost. *In vitro* studies conducted in rabbit ocular tissues demonstrated that AMA0076 was able to induce reversible changes in cell shape and decreased the number of actin filaments and focal adhesions that may facilitate AH outflow [35].

2.1.2. Adenosine receptor ligands

2.1.2.1. Description and biological function

Adenosine is an endogenous nucleoside modulator of both intracellular and extracellular origin. Adenosine half-life is very limited (~1.5 seconds) as it is rapidly metabolized to inosine and hipoxantine; this is why extracellular levels of adenosine, which usually range from 20 to 200 nM, are considered a good indicator of cellular homeostasis. Adenosine levels increase, even up to the micromolar range, in response to cellular stress conditions such as tissue hypoxia or ischemia. In fact, adenosine levels in AH are significantly elevated in ocular hypertensive individuals when compared to normotensive individuals [36, 37].

Adenosine receptors (ARs) belong to the family of G protein-coupled receptors (GPCR) [37]. Four subtypes of AR have been identified (A1, A2A, A2B and A3), and all of them are involved in regulation of cAMP production through different pathways: A1 and A3 down-regulate cAMP levels inhibiting adenylyl cyclase, whereas A2A and A2B receptors activate adenylyl cyclase, increasing cAMP production. ARs are expressed in numerous ocular tissues such as ciliary body, TM, SC and retina. Activation/inactivation of ARs impacts AH formation, outflow and consequently IOP homeostasis. Additionally, ARs are also involved in retinal function, impacting blood flow and neuronal survival [36].

2.1.2.2. Mechanism of action

Activation of A3 receptors results in activation of Cl^- channels in the non-pigmented ciliary epithelial (NPE) cells of the ciliary epithelium where AH is produced [38]. Studies conducted in A3AR knockout mice and in mice treated with A3AR antagonists showed that absence or inhibition of this receptor significantly decreases IOP when compared to native or untreated animals [39]. On the contrary, mice treated with A3AR agonists show enhanced chloride release resulting in increased AH production and rise in IOP. AR can also affect AH outflow; there are two pathways by which AR agonists increase conventional outflow through the TM and SC: cell volume modification mediated by ion transport and ECM remodelling [36]. A1, A2A and A3 AR agonists have shown to increase Ca^{2+} in the cells of the SC and to diminish

TM cell volume [40]. Outflow resistance in the TM is dependent on the composition of the ECM; activation of A1 ARs triggers signalling cascades that lead to the expression of high levels of metalloproteases such a MMP-2 and MMP-9, enzymes participating in ECM remodelling enhancing AH outflow and decreasing IOP. On the contrary, A2A and A2B AR activation increase ECM deposition and therefore difficult AH outflow increasing IOP [41].

In view of the previously exposed mechanisms, it can be concluded that AR ligands play a key role in IOP control. In general terms, adenosine binding to A1AR in the TM reduces outflow resistance. However, A2A AR stimulation may result in IOP increase or decrease depending on the alterations to the resistance in the SC. Finally, activation of A3 AR mediates activation of Cl^-channels in the NPE cells inducing AH production, while A3 AR antagonists prevent adenosine-induced activation of Cl^- channels decreasing IOP.

2.1.2.3. Drugs in development

Numerous AR ligands (both agonists and antagonists) are being developed with the purpose of exploiting their potential for modulation of IOP. The adenosine analogues that are currently in glaucoma clinical trials include trabodenoson (Inotek Pharmaceuticals, US), OPA-6566 (Acucela, US and Otsuka Pharmaceutical, Japan), ATL-313 (Santen Pharmaceutical) and CF-101 (Can-Fite Bio Pharma, US).

Trabodenoson, formerly known as INO-8875/PJ-875, is a highly selective A1 AR agonist administered in eye drops currently in Phase III clinical trials. The IOP-lowering effect of four different doses of trabodenoson ranging from 50 to 500 μg was evaluated when administered b.i.d during 28 consecutive days in a Phase II clinical trial [42]. Administration of trabodenoson resulted in a dose-related IOP reduction; the highest dose tested achieved a statistically significant IOP reduction in 25% (6.5 mmHg) when compared to placebo. All the doses tested showed a good tolerability profile. The proposed mechanism of action for trabodenoson involves activation of the A1 adenosine receptor that promotes phosphorylation of the extracellular signal-regulated kinases ERK1 and ERK2, resulting in increased secretion of MMP-2 and changes in the ECM that decrease TM resistance to the AH outflow.

OPA-6566 and **ATL-313** are two A2A agonists currently in Phase I clinical trials; at this point of development, little information on their clinical development is available. Both drugs are anticipated to increase AH outflow via the conventional pathway of the TM and SC rather than the uveoscleral pathway.

CF-101 is an A3 AR agonist orally administered presently in Phase II clinical trials. Recently, CF-1001 failed to meet its primary endpoint as no statistically significant differences in IOP were found between the CF101 group and the placebo group after 16 treatment weeks.

2.1.3. Nitric oxide donors

2.1.3.1. Description and biological function

Nitric oxide (NO) is a gaseous endogenous signalling molecule synthesized by nitric oxide synthases (NOS) that catalyse the oxidation of the amino acid L-arginine to form NO and

L-citrulline. There are three NOS isoforms: the neuronal NOS (nNOS or NOS-1), the endothelial NOS (eNOS or NOS-3) and the inducible NOS (iNOS or NOS-2). NOS-1 and NOS-3 are activated by the calcium/calmodulin complex in response to an increase in calcium and produce NO in the pico- or nanomolar scale. On the contrary, NOS-2 activation is calcium independent and produces NO in a micro- to millimolar scale [43].

NOS-3 is expressed in TM, SC, ciliary body and uveal vascular endothelium. NOS-1 is located in nerve fibres in the cornea and lens epithelium and iNOS is detected after directed stimulation in the TM and in the ciliary body and vessels. This expression pattern of NOS enzymes in the anterior segment of the eye suggests that NO plays a key role in the regulation of AH dynamics. In fact, levels of NO and NOS expression are diminished in glaucomatous human eyes. In addition, NOS-3 knock-out mice exhibit elevated IOP levels due to a reduction in the conventional outflow, whereas the opposite effect is observed in NOS-3 over expressing transgenic mice [43, 44].

2.1.3.2. Mechanism of action

NO stimulates soluble guanylatecyclase (sGC) leading to the elevation of intracellular cyclic guanosine monophosphate (cGMP levels), a secondary messenger that interacts with protein kinases and phosphodiesterases. Multiple studies indicate that the NO-cGMP pathway regulates IOP levels increasing AH outflow through the conventional route and by reducing AH secretion [43].

Cytoskeletal changes at the TM seem to be the underlying mechanism mediating the increase in AH outflow induced by NO. NO induces vascular smooth muscle cells (VSMC) relaxation by stimulation of cGMP synthesis that subsequently activates protein kinase G (PKG). This results in inhibition of the Rho-kinase cascade and leads to inhibition of the MLC-2 phosphorylation. Analogously to VSMCs, TM cells also exhibit contractile properties and modulation of these properties by NO is thought to mediate changes that result in a reduction in outflow resistance. Additionally, it has been demonstrated that inhibition of multi-drug resistance-associated protein-4 also induces TM cellular relaxation mediated by cGMP-PKG pathway [45]. NO could also mediate its IOP-lowering effects by targeting cells of the SC. In fact, Rho-kinase inhibition mediated by NO-cGMP regulates actin dynamics and cell contractility in cultured SC cells [46].

2.1.3.3. Drugs in development

Latanoprostene bunod (LBN; BOL-303259-X; Bausch & Lomb) is a novel nitric oxide-donating prostaglandin F2a analogue currently in Phase III clinical trials [47]. In the eye, LBN is metabolized to two moieties. The first, latanoprost acid, is an F2alpha prostaglandin analogue, while the second, butanediol mononitrate, releases nitric oxide, which activates the soluble cGMP signalling pathway. LBN achieves IOP control simultaneously enhancing AH outflow through the conventional and the uveoscleral routes. Doses ranging from 0.006 to 0.040% of LBN solution were administered once a day to patients with OAG or OHT for 28 consecutive days. LBN at 0.024 and 0.040% achieved statistically significant reductions in mean IOP when compared to latanoprost. During the Phase III clinical trial LBN 0.024% (QD) was not only non-inferior to timolol maleate 0.5% dosed twice daily (b.i.d) after 3 months of treatment but also provided significantly greater IOP reduction. LBN exhibited a similar safety profile than prostaglandins being conjunctival hyperaemia the most frequently reported AE.

2.2. New mechanisms of action

New drug targets are certainly playing an important part in modernising the way glaucoma will be treated in the future. But innovation in glaucoma is not only focused in the discovery of new drug targets, but it is also taking advantage of new and exciting mechanisms of action that seek to solve unmet needs that current treatments cannot solve. In the following section, we will give an overview of drugs using innovative mechanisms of action, focusing on those that have in the past few years entered in clinical development for glaucoma. It should be noted that although antibodies fall into this category of drugs using new mechanisms of action, they have not been included in this section since, up to the authors' knowledge, there are no clinical programmes currently developing antibodies for the treatment of glaucoma. A section on neuroprotective drugs has been included at the end of this section to highlight the importance these drugs are acquiring in the glaucoma pipeline.

2.2.1. Oligonucleotide-based compounds

Oligonucleotides have in the past decades turned out to be an interesting therapeutic approach, particularly due to their ability to address intracellular targets. Oligonucleotides can be designed to target specific genes or RNAs with the aim of altering gene expression or even exert a direct interaction by binding to molecules. The main classes of oligonucleotides that are currently being developed as therapeutic tools are aptamers, ASOs, siRNAs and microRNAs (miRNAs) [48].

2.2.1.1. Aptamers

Aptamers are RNA or DNA oligonucleotides that form a 3D structure designed to interact with large or small molecules. Aptamers typically bind to proteins but can be designed to act upon other types of molecules [49]. Aptamers, contrary to antibodies, are chemically synthetized products that do not require biological steps in their production processes; this results in products that are very well controlled without significant variability among batches. Aptamers have not been widely tested in the context of glaucoma. Pegaptanib, a first-in-class FDA-approved aptamer for the treatment of age-associated macular degeneration (AMD), has been briefly studied for the treatment of neovascular glaucoma [50]. This compound binds to a subtype vascular endothelial growth factor (VEGF), $VEGF_{165}$, hampering its ability to bind to its cell surface receptor thus impairing neovascularization [51]. In addition, ARC81, an anti-transforming growth factor-β (TGF-β) aptamer, has been studied for the reduction in corneal scaring, a common complication of glaucoma filtration surgery [52].

2.2.1.2. Antisense oligonucleotides (ASOs)

ASOs are single-strand RNA or DNA oligonucleotides, of approximately 15–25 bp, that mediate mRNA degradation by an RNaseH-mediated mechanism [53]. These compounds have been widely used to study cell function and lately applied to therapeutics. There are two FDA approved ASOs; vitravene, an intravireally administered ASO for the treatment of cytomegalovirus retinitis in AIDS patients and mipomersen, an intravenously administered ASO for the treatment of familiar hypercholesterolemia [54, 55]. The main advantage of this class of compounds is that they modulate gene expression without altering the genetic code, and that their action upon their target gene can be rapidly modified. In addition, as other oligonucleotides, ASOs are chemically synthetized, with all the advantages this entails. On the other hand, ASOs are labile products that require chemical modifications to increase their stability; these modifications can potentially increase their toxicity [48, 56].

There are two ASOs under development for treatment of different types of glaucoma; Aganirsen (GS-101) and ISTH0036. Aganirsen is a 25-bp ASO targeting insulin receptor substrate-1 (IRS-1) administered in eye drops; this compound is being developed for the treatment of corneal neovascularization and has also been tested in neovascular glaucoma [57]. ISTH0036 is a fully modified phosphorothioate 14-bp oligodeoxynucleotide with a 3 + 3 LNA-gapmer pattern targeting TGF-β2. TGF-β2 is an anti-proliferative and anti-inflammatory factor that is upregulated in the AH of POAG patients. Increases in TGF-β2 correlate with deposition of fibrillar extracellular matrix in the TM, one of the hallmarks of POAG [58]. These extracellular depositions in the TM hamper AH outflow and consequently result in IOP increase. ISTH0036 is currently being tested in a Phase I dose-finding clinical study in patients with advanced glaucoma undergoing filtration surgery due to uncontrollable elevated IOP. The compound is administered intravitreally (IVT) at the end of trabeculectomy; the outcomes of the study are safety, tolerability and effect on IOP.

2.2.1.3. *Short interfering RNAs (siRNAs)*

siRNAs are double-stranded RNA molecules of approximately 19–25 bp that mediate gene silencing by blocking translation of specific mRNAs into their corresponding protein [59]. These molecules, although usually larger than ASOs, are in general more potent and stable than ASOs. Depending on the target tissue and the level of expression of the target gene, these compounds can be administered in eye drops avoiding invasive administration methods, if deeper regions need to be accessed IVT administration may be required [60]. In addition, once the siRNA has entered the RISC complex its action lasts for quite some time, this means that a single molecule would be able to mediate the degradation of several mRNAs thus amplifying the effect of the compound. This prolonged action is particularly interesting in the case of glaucoma as it could avoid sudden increases in IOP due to skipped doses.

Bamosiran (SYL040012) is a 21-bp unmodified siRNA targeting adrenergic receptor β2 (ADRB2) for the treatment of glaucoma. This compound is administered in eye drops and penetrates the eye to reduce synthesis of AH by blocking the ADRB2 at the ciliary body and possibly also at the TM [61, 62]. In contrast to traditional beta-blockers, bamosiran acts only locally in the eye; this is because the molecule is rapidly degraded when it reaches systemic circulation, thus reducing the likelihood of systemic side effects. This characteristic makes bamosiran a safe compound for the treatment of individuals with risk of heart disease or other alterations in which beta-blockers are contraindicated.

QPI-1007 is a 19-bp siRNA targeting Caspase-2. This product, administered by IVT injection, is under development for the treatment of several optic neuropathies, including glaucoma [63]. Caspase-2 is specifically activated during ganglion cell death leading to irreversible loss of vision, thus reducing its expression could potentially protect retinal ganglion cells from apoptosis.

2.2.2. *Gene therapy*

Gene therapy is a technique that uses genetic material to modify the disease state, usually using a vector to transfer the genetic material. For ophthalmic affectations, distinct viral vectors can be used for the delivery of such genetic material. Most-studied vectors include adenovirus (AdV), adeno-associated virus (AAV), herpes simplex virus (HSV) and lentivirus; all of them offering distinct pros and cons [64]. While large advancement has been achieved in different eye diseases, gene therapy for glaucoma has faced substantial limitation due to the lack of obvious genetic alterations. Indeed, causative and risk factor genes such as myocilin (MYOC), optineurin (OPTN), Cytochrome P450 1B1 (CYP1B1), caveolin (CAV1/CAV2) and TANK-binding kinase 1 (TBK1), among others, represent less than 10% of glaucoma cases worldwide [65]. Up to date, only one gene therapy trial for glaucoma has been listed (Trial ID: US-0589). This Phase I study proposes to evaluate the safety of SCH-412499 (rAd-p21) after a single injection into the sub-conjunctival space of the eye in glaucoma subjects prior to trabeculectomy. The treatment uses an AdV vector for the expression of p21 WAF-1/Cip1, a potent cyclin-dependent kinase inhibitor to reduce wound healing process and fibroproliferation after filtering surgery [66]. No results have been disclosed yet; however, pre-clinical studies demonstrated a safe profile with strong anti-proliferative effect after filtration surgery in animal models [67, 68].

In collaboration with Mayo Clinic (Rochester, USA), Oxford BioMedica plc (Oxford, UK) is developing a novel gene therapy approach for the treatment of chronic glaucoma. Pre-clinical studies have been undertaken to determine the feasibility of the LentiVector® platform for the delivery and expression of cyclooxygenase (COX-2) and prostaglandin F2α (PGF-2α) genes to reduce IOP in glaucomatous patients. According to the company's announcement, pre-clinical studies demonstrated a good tolerance for the LentiVector® when used at high doses, with the ability to transduce proper target cells following transcorneal injection into the anterior chamber. Moreover, data showed a long-term gene expression for up to 5 months. Although pre-clinical efficacy studies on IOP have been planned, no additional results have been published.

Besides these two emerging gene therapy treatments for glaucoma, most investigational developments are still in pre-clinical phases, showing relative effect on IOP. For example, the COX-2 and PGF-2α gene therapy models previously described demonstrated a prolonged decrease in IOP in large animal models [69]. Similarly, using lentiviral-based dual expression vector to deliver prostaglandin F synthase, significant reduction in IOP has been achieved [70]. However, the overall reduction in IOP produced by these vectors was not as extensive as that observed for topical PG eye drops. Likewise, different gene therapy strategies to modulate the RhoA or Rho-kinase pathways showed an efficient but moderate IOP-lowering effect [71, 72]. In an elegant way, gene therapy has also been adapted to steroid-induced glaucoma.

In these patients, topical instillation of glucocorticoids is known to produce ocular hypertension by producing a downregulation of the matrix metalloproteinase 1 (MMP1) gene in the TM. Because the patients are under an on and off treatment schedule with glucocorticoids, a new self-complementary AAV has been generated for the expression of MMP1 under the control of a glucocorticoid response element. This allows for the induction of MMP1 expression only after the administration of glucocorticoids, a strategy that presents great advantages. Using this novel system, a reduction in IOP was detected in large animal model and would be highly beneficial in clinic [73].

In addition to cell transduction and adequate gene expression modulation, the route of administration is a critical factor for effective gene therapy. Interestingly, optimum delivery and transduction of AdV have been found through the TM and the SC, structures from where the AH flows [74]. However, the complexity of the whole outflow tract, which includes various cell-types harbouring different transduction properties, may impair the overall efficacy of gene therapy. Moreover, the possible systemic exposure with unwanted side effects is an important downside of direct release of viral vectors that can drain into the retinal venous circulation. Although we are still a long way from the instauration of gene therapy in glaucoma treatment, the advancement achieved in the field is encouraging and sustains the feasibility of such technique in human.

2.2.3. *Stem cell therapy*

Once glaucoma has reached advanced stages with irreversible vision loss, the nearly unique alternative is to replace the retinal ganglion cells of the optic nerve to restore functional vision. Hence, future objectives aim at regenerating the optic nerve in blind eyes using stem cell therapy. While the majority of clinical trials using stem cells have been conducted in neuroretinal degenerative diseases, trials in glaucoma are only starting to emerge. This is because the replacement of RGCs is a most tricky task and will depend on (1) cell engraftment, differentiation and migration to the ganglion cell layer, (2) the growth of axons into the optic disc and (3) the establishment of effective synapse connection [75]. To do so, cells can be implanted into different compartments of the eye, although most commonly tested sites are intravitreal or sub-retinal. The stem cells used can be of various sources and are often engineered *in vitro* through gene therapy [76]. Autologous transplantation of genetically modified cells that originate from the same patient has been favoured due to larger safety window, reducing host-defense mechanism and immune reaction such as those produced by AdV viral vectors. Because of the novelty of these methodologies, the primary goals of current registered clinical trials are towered first on safety outcomes (monitoring of adverse and serious adverse reaction), and secondary outcomes on efficacy (visual acuity, eye fundus and visual field improvement). In general, patients with advanced stages of glaucoma are recruited because of the lack of previous safety studies involving humans.

A novel Phase II trial aims to test the efficacy and safety of adipose-derived regenerative cells for the treatment of glaucomatous neurodegeration (NCT02144103). After liposuction, cells are harvested and isolated from fat tissues and injected into the same patient by subtenon administration. The rationale behind the use of adipose-derived mesenchymal stem cells is based on their capacity to differentiate into retinal pigment epithelium cells. Another promising treatment uses autologous bone marrow-derived stem cells (BMSC): after prior isolation and culture, these cells are injected intravitreally into the worst eye of the patient (NCT02330978). Safety parameters are the first objective of this Phase I trial, although an improvement in visual acuity and visual field are expected in secondary outcomes. Mechanisms for such potential effects remain uncertain. Surprisingly, in animal models, BMSCs have been shown to survive after intravitreal injection, although without showing any apparent differentiation ability. There are actual evidences that BMSC cannot pass the vitreoretinal interface, suggesting that BMSCs may act in a paracrine manner, most likely by providing neuroprotection, rather than by differentiating into RGCs [77]. A larger clinical trial is currently running to evaluate the efficacy of such BMSC therapy, comparing distinct injection sites for various ophthalmic diseases, including glaucoma (NCT01920867). Routes of injection include retrobulbar, subtenon, intravenous, intravitreal and intraocular, which may provide valuable information on the ability of BMSCs to improve visual acuity depending on the delivery site. Overall, big hopes are expected from these trials and their success would definitively represent important breakthrough.

Aside from clinical trials, numerous pre-clinical studies are underway to explore the capacity of different stem cell populations to provide neuroprotection or regeneration of optic nerves. For example, a novel stem cell therapy has been explored to prevent the loss of TM function and cell number observed in glaucoma. The TM and SC operate to drain out the AH and play pivotal role in sensing IOP fluctuation. In conjunction with the modulation of the extra-cellular matrix and enzymes activity, these two structures adapt to adjust the resistance to fluid flow. The aim of this new stem cell therapy, although still at pre-clinical stages, is to obtain new functional TM-like cells to restore functional outflow tract. Recently, in a mouse model of glaucoma, transplantation of induced pluripotent stem cells (iPSC) differentiated into TM cells was shown to reduce neuronal loss and IOP [78]. Surprisingly, the cell transplant led to increased proliferation of pre-existing TM cells. Obviously, further investigation will be needed to confirm the feasibility of these innovative therapies and to efficiently apply them to regular clinical practice.

2.2.4. Neuroprotective drugs

Transport of neurotrophic factors (NTFs) along RGCs axons is critical for cell survival, and unfortunately, this process is found altered in glaucoma. Indeed, the mechanical compression of the optic nerve hinders retrograde travelling of NFTs, leading to induction of the apoptotic cascade. Neuroprotective therapy thus aims to prevent RGCs cell death and damage of the optic nerve. Neuroprotective drugs have been initially developed for the treatment of various neuropathic diseases and their success raised the possible application for the prevention of vision loss in glaucoma. Pre-clinical studies have clearly demonstrated the efficacy of neuroprotective therapy for glaucoma; however, it has not yet been translated into clinic. When looking retrospectively, the development of such therapies has been hampered by the failure of Memantine to meet its primary outcome in Phase II trials, and consequently the drop from clinical development. This drug belongs to a new class of Alzheimer's disease medications that inhibits NMDA receptors to counteract the toxic effect of L-glutamate accumulation into the nervous system. It has been shown to strongly reduce RGCs loss in various animal species [79]. Unfortunately, Memantine failed to demonstrate any protective properties in glaucoma patients [80]. Consequently, companies became skeptical over undertaking such risky clinical trials. Up to date, the main difficulty relies on the fact that long-term efficacy for neuroprotection is extremely hard to prove. Nonetheless, the rationale behind this therapy remains valid and is still currently explored, mostly that a myriad of signalling pathways can be modulated to protect RGCs. The fact that many of these targets act through an IOP independent manner provides an appealing approach to treat patients with normal tension glaucoma. This chapter will explore some of these avenues, focusing on survival factors, apoptotic mechanisms and oxidative stress.

One of the best strategies to achieve neuroprotection focuses on the delivery of NTFs to RGCs using cell therapy. A Phase I clinical trial has been completed to evaluate the safety and efficacy of the NT-501 CNTF Implant after intravitreal injection into one selected eye (Neurotech Pharmaceuticals, Inc; NCT01408472). The implant contains human cells (designated NTC-201) that originate from a retinal pigment epithelial cell line genetically engineered to produce human ciliary neurotrophic factor (CNTF). A role for CNTF in neuroprotection of the retina has been established in a wide number of pre-clinical studies, which was shown to promote cell survival of RGCs in most animal models [81]. In human, such implant has been previously proved to release CNTF consistently over a 2-year period without producing systemic exposure, hence avoiding the need for multiple injections [82]. Outcomes have not been reported yet but studies suggest favourable pharmacokinetic of the implant with possible treatment of chronic retinal degenerative diseases. Overall, MSCs and BMDS transplant represent a valuable tool for long-term delivery of various NTFs as well as anti-inflammatory cytokines that may prevent apoptosis of RGCs.

Activation of apoptosis is a key mechanism in RGCs cell death and increasing amount of anti-apoptotic agents are currently being investigated for the treatment of glaucoma. Since apoptosis often occurs in early stages of the disease, its detection is of prime importance to prevent irreversible damage lost. A new Phase I study is evaluating the ability of ANX776 to identify RGC apoptosis as part of a new detection of apoptosing retinal cells (DARC) technique (NCT02394613). The primary purpose of the study is to develop a new diagnosis tool for glaucoma in healthy patients. As previously described, QPI-1007 is a promising candidate to achieve neuroprotection by reducing the expression of Caspase-2 (NCT01965106 and NCT01064505). Interestingly, brimonidine, a selective alpha2-adrenergic agonist, has been shown to protect against optic nerve damage independently of its IOP-lowering effect, most likely by inducing the production of the anti-apoptotic proteins Bcl-2 and Bcl-XL [83]. Effectively, in a clinical trial, normal tension glaucoma patients treated with brimonidine displayed preserved field function as compared to those that were given timolol [84]. Curiously, other classic IOP reducing agents have been proved to yield neuroprotective effect because of a dual mechanism of action. A different example is the beta adrenergic blocker Betaxolol. This drug interacts with other channels such as the sodium and L-type calcium channels, an affinity that was proposed to contribute to the protection of the visual field observed in treated patients [85]. Interestingly, a Phase III trial named 'Stop Retinal Ganglion Cell Dysfunction Study' is currently running to compare the protective effect of numerous hypotensive medications routinely used in clinic (NCT02390284). The trial recruits patients with normal vision and eyes are evaluated for changes in the pattern electroretinogram (PERG) and retinal nerve fibre layer (RNFL) thickness.

Therapy	Description	Phase/stage	Outcome	Trial ID
ASO	Intra-vitreal injection of ISTH0036 as an addition to filtration surgery	Phase I/recruiting	Safety and tolerability	NCT02406833
siRNA	Bamosiran eye drops for POAG	Phase II/completed	Safety, dose finding, IOP-lowering effect	NCT02250612
siRNA	QPI-1007 injection in primary angle closure glaucoma	Phase II completed	Safety and tolerability and pharmacokinetics	NCT01965106
Gene therapy	Intraocular delivery of p21 WAF-1/Cip1 gene before glaucoma surgery	PhaseI/unknown	Safety and tolerability, fibroproliferation and wound healing	US-0589
Gene therapy	LentiVector® platform for the delivery of COX-2 and PGF-2α to reduce IOP	Pre-clinical	Safety, IOP-lowering effect	
Stem cell therapy	Subtenon injection of adipose-derived regenerative cells	Phase II/recruiting	Safety, change in visual acuity, eye fundus, visual field	NCT02144103
Stem cell therapy	Intra-vitrial injection of BMSCs	Phase I/recruiting	Safety, change in visual acuity and visual field, optical coherence tomography, RGC function	NCT02330978
Stem cell therapy	Retro-bulbar, subtenon, intra-venous, intra-vitreal and intraocular injection of BMSCs	Phase II/recruiting	Change in visual acuity and visual field	NCT01920867
Stem cell therapy, neuroprotection	Delivery of NT-501 CNTF Implant	Phase I/completed	Safety, vision, visual field, nerve fibre layer, optic nerve topography	NCT01408472
Neuroprotection	RGCs protection by hypotensive eye drops	Phase III/recruiting	Change in PERG, RNFL	NCT02390284
Neuroprotection	Single intra-venous injection of ANX776 as new detection of apoptosing retinal cells (DARC) technique	Phase I/active	Safety and DARC count	NCT02394613

Table 1. Current clinical trials for new mechanisms of action for glaucoma.

Anti-oxidants also represent an attractive alternative to prevent long-term RGC damage. Due to high metabolic activity during visual transduction, retinal cells are particularly sensitive to oxidative stress, mainly in elderly. Increased levels of reactive oxygen species (ROS) and associated DNA damage have been reported in glaucoma patients [86]. Numerous pre-clinical studies in glaucoma animal models have shown a neuroprotective benefit for a large variety of anti-oxidant such as Vitamin E, Coenzyme Q10, Ginkgo biloba extract and other Chinese medicines [79]. One clinical trial previously addressed the impact of oral versatile anti-oxidants on glaucoma progression, comparing Ginkgo biloba and α-tocopherol for 3 months (NCT01544192), however no clear benefits have been reported, and other similar studies failed to find differences among treatments (**Table 1**) [87].

3. Innovation in medical devices and surgical procedures

There are two types of surgical procedures aimed at lowering IOP, trabeculoplasty and trabeculectomy. The former is aimed towards treating the TM with LASER to diminish AH resistance and increase drainage into collecting channels or into the outside of the eye. In the latter, a part of the TM is removed to reduce resistance to outflow. These approaches usually reduce IOP for a period of up to 5 years, but additional medical or surgical interventions are commonly required after this period due to scaring or secondary complications. Improvements in surgery thus seek using artificial channels that enlarge drainage routes or shunts that bypass the TM draining the AH directly to the SC or to the suprachoroidal space [88]. In the last decade, minimally invasive glaucoma surgery (MIGS) has gained popularity due to its minimal tissue destruction, short surgery time and fast post-operative recovery. Here, we present an overview of glaucoma draining devices that are in development for these procedures.

3.1. Drainage devices to the SC or to the sub-conjunctival space

The SC is an endothelium-lined channel derived from the TM located at the joining point of the sclera and cornea. The TM is composed of three layers: the innermost uveal meshwork, the middle layer section composed of connective tissue called the corneoscleral meshwork and the third layer, also known as juxtacanalicular tissue. The juxtacanicular tissue is a non-fenenstrated endothelial layer immersed in fibres and a rich extra-cellular matrix that lines the inner wall of the SC. In humans, 75% of the resistance to AH outflow is exerted by the TM, mainly by the juxtacanalicular portion and the deposition of glycosaminoglycans in the TM ECM [89]. As such, bypassing the TM draining the liquid to the SC has been widely used as an approach to alleviate elevated IOP. Several devices are currently under development with the aim of improving the outflow through the TM.

3.1.1. Devices in development

The Glaukos iStent (Glaukos Corporation, Laguna Hills, CA, USA) is a heparin-coated micro stent that bypasses the TM by creating a pathway from the anterior chamber to the SC [90]. Implantation of this device in patients undergoing cataract surgery resulted in a sustained decrease in IOP (IOP ≤ 21 mmHg) in 72% of patients 12 months after implantation compared to 50% in the control group. Twenty-four months after surgery 61% still had IOP levels below 21 mmHg whereas in the control group 50% of patients maintained the targeted IOP. Other outcomes included in the study, such as decrease in IOP ≥ 20% and medications reduction, were also positive for the device-implanted patient group. Further studies have shown that sustained elevated IOP may affect the shape of the SC and therefore implanting one iStent may not be sufficient to achieve a sustained decrease in IOP. To solve this issue studies implanting several iStents have been performed showing promising data [91].

The Hydrus microstent (Ivantis Inc., Irvine, CA, USA) is an intra-canalicular scaffold made of nitinol that is surgically implanted into the SC during cataract surgery. This device is manufactured to follow the curve of the SC and widens the opening of the canal avoiding its collapse. The efficacy of this device has been studied in patients undergoing cataract surgery and the results of these studies show that reduction in washed out diurnal IOP ≥ 20% was higher in the implanted group compared to the cataract surgery alone group 24 months after surgery (80 vs. 46%). Implantation of the device was also able to reduce the use of hypotensive medications [92].

InnFocus Microsunt, previously known as the MIDI Arrow (InnFocus Inc., Miami, FL, USA), is made of poly(styrene-block-isobutylene-block-styrene) SIBS, a synthetic thermoplastic elastomeric biomaterial that does not cause inflammation. The implant is used in conjunction with Mitomycin C to modulate would healing post-surgery. This device is placed in the anterior chamber and drains into the scleral surface [93]. The device was implanted in 23 eyes that had failed maximum tolerated glaucoma medication. The patients were followed for a period of 3 years; 14 patients received the implant alone whereas the rest were implanted concomitantly to cataract surgery. Years 1, 2 and 3 after the procedure 100, 91 and 95% of the patients fulfilled the success criteria of the study (IOP ≤ 14 mm Hg and IOP reduction ≥20%), and the mean number of glaucoma medications was reduced from 2.4 ± 0.9 to 0.3 ± 0.8, 0.4 ± 1.0 and 0.7 ± 1.1, respectively. Adverse events of the procedure included transient hypotony (13%) and transient choroidal effusion (8.7%); both adverse events resolved spontaneously [94].

The XEN45 Gel Stent (Allergan, Dublin, Ireland) is a soft flexible implant initially developed by AqueSys but later acquired by Allergan. The device is manufactured in collagen-derived gelatine cross-linked with glutaraldehyde and is injected through the anterior chamber into the sub-conjunctival space. The device swells upon hydration creating the channel. The XEN45 is approved in Europe, Turkey, Canada and Switzerland for reduction in IOP in patients with POAG where previous medical treatments have failed and is in late stage development in the USA. In Europe, the device can be used in conjunction with cataract surgery or as a standalone procedure. The data obtained from clinical trials show a mean drop of 47% from preoperative IOP in the standalone procedure and a 40% decrease when combined with cataract surgery. The main adverse events of this procedure include intra-operative sub-conjunctival or anterior chamber bleeding (1.2%), cataract-related complications (0.8%), post-operative hyphema (2.6%), self-limiting choroidal effusion (1%) shallow anterior chamber (0.8%), viscoelastic injection into the anterior chamber (0.6%) and anterior chamber tap to release retained viscoelastic (0.4%).

3.2. Drainage devices to the suprachoroidal space

There are several devices designed to drain AH from the anterior chamber to the suprachoroidal space, where the fluid is reabsorbed by the scleral channels of the choriocapillaries. These devices are based on the existence of a difference in hydrostatic pressure between the supra-choroidal space and the anterior chamber; this difference favours unidirectional flow from the anterior chamber to the suprachoroidal space reducing IOP. The materials used to manufacture these devices vary from gold to non-biodegradable polymers; materials that are inert, non-biodegradable and biocompatible to ensure proper function of the device.

3.2.1. Devices in development

The CyPass (Transcend Medical, Menlo Park, CA, USA) is a fenestrated polyamide supraciliary device that connects the anterior chamber with the suprachoroidal space. The device is implanted during cataract surgery and its efficacy has been tested in a multi-centre, prospective study enrolling 136 subjects with two cohorts. Cohort 1 was composed of subjects with OAG requiring cataract surgery that had uncontrolled IOP (IOP; ≥21 mmHg, $n = 51$), whereas cohort 2 was composed of subjects with OAG requiring cataract surgery with controlled IOP (<21 mmHg, $n = 85$). Glaucoma medications were stopped post-surgery but could be restarted if needed. The results of the study indicate that there was a reduction of 37% in mean IOP 24 months after surgery. There was a statistically significant decrease in the need for glaucoma medications in both cohorts [95]. Further development of this device includes a randomized controlled trial that is currently underway (**Table 2**).

	Device	Manufacturer	Material	Status	Trial ID
Devices draining to the SC or to the sub-conjunctival space	iSTENT	Glaukos Corporation	Non-ferromagnetic titanium	FDA approved in patients undergoing cataract surgery. Phase IV	NCT00326066
	Hydrus microstent	Ivantis	Nitinol (alloy of nickel and titanium)	Phase III	NCT01539239
	InnFocus Microshunt	InnFocus	Poly(styrene-block-isobutylene-block-styrene) SIBS	Phase IV	NCT02177123
	XEN45	Allergan (AqueSys)	Collagen-derived gelatine	Phase IV	NTC02006693
Devices draining to the suprachoroidal space	CyPass	Transcend Medical	Non-biodegradable polyimide	Safety and Efficacy	NCT01085357
	SOLX gold shunt	SOLX	Gold	Phase III	NCT01282346
	Aquashunt	OPKO health	Polypropylene	Safety and Efficacy	NCT00834223
	STARflo	iSTAR Medicals	Silicone microporus material	Safety and Efficacy	NCT02272569

Table 2. Devices in development for glaucoma.

The SOLX gold shunt (SOLX Inc., Waltham, MA, USA) communicates the anterior chamber with the suprachoroidal space via 19 channels formed between the two 24-karat medical-grade gold plates that form the shunt. The device is approved in Europe but still investigational in the USA. Several clinical trials have been conducted for this device with different outcomes. Success for this device was defined as a target IOP between 5 and 22 mmHg and an IOP decrease ≤20%. Most clinical studies for this device have yielded a success rate around 80%. In contrast, in a study performed by Hueber and co-workers enrolling 31 patients implanted with the device and followed up for a period of 4 years most patients (97%) failed the established success criteria. This difference outcome may be due to a fibrotic reaction to the device in this particular trial [96].

The Aquashunt (OPKO Health Inc., Miami, FL, USA) is a device made of polypropylene curved to accommodate the eye's shape. The results from a clinical study enrolling 15 patients with uncontrolled IOP indicate that eight of the patients achieved an IOP reduction of 31%, four of which needed concurrent medical therapy to reach satisfactory IOP after a period of 12 months. Further clinical studies have not been initiated [96].

The STARflo glaucoma implant (iSTAR Medical SA, Wavre, Belgium) is made of a microporous silicon elastomer and implanted intrascleraly into the suprachoroidal space. Clinical data are available from a limited number of cases, and it shows a reduction in the pre-operative IOP of 37.0 mmHg to a post-operative IOP of 14.3 mmHg 12 months after implantation. The reduction in glaucoma medication intake went from 3.25 medications/day to 1.5 intake/day.

4. Conclusions

Current medical therapy for glaucoma is insufficient to avoid the deleterious effects of this progressive ophthalmic neuropathy. In the last decade, significant efforts have been made in order to develop new products that use novel approaches to address the unmet needs of a disease that is still the second cause of blindness. This review gives an overview of these approaches, focusing on new targets that regulate AH balance in the eye or that are involved in fibrosis and scaring; processes that complicate the long-term success of glaucoma filtration surgery.

New mechanism of actions such as therapies based on oligonucleotides, gene therapy and stem cells is also reviewed. Products based on these mechanisms of action are already showing promising results in the clinical setting and may represent new options for patients that have uncontrolled IOP and that do not respond to current therapy.

A brief overview of neuroprotective approaches is also given; products based on this approach represent an excellent complementary option for IOP reduction strategies.

Finally, improvements in medical devices used to increase AH outflow are also reviewed. New devices achieve significant reduction in IOP and many can be used as stand-alone procedures offering an option to patients and settings where glaucoma medications are not a medically viable option.

Innovation in glaucoma may eventually change current disease treatment paradigms in order to offer solutions to a wider number of patients for whom current treatment options cannot stall disease progression. Achieving a sustained IOP reduction that warrants optic nerve protection over time is the main goal to be achieved, and some of these products may contribute towards that goal. As it has been the case for current glaucoma therapy, significant advances in quality of life of glaucoma patients may come from combining different approaches together to treat glaucoma in a comprehensive way.

Author details

Bleau Anne-Marie, Vargas Beatriz, Jiménez Ana Isabel and Pañeda Covadonga*

*Address all correspondence to: cpaneda@sylentis.com

Sylentis c/Santiago Grisolía, Tres Cantos, Madrid, Spain

References

[1] King A, Azuara-Blanco A, Tuulonen A: Glaucoma. B M J. 2013;346:f3518.

[2] Heijl A, Leske MC, Bengtsson B, Hyman L, Hussein M: Reduction of intraocular pressure and glaucoma progression: results from the early manifest glaucoma trial. Arch Ophthalmol. 2002;120:1268–79.

[3] Zhou EH, Krishnan R, Stamer WD, Perkumas KM, Rajendran K, Nabhan JF, Lu Q, Fredberg JJ, Johnson M: Mechanical responsiveness of the endothelial cell of Schlemm's canal: scope, variability and its potential role in controlling aqueous humour outflow. J R Soc Interface. 2012;9:1144–55. DOI:10.1098/rsif.2011.0733

[4] Bishop AL, Hall A: Rho GTPases and their effector proteins. Biochem J. 2000;348 Pt 2:241–55.

[5] Smithers CC, Overduin M: Structural mechanisms and drug discovery prospects of Rho GTPases. Cell. 2016;5. DOI:10.3390/cells5020026

[6] Bos JL, Rehmann H, Wittinghofer A: GEFs and GAPs: critical elements in the control of small G proteins. Cell. 2007;129:865–77. DOI:10.1016/j.cell.2007.05.018

[7] Chi X, Wang S, Huang Y, Stamnes M, Chen J-L: Roles of Rho GTPases in intracellular transport and cellular transformation. Int J Mol Sci. 2013;14:7089–108. DOI:10.3390/ijms14047089

[8] Goldhagen B, Proia AD, Epstein DL, Rao PV: Elevated levels of RhoA in the optic nerve head of human eyes with glaucoma. J Glaucoma. 2012;21:530–8. DOI:10.1097/IJG.0b013e318241b83c

[9] Riento K, Ridley AJ: Rocks: multifunctional kinases in cell behaviour. Nat Rev Mol Cell Biol. 2003;4:446–56. DOI:10.1038/nrm1128

[10] Fukiage C, Mizutani K, Kawamoto Y, Azuma M, Shearer TR: Involvement of phosphorylation of myosin phosphatase by ROCK in trabecular meshwork and ciliary muscle contraction. Biochem Biophys Res Commun. 2001;288:296–300. DOI:10.1006/bbrc.2001.5751

[11] Pattabiraman PP, Maddala R, Rao PV: Regulation of plasticity and fibrogenic activity of trabecular meshwork cells by Rho GTPase signaling. J Cell Physiol. 2014;229:927–42. DOI:10.1002/jcp.24524

[12] Whitlock NA, Harrison B, Mixon T, Yu XQ, Wilson A, Gerhardt B, Eberhart DE, Abuin A, Rice DS: Decreased intraocular pressure in mice following either pharmacological or genetic inhibition of ROCK. J Ocul Pharmacol Ther. 2009;25:187–94. DOI:10.1089/jop.2008.0142

[13] Kaneko-Kawano T, Takasu F, Naoki H, Sakumura Y, Ishii S, Ueba T, Eiyama A, Okada A, Kawano Y, Suzuki K: Dynamic regulation of myosin light chain phosphorylation by Rho-kinase. PLoS One. 2012;7:e39269. DOI:10.1371/journal.pone.0039269

[14] Boland S, Bourin A, Alen J, Geraets J, Schroeders P, Castermans K, Kindt N, Boumans N, Panitti L, Vanormelingen J, Fransen S, Van de Velde S, Defert O: Design, synthesis and biological characterization of selective LIMK inhibitors. Bioorg Med Chem Lett. 2015;25:4005–10. DOI:10.1016/j.bmcl.2015.07.009

[15] Wang SK, Chang RT: An emerging treatment option for glaucoma: Rho kinase inhibitors. Clin Ophthalmol. 2014;8:883–90. DOI:10.2147/opth.s41000

[16] Rao PV, Deng PF, Kumar J, Epstein DL: Modulation of aqueous humor outflow facility by the Rho kinase-specific inhibitor Y-27632. Invest Ophthalmol Vis Sci. 2001;42:1029–37.

[17] Van de Velde S, Van Bergen T, Vandewalle E, Kindt N, Castermans K, Moons L, Stalmans I: Rho kinase inhibitor AMA0526 improves surgical outcome in a rabbit model of glaucoma filtration surgery. Prog Brain Res. 2015;220:283–97. DOI:10.1016/bs.pbr.2015.04.014

[18] Sugiyama T, Shibata M, Kajiura S, Okuno T, Tonari M, Oku H, Ikeda T: Effects of fasudil, a Rho-associated protein kinase inhibitor, on optic nerve head blood flow in rabbits. Invest Ophthalmol Vis Sci. 2011;52:64–9. DOI:10.1167/iovs.10-5265

[19] Tokushige H, Waki M, Takayama Y, Tanihara H: Effects of Y-39983, a selective Rho-associated protein kinase inhibitor, on blood flow in optic nerve head in rabbits and axonal regeneration of retinal ganglion cells in rats. Curr Eye Res. 2011;36:964–70. DOI:10.3109/02713683.2011.599106

[20] Van de Velde S, De Groef L, Stalmans I, Moons L, Van Hove I: Towards axonal regeneration and neuroprotection in glaucoma: Rho kinase inhibitors as promising therapeutics. Prog Neurobiol. 2015;131:105–19. DOI:10.1016/j.pneurobio.2015.06.002

[21] Tanihara H, Inatani M, Honjo M, Tokushige H, Azuma J, Araie M: Intraocular pressure-lowering effects and safety of topical administration of a selective ROCK inhibitor, SNJ-1656, in healthy volunteers. Arch Ophthalmol. 2008;126:309–15. DOI:10.1001/archophthalmol.2007.76

[22] Inoue T, Tanihara H, Tokushige H, Araie M: Efficacy and safety of SNJ-1656 in primary open-angle glaucoma or ocular hypertension. Acta Ophthalmol. 2015;93:e393–5. DOI:10.1111/aos.12641

[23] Garnock-Jones KP: Ripasudil: first global approval. Drugs. 2014;74:2211–5. DOI:10.1007/s40265-014-0333-2

[24] Yamamoto K, Maruyama K, Himori N, Omodaka K, Yokoyama Y, Shiga Y, Morin R, Nakazawa T: The novel Rho kinase (ROCK) inhibitor K-115: a new candidate drug for neuroprotective treatment in glaucoma. Invest Ophthalmol Vis Sci. 2014;55:7126–36. DOI:10.1167/iovs.13-13842

[25] Tanihara H, Inoue T, Yamamoto T, Kuwayama Y, Abe H, Araie M: Phase 1 clinical trials of a selective Rho kinase inhibitor, K-115. JAMA Ophthalmol. 2013;131:1288–95. DOI:10.1001/jamaophthalmol.2013.323

[26] Tanihara H, Inoue T, Yamamoto T, Kuwayama Y, Abe H, Araie M: Phase 2 randomized clinical study of a Rho kinase inhibitor, K-115, in primary open-angle glaucoma and ocular hypertension. Am J Ophthalmol. 2013;156:731–6. DOI:10.1016/j.ajo.2013.05.016

[27] Isobe T, Mizuno K, Kaneko Y, Ohta M, Koide T, Tanabe S: Effects of K-115, a rho-kinase inhibitor, on aqueous humor dynamics in rabbits. Curr Eye Res. 2014;39:813–22. DOI:10.3109/02713683.2013.874444

[28] Kaneko Y, Ohta M, Inoue T, Mizuno K, Isobe T, Tanabe S, Tanihara H: Effects of K-115 (Ripasudil), a novel ROCK inhibitor, on trabecular meshwork and Schlemm's canal endothelial cells. Sci Rep. 2016;6:19640. DOI:10.1038/srep19640

[29] Sturdivant JM, Royalty SM, Lin CW, Moore LA, Yingling JD, Laethem CL, Sherman B, Heintzelman GR, Kopczynski CC, deLong MA: Discovery of the ROCK inhibitor netarsudil for the treatment of open-angle glaucoma. Bioorg Med Chem Lett. 2016;26:2475–80. DOI:10.1016/j.bmcl.2016.03.104

[30] Bacharach J, Dubiner HB, Levy B, Kopczynski CC, Novack GD: Double-masked, randomized, dose-response study of AR-13324 versus latanoprost in patients with elevated intraocular pressure. Ophthalmology. 2015;122:302–7. DOI:10.1016/j.ophtha.2014.08.022

[31] Li G, Mukherjee D, Navarro I, Ashpole NE, Sherwood JM, Chang J, Overby DR, Yuan F, Gonzalez P, Kopczynski CC, Farsiu S, Stamer WD: Visualization of conventional outflow tissue responses to netarsudil in living mouse eyes. Eur J Pharmacol. 2016;787:20-31. DOI:10.1016/j.ejphar.2016.04.002

[32] Wang RF, Williamson JE, Kopczynski C, Serle JB: Effect of 0.04% AR-13324, a ROCK, and norepinephrine transporter inhibitor, on aqueous humor dynamics in normotensive monkey eyes. J Glaucoma. 2015;24:51–4. DOI:10.1097/IJG.0b013e3182952213

[33] Lewis RA, Levy B, Ramirez N, Kopczynski CC, Usner DW, Novack GD: Fixed-dose combination of AR-13324 and latanoprost: a double-masked, 28-day, randomised, controlled study in patients with open-angle glaucoma or ocular hypertension. Br J Ophthalmol. 2016;100:339–44. DOI:10.1136/bjophthalmol-2015-306778

[34] Winkler NS, Fautsch MP: Effects of prostaglandin analogues on aqueous humor outflow pathways. J Ocul Pharmacol Ther. 2014;30:102–9. DOI:10.1089/jop.2013.0179

[35] Van de Velde S, Van Bergen T, Sijnave D, Hollanders K, Castermans K, Defert O, Leysen D, Vandewalle E, Moons L, Stalmans I: AMA0076, a novel, locally acting Rho kinase inhibitor, potently lowers intraocular pressure in New Zealand white rabbits

with minimal hyperemia. Invest Ophthalmol Vis Sci. 2014;55:1006–16. DOI:10.1167/iovs.13-13157

[36] Zhong Y, Yang Z, Huang WC, Luo X: Adenosine, adenosine receptors and glaucoma: an updated overview. Biochim Biophys Acta. 2013;1830:2882–90. DOI:10.1016/j.bbagen.2013.01.005

[37] Daines BS, Kent AR, McAleer MS, Crosson CE: Intraocular adenosine levels in normal and ocular-hypertensive patients. J Ocul Pharmacol Ther. 2003;19:113–9. DOI:10.1089/108076803321637645

[38] Mitchell CH, Peterson-Yantorno K, Carre DA, McGlinn AM, Coca-Prados M, Stone RA, Civan MM: A3 adenosine receptors regulate Cl-channels of nonpigmented ciliary epithelial cells. Am J Physiol. 1999;276:C659–66.

[39] Avila MY, Stone RA, Civan MM: Knockout of A3 adenosine receptors reduces mouse intraocular pressure. Invest Ophthalmol Vis Sci. 2002;43:3021–6.

[40] Fleischhauer JC, Mitchell CH, Stamer WD, Karl MO, Peterson-Yantorno K, Civan MM: Common actions of adenosine receptor agonists in modulating human trabecular meshwork cell transport. J Membr Biol. 2003;193:121–36. DOI:10.1007/s00232-002-2013-5

[41] Li A, Leung CT, Peterson-Yantorno K, Stamer WD, Civan MM: Cytoskeletal dependence of adenosine triphosphate release by human trabecular meshwork cells. Invest Ophthalmol Vis Sci. 2011;52:7996–8005. DOI:10.1167/iovs.11-8170

[42] Myers JS, Sall KN, DuBiner H, Slomowitz N, McVicar W, Rich CC, Baumgartner RA: A dose-escalation study to evaluate the safety, tolerability, pharmacokinetics, and efficacy of 2 and 4 weeks of twice-daily ocular trabodenoson in adults with ocular hypertension or primary open-angle glaucoma. J Ocul Pharmacol Ther. 2016;10:555-62. DOI:1089/jop.2015.0148

[43] Cavet ME, Vittitow JL, Impagnatiello F, Ongini E, Bastia E: Nitric oxide (NO): an emerging target for the treatment of glaucoma. Invest Ophthalmol Vis Sci. 2014;55:5005–15. DOI:10.1167/iovs.14-14515

[44] Nathanson JA, McKee M: Identification of an extensive system of nitric oxide-producing cells in the ciliary muscle and outflow pathway of the human eye. Invest Ophthalmol Vis Sci. 1995;36:1765–73.

[45] Pattabiraman PP, Pecen PE, Rao PV: MRP4-mediated regulation of intracellular cAMP and cGMP levels in trabecular meshwork cells and homeostasis of intraocular pressure. Invest Ophthalmol Vis Sci. 2013;54:1636–49. DOI:10.1167/iovs.12-11107

[46] Stamer WD, Lei Y, Boussommier-Calleja A, Overby DR, Ethier CR: eNOS, a pressure-dependent regulator of intraocular pressure. Invest Ophthalmol Vis Sci. 2011;52:9438–44. DOI:10.1167/iovs.11-7839

[47] Krauss AH, Impagnatiello F, Toris CB, Gale DC, Prasanna G, Borghi V, Chiroli V, Chong WK, Carreiro ST, Ongini E: Ocular hypotensive activity of BOL-303259-X, a nitric oxide donating prostaglandin F2alpha agonist, in preclinical models. Exp Eye Res. 2011;93:250–5. DOI:10.1016/j.exer.2011.03.001

[48] Pañeda C, Martinez T, Wright N, Jimenez AI: Recent advances in ocular nucleic acid-based therapies: the silent era. In: Adio A, editor. Ocular Diseases. Croatia: InTech; 2012. pp. 157–85. DOI:10.5772/48454

[49] Ellington AD, Szostak JW: In vitro selection of RNA molecules that bind specific ligands. Nature. 1990;346:818–22. DOI:10.1038/346818a0

[50] Filippopoulos T, Ducharme JF, Loewenstein JI, Krzystolik MG: Antiangiogenic agents as an adjunctive treatment for complicated neovascular glaucoma. Invest Ophthalmol Vis Sci. 2006;47:4476.

[51] Gragoudas ES, Adamis AP, Cunningham ET, Jr., Feinsod M, Guyer DR: Pegaptanib for neovascular age-related macular degeneration. N Engl J Med. 2004;351:2805–16. DOI:10.1056/NEJMoa042760

[52] McCauley TG, Kurz JC, Merlino PG, Lewis SD, Gilbert M, Epstein DM, Marsh HN: Pharmacologic and pharmacokinetic assessment of anti-TGFbeta2 aptamers in rabbit plasma and aqueous humor. Pharm Res. 2006;23:303–11. DOI:10.1007/s11095-005-9305-2

[53] Persidis A: Antisense therapeutics. Nat Biotechnol. 1999;17:403–4. DOI:10.1038/7973

[54] Jabs DA, Griffiths PD: Fomivirsen for the treatment of cytomegalovirus retinitis. Am J Ophthalmol. 2002;133:552–6.

[55] Geary RS, Baker BF, Crooke ST: Clinical and preclinical pharmacokinetics and pharmacodynamics of mipomersen (kynamro((R))): a second-generation antisense oligonucleotide inhibitor of apolipoprotein B. Clin Pharmacokinet. 2015;54:133–46. DOI:10.1007/s40262-014-0224-4

[56] Levin AA, Henry S: Toxicology of oligonucleotide therapeutics and understanding the relevance of the toxicities. In: Cavagnaro JA, editor. Preclinical Safety Evaluation of Biopharmaceuticals: A Science-Based Approach to Facilitating Clinical trials. Hoboken, New Jersey, USA. John Wiley & Sons, Inc.; 2008. pp. 537–75.

[57] Kain H, Goldblum D, Geudelin B, Thorin E, Beglinger C: Tolerability and safety of GS-101 eye drops, an antisense oligonucleotide to insulin receptor substrate-1: a 'first in man' phase I investigation. Br J Clin Pharmacol. 2009;68:169–73. DOI:10.1111/j.1365-2125.2009.03450.x

[58] Fleenor DL, Shepard AR, Hellberg PE, Jacobson N, Pang IH, Clark AF: TGFbeta2-induced changes in human trabecular meshwork: implications for intraocular pressure. Invest Ophthalmol Vis Sci. 2006;47:226–34. DOI:10.1167/iovs.05-1060

[59] Ghildiyal M, Zamore PD: Small silencing RNAs: an expanding universe. Nat Rev Genet. 2009;10:94–108. DOI:10.1038/nrg2504

[60] Martinez T, Gonzalez MV, Vargas B, Jimenez AI, Pañeda C: Preclinical development of RNAi-inducing oligonucleotide therapeutics for eye diseases. In: Abdurakhmonov IY, editor. RNA Interference. Croatia: InTech; 2016. pp. 245–72. DOI:10.5772/60631

[61] Martinez T, Gonzalez MV, Roehl I, Wright N, Paneda C, Jimenez AI: In vitro and in vivo efficacy of SYL040012, a novel siRNA compound for treatment of glaucoma. Mol Ther. 2014;22:81–91. DOI:10.1038/mt.2013.216

[62] Moreno-Montanes J, Sadaba B, Ruz V, Gomez-Guiu A, Zarranz J, Gonzalez MV, Paneda C, Jimenez AI: Phase I clinical trial of SYL040012, a small interfering RNA targeting beta-adrenergic receptor 2, for lowering intraocular pressure. Mol Ther. 2014;22:226–32. DOI:10.1038/mt.2013.217

[63] Solano EC, Kornbrust DJ, Beaudry A, Foy JW, Schneider DJ, Thompson JD: Toxicological and pharmacokinetic properties of QPI-1007, a chemically modified synthetic siRNA targeting caspase 2 mRNA, following intravitreal injection. Nucleic Acid Ther. 2014;24:258–66. DOI:10.1089/nat.2014.0489

[64] Dang Y, Loewen R, Parikh HA, Roy P, Loewen NA: Gene transfer to the outflow tract. Exp Eye Res. 2016. DOI:10.1016/j.exer.2016.04.023

[65] Khan AO: Genetics of primary glaucoma. Curr Opin Ophthalmol. 2011;22:347–55. DOI:10.1097/ICU.0b013e32834922d2

[66] Heatley G, Kiland J, Faha B, Seeman J, Schlamp CL, Dawson DG, Gleiser J, Maneval D, Kaufman PL, Nickells RW: Gene therapy using p21WAF-1/Cip-1 to modulate wound healing after glaucoma trabeculectomy surgery in a primate model of ocular hypertension. Gene Ther. 2004;11:949–55. DOI:10.1038/sj.gt.3302253

[67] Veneziale RW, Bral CM, Sinha DP, Watkins RW, Cartwright ME, Rosenblum IY, Treinen KA, Kishnani NS, Nelson J, Chen Z, Faha B, Maneval D, Munger RJ, Cai XY, Cullen C, Arezzo JC: SCH 412499: Biodistribution and safety of an adenovirus containing P21(WAF-1/CIP-1) following subconjunctival injection in cynomolgus monkeys. Cutan Ocul Toxicol. 2007;26:83–105. DOI:10.1080/15569520701212167

[68] Perkins TW, Faha B, Ni M, Kiland JA, Poulsen GL, Antelman D, Atencio I, Shinoda J, Sinha D, Brumback L, Maneval D, Kaufman PL, Nickells RW: Adenovirus-mediated gene therapy using human p21WAF-1/Cip-1 to prevent wound healing in a rabbit model of glaucoma filtration surgery. Arch Ophthalmol. 2002;120:941–9.

[69] Barraza RA, McLaren JW, Poeschla EM: Prostaglandin pathway gene therapy for sustained reduction of intraocular pressure. Mol Ther. 2010;18:491–501. DOI:10.1038/mt.2009.278

[70] Lee ES, Rasmussen CA, Filla MS, Slauson SR, Kolb AW, Peters DM, Kaufman PL, Gabelt BT, Brandt CR: Prospects for lentiviral vector mediated prostaglandin F synthase gene delivery in monkey eyes in vivo. Curr Eye Res. 2014;39:859–70. DOI:10.3109/02713683.2014.884593

[71] Rao PV, Deng P, Maddala R, Epstein DL, Li CY, Shimokawa H: Expression of dominant negative Rho-binding domain of Rho-kinase in organ cultured human eye anterior segments increases aqueous humor outflow. Mol Vis. 2005;11:288–97.

[72] Borras T, Buie LK, Spiga MG, Carabana J: Prevention of nocturnal elevation of intraocular pressure by gene transfer of dominant-negative RhoA in rats. JAMA Ophthalmol. 2015;133:182–90. DOI:10.1001/jamaophthalmol.2014.4747

[73] Borras T, Buie LK, Spiga MG: Inducible scAAV2.GRE.MMP1 lowers IOP long-term in a large animal model for steroid-induced glaucoma gene therapy. Gene Ther. 2016;23:438–49. DOI:10.1038/gt.2016.14

[74] Borras T: Advances in glaucoma treatment and management: gene therapy. Invest Ophthalmol Vis Sci. 2012;53:2506–10. DOI:10.1167/iovs.12-9483o

[75] Mead B, Berry M, Logan A, Scott RA, Leadbeater W, Scheven BA: Stem cell treatment of degenerative eye disease. Stem Cell Res. 2015;14:243–57. DOI:10.1016/j.scr.2015.02.003

[76] Quigley HA, Iglesia DS: Stem cells to replace the optic nerve. Eye (Lond). 2004;18:1085–8. DOI:10.1038/sj.eye.6701577

[77] Mesentier-Louro LA, Zaverucha-do-Valle C, Rosado-de-Castro PH, Silva-Junior AJ, Pimentel-Coelho PM, Mendez-Otero R, Santiago MF: Bone marrow-derived cells as a therapeutic approach to optic nerve diseases. Stem Cells Int. 2016;2016:5078619. DOI:10.1155/2016/5078619

[78] Zhu W, Gramlich OW, Laboissonniere L, Jain A, Sheffield VC, Trimarchi JM, Tucker BA, Kuehn MH: Transplantation of iPSC-derived TM cells rescues glaucoma phenotypes in vivo. Proc Natl Acad Sci U S A. 2016. DOI:10.1073/pnas.1604153113

[79] Gossman CA, Christie J, Webster MK, Linn DM, Linn CL: Neuroprotective strategies in glaucoma. Curr Pharm Des. 2016;22:2178–92.

[80] Sena DF, Lindsley K: Neuroprotection for treatment of glaucoma in adults. Cochrane Database Syst Rev. 2013;2:CD006539. DOI:10.1002/14651858.CD006539.pub3

[81] Wen R, Tao W, Li Y, Sieving PA: CNTF and retina. Prog Retin Eye Res. 2012;31:136–51. DOI:10.1016/j.preteyeres.2011.11.005

[82] Kauper K, McGovern C, Sherman S, Heatherton P, Rapoza R, Stabila P, Dean B, Lee A, Borges S, Bouchard B, Tao W: Two-year intraocular delivery of ciliary neurotrophic factor by encapsulated cell technology implants in patients with chronic retinal degenerative diseases. Invest Ophthalmol Vis Sci. 2012;53:7484–91. DOI:10.1167/iovs.12-9970

[83] Tatton W, Chen D, Chalmers-Redman R, Wheeler L, Nixon R, Tatton N: Hypothesis for a common basis for neuroprotection in glaucoma and Alzheimer's disease: anti-apoptosis by alpha-2-adrenergic receptor activation. Surv Ophthalmol. 2003;48 Suppl 1:S25–37.

[84] Krupin T, Liebmann JM, Greenfield DS, Ritch R, Gardiner S: Low-Pressure Glaucoma Study G: a randomized trial of brimonidine versus timolol in preserving visual function: results from the Low-Pressure Glaucoma Treatment Study. Am J Ophthalmol. 2011;151:671–81. DOI:10.1016/j.ajo.2010.09.026

[85] Osborne NN, Wood JP, Chidlow G: Invited review: neuroprotective properties of certain beta-adrenoceptor antagonists used for the treatment of glaucoma. J Ocul Pharmacol Ther. 2005;21:175–81. DOI:10.1089/jop.2005.21.175

[86] Payne AJ, Kaja S, Naumchuk Y, Kunjukunju N, Koulen P: Antioxidant drug therapy approaches for neuroprotection in chronic diseases of the retina. Int J Mol Sci. 2014;15:1865–86. DOI:10.3390/ijms15021865

[87] Guo X, Kong X, Huang R, Jin L, Ding X, He M, Liu X, Patel MC, Congdon NG: Effect of Ginkgo biloba on visual field and contrast sensitivity in Chinese patients with normal tension glaucoma: a randomized, crossover clinical trial. Invest Ophthalmol Vis Sci. 2014;55:110–6. DOI:10.1167/iovs.13-13168

[88] Roy Chowdhury U, Hann CR, Stamer WD, Fautsch MP: Aqueous humor outflow: dynamics and disease. Invest Ophthalmol Vis Sci. 2015;56:2993–3003. DOI:10.1167/iovs.15-16744

[89] Goel M, Picciani RG, Lee RK, Bhattacharya SK: Aqueous humor dynamics: a review. Open Ophthalmol J. 2011;4:52–9. DOI:10.2174/1874364101004010052

[90] Arriola-Villalobos P, Martinez-de-la-Casa JM, Diaz-Valle D, Fernandez-Perez C, Garcia-Sanchez J, Garcia-Feijoo J: Combined iStent trabecular micro-bypass stent implantation and phacoemulsification for coexistent open-angle glaucoma and cataract: a long-term study. Br J Ophthalmol. 2012;96:645–9. DOI:10.1136/bjophthalmol-2011-300218

[91] Katz LJ, Erb C, Carceller GA, Fea AM, Voskanyan L, Wells JM, Giamporcaro JE: Prospective, randomized study of one, two, or three trabecular bypass stents in open-angle glaucoma subjects on topical hypotensive medication. Clin Ophthalmol. 2015;9:2313–20. DOI:10.2147/opth.s96695

[92] Manasses DT, Au L: The new era of glaucoma micro-stent surgery. Ophthalmol Ther. 2016;113(25):E492-500. DOI:10.1007/s40123-016-0054-6

[93] Pinchuk L, Riss I, Batlle JF, Kato YP, Martin JB, Arrieta E, Palmberg P, Parrish RK, Weber BA, Kwon Y, Parel J-M: The development of a micro-shunt made from poly(styrene-block-isobutylene-block-styrene) to treat glaucoma. J Biomed Mater Res Part B: Appl Biomater. 2015. DOI:10.1002/jbm.b.33525

[94] Batlle JF, Fantes F, Riss I, Pinchuk L, Alburquerque R, Kato YP, Arrieta E, Peralta AC, Palmberg P, Parrish RKI, Weber BA, Parel J-M: Three-year follow-up of a novel aqueous humor microshunt. J Glaucoma. 2016;25:e58–65. DOI:10.1097/ijg.0000000000000368

[95] Höh H, Grisanti S, Rau M, Ianchulev S: Two-year clinical experience with the CyPass micro-stent: safety and surgical outcomes of a novel supraciliary micro-stent. Klin Monatsbl Augenheilkd. 2014;231:377–81. DOI:10.1055/s-0034-1368214

[96] Gigon A, Shaarawy T: The suprachoroidal route in glaucoma surgery. J Curr Glaucoma Pract. 2016;10:13–20. DOI:10.5005/jp-journals-10008-1197

7

Combined Glaucoma and Cataract

Jesús Jiménez-Román, Carolina Prado-Larrea,
Luis Laneri-Pusineri and Roberto Gonzalez-Salinas

Abstract

Glaucoma and cataract frequently coexist in our elderly population regardless of geographical location or ethnicity. Cataract extraction alone has demonstrated to reduce intraocular pressure in eyes either with or without glaucoma. However, this chapter focuses on how cataract surgery might be combined with different glaucoma surgical procedures, such as trabeculectomy, non-penetrating procedures and minimally invasive procedures (MIGS), as well as implantation of drainage devices like the Trabectome® and the iStent®, both used for trabecular flow increase; the CyPass® implant, which acts by increasing the uveoscleral flow; the XEN® implant that facilitates the drainage of the aqueous humor from the anterior chamber to the subconjunctival space and finally the endocyclophotocoagulation that decreases the aqueous humor production. Current surgical options will be discussed, focusing on recently reported studies, analyzing the clinical aspects that influence the choice for each surgical treatment.

Keywords: MIGS, glaucoma, cataract, IOP, combined surgery, novel glaucoma procedures

1. Introduction

Cataract and glaucoma are ranked as the leading causes of blindness worldwide (51 and 8%, respectively). Cataract and glaucoma frequently coexist in our patient population. Phacoemulsification combined with trabeculectomy has historically been the preferred surgical approach for concurrently managing cataract and glaucoma. The severity of glaucoma must be taken into account for all cases of cataract surgery in glaucoma patients. In case of a refractory glaucoma; when more than three types of medication are required, with associated early stage cataract; it is advisable to postpone any phacoemulsification procedure until after glaucoma surgery. However, all cases most be evaluated individually, and cataractogenous effect of the procedure should be considered in this situation. Moreover, cataract extraction performed after a filtering surgery may lead to a reduction of the bleb function.

2. When to combine surgeries and how to minimize complications

In the last few years, glaucoma surgery has undergone great advances when we are talking about surgical treatment of the glaucoma, one of the main points about this is combining cataract and glaucoma surgery [1].

We can combine cataract surgery with different glaucoma surgeries, such as trabeculectomy, implantation of drainage devices, non-penetrating procedures and minimally invasive procedures (MIGS) to mention a few [1].

The success of them depends on several factors among which they can mention:

- Type of glaucoma
- Severity of damage
- Amount and time of use of topical medicine
- Previous surgery/s
- Type of surgery to be performed

Within this last group of surgeries are procedures and devices that seek to derive the aqueous humor toward the Schlemm's channel, the suprachoroidal space, to the subconjunctival space and that reduce the aqueous humor production [1].

This opens a range of possibilities for the treatment of glaucoma, mainly in early stages of the disease, which turns it into a useful resource for the control of glaucoma and making it an option with fewer risks and complications than the classic procedures [1].

2.1. Newer surgical alternatives

Among the methods that can be used, FDA-approved, are Trabectome® and iStent® for use since 2006 and 2012, respectively, both used for trabecular flow increase, the recently approved CyPass® implant in 2016, acts by increasing the uveoscleral flow, the XEN® implant that facilitates the drainage of the aqueous humor from the anterior chamber to the subconjunctival space and finally the endocyclophotocoagulation that decreases the aqueous humor production [2].

It has now been established that the MIGS techniques are prepared for a decrease in intraocular pressure (IOP) at least 20% to be considered effective. In addition to being considered as safe, this means a very low incidence of adverse effects and complications, especially those that affect the patient's vision.

The efficacy and safety of some devices have been demonstrated by many multicenter studies [2].

The hypotensive effect of these techniques may be additional if combined with cataract surgery, phacoemulsification specifically, with this combination is reporting the IOP description up to 40% [4]. The fact that those are techniques with a lower IOP decrease should not be seen as a problem and it is a mistake to compare these techniques with the standard surgery of glaucoma, trabeculectomy with mitomycin C, since they are not designed to replace the latter to fill the gap between medical treatment and more aggressive surgeries [3].

Any patient who undergo phacoemulsification of the lens gives us an opportunity to combine the surgery with a minimally invasive procedure of glaucoma. Due to the efficacy and safety profile, these procedures should be used in cases of mild-to-moderate glaucoma. Regarding the type of glaucoma, they are performed in open-angle primary and secondary to pseudoexfoliation and pigment, except for endocyclophotocoagulation that can be used in other types of glaucoma. With all this, MIGS would help us gain time and delay, as far as possible, more aggressive surgery [3].

In situations in which we combine cataract surgery with some minimally invasive procedure, it is not easy to differentiate what proportion of the hypotensive effect is due to cataract surgery and how much is due to the MIGS procedure. We can say that the hypotensive effect of cataract surgery alone reported by different authors is 2–4 mmHg in a variable period of time (1–7 years) [2, 3].

Some recommendations to facilitate the procedure or implantation of devices and to reduce the rate of intra and postoperative complications are: familiarization with the technique and/or device to be implanted, use of the surgical microscope with different viewing angles, correct use of surgical goniolens and previous experience in procedures or surgeries involving surgical manipulation of the angle [2].

According to a meta-analysis, comparing the efficacy of iStent combined with cataract surgery versus phacoemulsification alone in patients with glaucoma and cataract, the decrease in IOP was greater in the group in whom iStent was placed and this effect is even greater if more implantation is performed of a device [4].

2.2. Combined phacoemulsification and canaloplasty

Mention will be made of some of the minimally invasive procedures currently performed, beginning with canaloplasty. This procedure consists in the creation of two overlapping scleral flaps, the probing of the Schlemm's canal with a catheter designed for that effect and the introduction of a suture with the aid of the same catheter and then knotted at its free ends to achieve a canal distension and a tension in the tissues of the trabecular meshwork with the consequent opening of the trabecular meshwork, ending with a watertight suture of the superficial flap. Better results are obtained when this procedure is combined with phacoemulsification of the lens. The reduction obtained is approximately 40% to 3 years with a success of up to 65–82% [5, 6].

2.3. Combined phacoemulsification and iStent®

Another available procedure is the iStent implant, which consists of a metal device that is implanted at the level of the trabecular meshwork to create a bypass between the anterior chamber and the Schlemm's canal. It is the smallest device that is implanted throughout the body as depicted in **Figure 1**. The method may be done in isolation or in combination with phacoemulsification of the lens; if implanted in conjunction with surgery of the lens, the moment in which it is implanted is variable, being able to be before or after the extraction of the lens, taking into account that it must be done with the pupil in miosis and under the direct visualization of the angle through a goniolens. The hypotensive effect of this device increases when it is associated with cataract surgery in the same surgical act, as well as with the number of implanted devices [4].

If we compare the IOP results, between cataract surgery and cataract surgery plus iStent implantation in PAOG patients with at least one medication and IOP ≥ 19 mmHg, at 15 months the IOP reduction was 17.3% and a 80% medication reduction in the iStent group, compared to 9% IOP reduction and 32% medication reduction (cataract surgery alone) [8].

Almost all of the randomized controlled trials show a mild IOP reduction (between 10 and 20%). But when multiple iStents are implanted with cataract extraction, the IOP reduction is up to 40% with three stents, attention has turned toward using multiple iStents [7].

For multiple iStents alone (without cataract surgery), using the second-generation iStent inject among phakic and pseudophakic subjects, the results show a 29–48% IOP reduction from medicated baseline. At 1 year after implantation of two stents, 66% had IOP ≤18 mmHg off of medication, and the mean IOP reduction among all was 40% [8].

2.4. Combined phacoemulsification and CyPass®

One device used to increase drainage through the uveoscleral pathway is the CyPass Micro-stent, which creates a communication between the suprachoroidal space and the anterior chamber. The CyPass Micro-stent is a fenestrated micro-stent made with a biocompatible

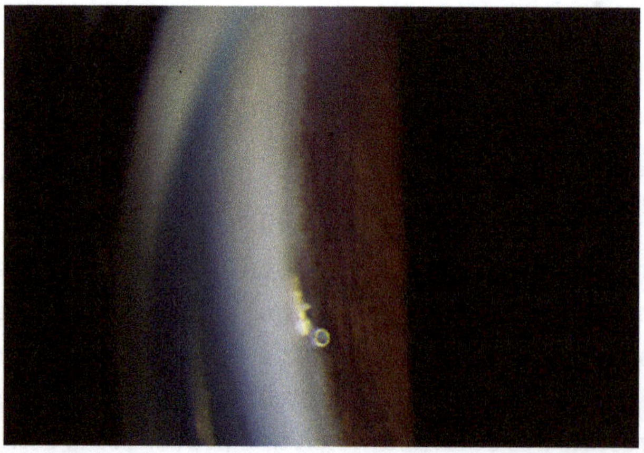

Figure 1. iStent implant at the level of the trabecular meshwork to create a bypass between the anterior chamber and the Schlemm's canal.

polyamide, 6.35 mm in length and an external diameter of 510 μm. It is introduced under gonioscopic visualization at the level of the union of the scleral spur with the band of the ciliary body by a curved guide to follow the contour of the sclera along the supraciliar space. Trough physical and mechanical properties and a series of retaining rings at the proximal end of the device, the stability of the device is ensured in the supraciliar space. Different studies have shown that the implantation of this device decreases IOP both in isolation and in combination with cataract surgery, with an IOP decrease of approximately 30–35%, and this effect is maintained over time, as well as in the use of hypotensive medication from 1.4 drugs to 0.2 on average. The complications that can be observed after the implantation of this device are few and include loss of visual acuity, corneal edema, iris inflammation, cyclodialysis, hypotonia, migration or obstruction of the device and increase of IOP [9, 10].

CyPass with cataract extraction demonstrate a favorable safety profile. The mean IOP reduction was 5.5 mmHg (from 21.1 ± 5.91 to 15.6 ± 0.53 mmHg) which means a 37% decrease from baseline IOP and a 50% reduction in glaucoma medications [11].

This are the results at one-year follow-up from CyPass implantation alone in a recent multicenter interventional study. Baseline IOP was reduced from 24.5 ± 2.8 mmHg with 2.2 ± 1.1 medications to 16.4 ± 5.5 mmHg with 1.4 ± 1.3 medications at 12 months. This was a 34.7% reduction in IOP. About 83% of eyes avoided conventional incisional glaucoma surgery [11].

2.5. Combined phacoemulsification and endocyclophotocoagulation

Cyclophotocoagulation, initially with a transscleral probe, typically used in refractory glaucoma. Recent reports demonstrate the safety and efficacy of endocyclophotocoagulation (ECP) in the treatment of mild-to-moderate glaucoma. Similar to other MIGS, it is conjunctival-sparing, blebless, and can be combined with cataract surgery. The laser endoscope probe can be inserted through a temporal 2.4 mm clear corneal wound into the anterior chamber and sulcus (filled with OVD). With direct visualization of the ciliary processes, the visible portion of the ciliary process are treated with the diode laser (Iridex Oculight, Mountain View) at 200 mW mean power and continuous duration. Approximately 270° of ciliary processes must be treated to the point of blanching and shrinking of the tissue. Overtreatment is defined by extreme blanching and a popping sound, which indicates an air-bubble explosion [12].

A 3-year outcomes of a prospective nonrandomized matched-control study comparing ECP with cataract extraction versus cataract extraction alone in medically controlled OAG, showed a 10.1% IOP reduction and a 73% medication reduction at 2 years in the treatment group. The control group (cataract surgery alone) showed a 0.8% IOP reduction and a 17% medication reduction at 2 years [12].

Another author reported retrospective results of endocyclophotocoagulation and cataract extraction versus cataract extraction alone in mild-to-moderate glaucoma patients, the combined group had a 14.5% IOP reduction with 85% medication reduction at 36 months. The control group (phacoemulsification alone) 12.4% IOP reduction and a 13.3% medication reduction at 36 months. While there was no significant difference in the IOP reduction between groups, there was a significant difference in medication reduction. At 36 months, the 61.4% of the combined group versus 23.3% of the control group achieved an outcome of 20% IOP reduction with a decrease of at least one ocular hypotensive medication [13].

2.6 Combined phacoemulsification and Ex-PRESS®

The Ex-PRESS Glaucoma Filtration Device (Alcon Laboratories Inc., Fort Worth, TX) is a biocompatible [14], non-valved stainless steel device, designed to offer a fast an simple glaucoma filtering device [15] and to provide a lower complication rate with a more stable early postoperative course [16]. Initially it was implanted through full-thickness sclera, directly under the conjunctiva, allowing aqueous drainage into the subconjunctival space [17], alone or in a combined procedure including phacoemulsification, as depicted in **Figure 2**. This technique however, was associated with a higher rate of complications: persistent hypotony, flat anterior chamber, choroidal detachment, suprachoroidal hemorrhage, conjunctival scarring and implant extrusion [18–21]. In 2005, Dahan and Carmichael [15] described an alternative device to be implanted under a scleral flap; these modifications provided satisfactory IOP control and reduced postoperative complications rates.

In a retrospective study by Lan et al. [22] that described the long-term outcomes of the Ex-Press Device combined with phacoemulsification in patients with primary open-angle glaucoma (POAG) and primary angle-closure glaucoma (PACG) and founded a lower postoperative IOP on the POAG group, in addition to more hypotony when compared to the PACG group. Three years after surgery the cumulative complete and qualified success rates were 63.3 and 83.3% (POAG) and 53.3 and 73.3% (POAG), respectively.

Huerva et al. [23] evaluated the efficacy and safety of the Ex-Press device in combination with cataract surgery. After 1-year follow-up, 59.5% of patients had IOP control without medications and 10.8% with one medication. Complications in the early period included ocular hypotony and uveal effusion in 5%, as well as one case of re-intervention after 1-year due to uncontrolled IOP.

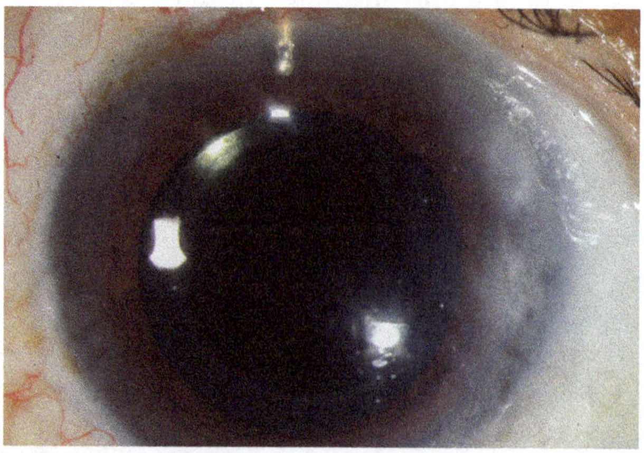

Figure 2. The Ex-PRESS Glaucoma Filtration Device implanted through full-thickness sclera in to the anterior chamber.

3. Impact of cataract surgery on intraocular pressure

The leading cause of age-related, reversible blindness is cataract and the leading cause of irreversible blindness worldwide is glaucoma, the incidence of both cataract and elevated intraocular pressure, with or without glaucoma, increases with age [24]. There have been various reports of the effect of cataract surgery on intraocular pressure (IOP) in glaucomatous and non-glaucomatous eyes, however, the magnitude and clinical significance of these changes continues to be debated. Some studies found a significant IOP reduction whereas others reported no significant change [25], depending on the type of glaucoma.

Intraocular pressure is the only known modifiable risk factor for the development and progression of glaucoma and intraocular pressure-lowering therapy delays its progression [26]. In glaucoma patients, the indication of cataract surgery differs from other patients, depending on various factors such as disease stage, preoperative IOP, number of medications, gonioscopy appearance, age and the experience and skills of the surgeon. Therefore every surgeon should recognize the influence of cataract surgery on IOP control in each type of glaucoma [27].

Previous reports of the effect of cataract surgery in IOP have reflected great variability in IOP reduction, related to angle anatomy, preoperative IOP and anterior chamber depth [28–30]. Identify which patient would experience an IOP-lowering response with cataract surgery alone could modify surgical decision-making.

3.1. Cataract surgery and open-angle glaucoma

In glaucomatous and normal eyes, cataract surgery produces a reduction in IOP, although these effects are more pronounced in patients with primary angle-closure glaucoma (PACG), there has been noticed a reduction in IOP also in POAG.

In a prospective study, Elgin et al. [31] compared the effect of cataract surgery on anterior segment parameters measured by optical biometry in patients with primary open-angle glaucoma (POAG) and pseudoexfoliation glaucoma (PSX), IOP decreased postoperatively 1.9 mmHg and 3.1 mmHg in each group, they also observed a significant increase in anterior chamber depth in both groups with a greater increase in PSX patients probably related to ciliary zonular laxity.

In a retrospective study of the Swedish National Cataract Register Data, Charlotta Zetterström et al. [24] found that after cataract surgery, patients with glaucoma had a larger reduction in IOP than the group of patients who did not have glaucoma and patients with glaucoma and PSX had significantly greater IOP reduction than patients without these diagnoses. They also found that when high IOP was given as an indication for surgery, the IOP reduction after cataract surgery was greater.

Shingleton et al. [32] retrospectively evaluated the change in IOP and glaucoma medications after cataract surgery in glaucoma patients, glaucoma suspects and normal patients. At 3 years follow-up IOP decreased 1.4 mmHg in glaucoma patients and glaucoma suspects and 1.7 mmHg in normal patients, the number of glaucoma medications in the glaucoma group did not show any significant change at follow-up and they found that after 3 years, 85% of the glaucoma patients had IOP less than or equal to their preoperative IOP, with the same number of glaucoma medications or less. Despite being a retrospective study it demonstrated a sustained reduction in IOP after cataract removal.

Slabaugh et al. [33] in a retrospective study of 157 patients with POAG found a decrease in IOP by a mean of 1.8 mmHg after phacoemulsification at 1 year follow-up but 38% had worsening of IOP control including 24% that needed additional medications or laser trabeculoplasty and 0.6% that required trabeculectomy. Among patients that did not have any change in medications, higher preoperative IOP, older age and deeper anterior chamber depth were associated with lower postoperative IOP.

The American Academy of Ophthalmology in a recent assessment investigated the long-term effect of phacoemulsification on IOP in patients with POAG, PSX and PACG [34]. They found that higher IOP before phacoemulsification is the single most common significant factor associated with a greater drop in IOP after phacoemulsification and concluded that for patients with POAG controlled with 1 or 2 medications, phacoemulsification alone results in a decrease in IOP (−13%) and medication requirement (−12%) although 26% of patients experience worse IOP control after phacoemulsification and may require additional medications, laser treatment or both.

3.2. Cataract surgery and angle-closure glaucoma

The prevalence of primary angle-closure glaucoma is highest in Asia (1.09%) and there is an estimated of 23.4 million cases worldwide for 2020 [35].

Patients with chronic primary angle-closure glaucoma (PACG) have an altered trabecular meshwork architecture with fewer spaces and fused trabecular beams, these changes are the result of mild, recurrent subacute attacks of angle closure that lead to chronic angle-closure glaucoma [36].

In a large percent of patients, there are multiple mechanisms for angle-closure glaucoma as pupillary blocking and plateau iris, in those patents residual angle-closure post iridotomy would result in poor control of IOP, in those patients lens extraction may resolve residual angle closure [37]. Previous studies demonstrated that lens extraction has the ability to lower IOP, lens extraction would widen the angle even without structural alterations of plateau iris because the lens plays a central role in the pathogenesis of PACG, its increased thickness, relative anterior positioning and progression of its thickness result in narrowing of the anterior chamber.

Lens extraction reduces diurnal IOP fluctuations, IOP levels and the number of anti glaucoma medication in PACG with previous laser iridotomy, the change in IOP fluctuation values correlates positively with the change in anterior chamber deep an preoperative IOP fluctuation [38]. Thus patients with narrowest angles might experience a greater benefit from cataract surgery alone depending on the proportion of the angle that has been permanently closed by peripheral anterior synechiae.

In 1998, Gunning and Greve [39] retrospectively evaluated the long-term effects of extraction of incipient cataracts or clear lenses in patients with subacute or chronic angle-closure glaucoma, after a mean follow-up of 52.6 months glaucoma control was achieved in 68% of patients, they concluded that the choice of first a cataract procedure with the option of a future trabeculectomy may be a more attractive approach in patients with subacute or chronic angle-closure glaucoma than trabeculectomy followed by an optional cataract procedure.

In the EAGLE trial, they assessed the efficacy and of clear lens extraction versus laser peripheral iridotomy and topical medical treatment as first-line therapy in people with newly diagnosed primary angle closure and intraocular hypertension or primary angle-closure glaucoma. After a mean follow-up of 36 months, clear lens extraction showed greater efficacy and was more cost-effective than laser peripheral iridotomy, they concluded that clear lens extraction should be considered as an option for first-line treatment [40].

In a prospective study, Tham et al. [41] compared phacoemulsification alone versus combined phacotrabeculectomy in patients with PACG medically controlled, after 2 years follow-up combined surgery resulted in less topical glaucoma drugs but there were no differences in glaucomatous progression, also combined surgery was associated with more postoperative complications.

In another prospective study, Tham et al. [42] also compared phacoemulsification versus trabeculectomy in patients with PACG medically uncontrolled, alter 1 year follow-up, there was a significant and comparable reduction in IOP in both groups but trabeculectomy was more effective in reducing dependence on glaucoma drugs also with more postoperative complications. In the phacoemulsification group, only 27% did not require IOP-lowering medications or further surgery after 24 months.

The decision of a cataract surgery alone versus a combined surgery should be made taking account of the type of glaucoma, the severity of the disease and the IOP. Patients with a mild damage and a controlled IOP with topical medications are good candidates for cataract surgery alone.

4. Surgical complications in combined surgery

Patients after glaucoma surgery have an increased risk of cataract formation or progression, approximately 50% of patients will require cataract surgery within the first years after trabeculectomy surgery [43].

Phacoemulsification in presence of a functioning filtration bleb increases the risk of bleb failure in 33%, there are changes in bleb morphology that results in elevations in intraocular pressure (IOP), increased glaucoma medications or additional surgical treatment [44, 45].

The coexistence of cataract and glaucoma in the same patient can follow different strategies such as glaucoma surgery first, cataract surgery first or combined surgery, it depends of the type of glaucoma, the severity of the disease, target intraocular pressure, patients age and the preference of the surgeon.

4.1. Phacotrabeculectomy

Although a staged approach of trabeculectomy followed by cataract surgery has demonstrated successful refractive results, with the last improvements in phacoemulsification and trabeculectomy, phacotrabeculectomy stills a surgical option for some patients with cataract and glaucoma. The indications for phacotrabeculectomy are the simultaneous presence of a visually significant cataract and medically uncontrolled glaucoma, advanced glaucomatous optic nerve damage or visual field loss. A combined approach has the advantages of reduced overall cost, reduced anesthesia and surgery time and less recovery time.

In a retrospective study, Jin et al. [46] evaluated the outcomes after phacotrabeculectomy in consecutive patients. Over 60 patients included in the study, hyphema and hypotony developed in three eyes in the early postoperative period. Bleb hemorrhage occurred in two eyes and cleared within 2 weeks without incident, one eye had a bleb leak that resolved after conservative treatment. The most frequent late complication was posterior capsule opacification requiring capsulotomy in six eyes. Bleb revision was performed in two eyes for dysesthetic bleb 2–3 years after surgery. A second trabeculectomy and an injection of 5-fluorouracil were performed each in one eye, for poor filtration. In this study, the rate of complications was remarkable lower compared with other reports.

In another retrospective study in Singapore [47], the complications after phacotrabeculectomy with Mitomycin C were evaluated, the mean follow-up was 47 months. Most of the postoperative complications occurred within the first month: hypotony in 25.6%, hyphema and shallow anterior chamber in 10% each one. About 11.3% of patients required surgical intervention: bleb needling with antimetabolite use in 4.4%, implant of glaucoma drainage device 1.3%, anterior chamber reformation 1.3% and lens repositioning 0.6%, the majority of complications were transient and self-limiting. They concluded that close and active monitoring is critical in the early postoperative period to prevent complications and surgical failure.

There are reports of tilt and decentration of intraocular lens (IOLs) after phacoemulsification in patients with glaucoma; those are more common in eyes with pseudoexfoliation syndrome or closed-angle glaucoma.

In combined surgery, the changes in anterior chamber depth, axial length, changes in corneal curvature, iridectomy and fluctuations of IOP could affect the accuracy of the IOL power calculation and its position. Ong et al. [48] in a retrospective study investigated the refractive outcome of phacotrabeculectomy compared with a sequential approach, they found a greater myopic refractive prediction error and mean absolute error in the combined group. They advocate the surgeon aim for a slightly more hyperopic result for the combined approach to achieve results closer to emmetropia.

4.2. Combined phacoemulsification and glaucoma drainage implant

In the case of phacoemulsification combined with a glaucoma drainage device operative complications include anterior and/or posterior capsule tears, vitreous loss and IOL-capsular bag subluxation. Cataract extraction combined with implant insertion produce a moderate to severe reduction in IOP (hypotony) lasting for 1–14 days or more, after which the IOP return to safe levels. Other complications include hyphema, anterior chamber shallowing, choroidal detachment associated with varying degrees of hypotony and IOP spikes [49]. Distended and symptomatic blebs could be seen in these patients and, most infrequently, diplopia.

Corneal decompensation after insertion of drainage devices and cataract extraction was likely to be due to pre-existing endothelial loss caused by previously uncontrolled IOP, but it is possible that endothelial injury may also be aggravated during phacoemulsification [39]. The hypertensive phase defined as elevated IOP in the presence of a functioning bleb and a patent tube and occurring up to 9 months after surgery was found to occur in similar rate than in the isolated drainage implant surgery (22–50%) [49–51]. Tube erosion and occlusion show no difference between tube implant alone and when it is combined with cataract extraction [49–51].

4.3. Phacoemulsification and non-penetrating surgeries

There are several options to manage patients with both cataract and open-angle glaucoma and the rates of complications are different in non-penetrating surgeries compared with trabeculectomy. One of the advantages of phacoemulsification with non-penetrating surgeries versus phacotrabeculectomy is a lower incidence of postoperative inflammation and other immediate complications like hyphema and shallow anterior chamber.

In a retrospective study, Schoenberg et al. [52] compared the surgical outcomes between phaco canaloplasty and phacotrabeculectomy. There were no differences in overall failure rates between the two groups, in the phacotrabeculectomy group two patients had a decrease in vision but only one was related to the surgery. Five patients in each group required revision of the surgical site at the slit lamp for management of elevated IOP.

The most common complication in the phacocanaloplasty group was hyphema (27.7%) and resolved over a 2 week period in all patients. There were some serious complications during follow-up, one patient in each group developed choroidal effusion, one patient had a suprachoroidal hemorrhage and two developed hypotony maculopathy in the phacotrabeculectomy group. They concluded than phacocanaloplasty is an excellent option in patients with mild-to-moderate open-angle glaucoma but despite the higher risks of serious complications phacotrabeculectomy may be a good choice in patients with advanced glaucoma requiring greater IOP reduction.

A retrospective study [53] compared the outcomes of phacotrabeculectomy versus phacoemulsification-deep sclerectomy, there were no cases of bleb infections or endophthalmitis, hypotony occurred in only two patients who underwent laser goniopuncture after phacoemulsification-deep sclerectomy. The frequency of late bleb leaks was significantly higher in the phacotrabeculectomy group, there was a low incidence of immediate side effects in both groups but there was a high incidence of intraoperative perforations (15.7%) in the phacoemulsification-deep sclerectomy group.

A recent survey of the American Glaucoma Society [54] assessed the surgical practice patterns among their members in various clinical settings. In the case of a patient without prior incisional surgery and with a visually significant cataract, 24% of surgeons performed phacotrabeculectomy with mitomycin C, 22% phacoemulsification with minimally invasive glaucoma surgery and 9% phacoemulsification with a glaucoma drainage device versus 44% of surgeons that preferred phacoemulsification alone.

The surgical approach for a patient with cataract and glaucoma has evolved over the years, improvements in previous surgical techniques and new available surgical options with less rates of complications has changed practice patterns among glaucoma surgeons.

5. Novel surgical approaches in cataract surgery

Cataract and glaucoma are ranked as the leading causes of blindness worldwide (51 and 8%, respectively) [55]. Both the cataract and glaucoma can coexist in elderly patient population. An estimate of 20% of cataract procedures performed annually in the USA has glaucoma or ocular hypertension. A combined cataract extraction with trabeculectomy has been the preferred surgical approach for managing cataract and glaucoma [56].

In developed countries, glaucoma is the second leading cause of irreversible blindness and this burden tends to increase as the population ages [57]. Similarly, for cataract, whose prevalence is also age-related the global prevalence of 15.5% increases to 45.9% in those over 75 years and is expected to duplicate by 2020 [58].

Cataract surgery has been demonstrated to reduce IOP in glaucoma patients as well as in non-glaucomatous eyes, with variable magnitude depending on anterior chamber depth, angle configuration or the presence of concomitant pathology as pseudoexfoliation syndrome [34]. Additionally, several series have demonstrated a greater IOP reduction postoperatively in elderly patients, females, eyes with an axial length ≤21 mm, and PXF patients [59]. Also, another beneficial effect of cataract removal can be observed in the capacity to increase the accuracy of functional and structural analyses currently used for diagnosing and evaluating glaucoma and its progression, since a visually significant cataract may act as an obstacle to these tests. Therefore, we can presume that combined treatment could be established, with cataract surgery being part of glaucoma treating standardized procedures.

5.1. Simultaneous or sequential cataract and glaucoma surgery

Currently, a variety of surgical procedures are available: first, phacoemulsification cataract extraction alone. Second, sequential glaucoma surgery and cataract extraction, and finally combined surgery. Phacoemulsification alone is suggested for controlled glaucoma patients with moderate and non-progressive visual field defect [59].

The severity of glaucoma must be taken into account for all cases of cataract surgery in glaucoma patients'. In case of a refractory glaucoma, when more than three types of medication are required, with associated early stage cataract, it is advisable to postpone any phacoemulsification procedure until after glaucoma surgery [61]. Moreover, when phacoemulsification cataract extraction is performed after glaucoma surgery, it is advisable to verify bleb function, which could be reduced. For these cases, combined surgery is more beneficial due to an improvement on intraocular pressure decrease when compared to phacoemulsification alone [60, 61].

5.2. Femtosecond-assisted cataract surgery in glaucoma

Femtosecond laser-assisted cataract surgery (FLACS), a new technology that was firstly introduced in 2008 has shown promising treatment outcomes, has realized increasing popularity [62]. Non-inferiority has been established relative to manual cataract surgery, and some reports have suggested superiority relative to manual methods [63]. Potential advantages include customized corneal incisions and capsulotomy position, precision in shape and size of capsulotomy, custom lens fragmentation patterns, endothelial cell loss reduction and better refractive stability and predictability [63].

To date, many studies have attempted to compare the outcome and complications of FLACS and conventional phacoemulsification cataract surgery. Some studies have shown better visual acuity recovery and lower endothelial cell loss after FLACS when compared with conventional phacoemulsification, in non-glaucoma patients [64, 65]. However, in glaucoma patients, the use of FLACS alone or in combination to filtering glaucoma surgery have been optimal, when taking into account postoperative visual recovery, corneal cell integrity and functionality [65].

With femtosecond laser technology and intraoperative image guidance, options for overcoming major challenges in otherwise difficult cataract cases are now available [66]. Preoperative assessment of pupil dilation (4.0 mm or greater) and presence of iridocorneal or iridolenticular adhesions is important in determining whether a patient with Peters anomaly is a candidate for femtosecond laser-assisted cataract extraction. Iridocorneal or iridolenticular adhesions that encroach on the central 4.0 mm of the visual axis may interrupt the laser capsulotomy and may necessitate decentration of the capsulotomy or exclusion of the patient [62].

During femtosecond laser pretreatment in cataract surgery, suction is applied to stabilize the eye before laser anterior capsulotomy, main incision construction and lens fragmentation [67]. Recently reported data from femtosecond pretreatment in cataract surgery suggest that the above-mentioned vacuum application transiently increases intraocular pressure (IOP) [62, 67]. Moreover, large increases in IOP can cause vascular or rhegmatogenous events; however, Schultz et al., reported recently that during femtosecond pretreatment, the IOP increase in healthy eyes is small (mean peak increase 18.5 mmHg from baseline) and appears to be well tolerated [68]. Currently, it is not known whether glaucoma patients are more predisposed to the acute complications or whether their response to vacuum applied during femtosecond laser pretreatment differs from that of patients without glaucoma [69]. Furthermore, a significant increase in IOP during laser pretreatment could result in nerve fiber damage and glaucoma progression.

5.3. Combined FLACS and glaucoma

5.3.1. Preoperative assessment

Laser-assisted cataract surgery patients should be evaluated for glaucoma. Therefore, a number of factors should be taken into account.

1. Glaucoma family history: it has been shown that people with familiar predisposition for glaucoma have increased risk of developing ocular hypertension and glaucoma. In

addition, these patients can develop glaucoma/OHT at a younger age. Therefore, glaucoma and visual field assessment is mandatory for patient's undergoing cataract surgery [70].

2. Elevated IOP remains the most important, modifiable, risk factor for developing glaucoma. However, a single IOP measurement is not sufficient to assess the actual risk of glaucoma, especially when there are other coexisting risk factors, taking into account that transient increase on intraocular pressure is going to be induced by the docking procedure during laser pretreatment [71].

3. Other ophthalmic diseases: pigment dispersion as well as pseudoexfoliation syndrome have been associated to secondary open-angle glaucoma [72, 73]. Previous reports have demonstrated that the presence of pigment dispersion syndrome does not affect the results of refractive surgery; however, topical antiglaucoma medication before surgery can modify the healing process thus the corneal wound can last longer [74].

4. Hypermetropia: hypermetropes are more likely to have narrow anterior chamber angles and a case of acute angle closure after LASIK in a hypermetropic patient has been reported. Preoperative gonioscopy will help the surgeon to recognize patients with narrow angles [75].

5.4. Toric IOL in glaucoma patients

Cataract surgery has gradually changed from vision rehabilitation to refractive surgery, which aims to achieve the best visual quality with minimal surgical trauma. With improvements of surgical techniques, postoperative corneal astigmatism has become a key factor affecting postoperative visual quality. Surgical astigmatism is caused by many factors, of which surgical incision is the main factor. The application of phacoemulsification on a clear corneal incision can cause slight reverse astigmatism, suggesting that the healing process of clear corneal incision directly affects changes of corneal astigmatism. This astigmatism is caused by the structure of the corneal incision, and corneal biomechanical changes.

Femtosecond laser-assisted cataract surgery (FLACS), which includes lens fragmentation, clear corneal incisions, and limbal relaxing incisions, was first reported by Nagy et al. [64]. The clinical application of the femtosecond laser has led to new developments for cataract surgery. The femtosecond laser system can make ladder-like multi-plane incisions in which the inner surface is enclosed. That is, the ladder between the corneal surface and matrix is made first to improve the impermeability of the incision, maintain intraocular pressure (IOP) and anterior chamber stability and prevent leakage of aqueous humor, thus reducing the incidence of endophthalmitis. The femtosecond laser system was first used to complete the phacoemulsification steps including capsulorhexis, nucleus fragmentation and clear corneal incision. The patients were then subjected to phacoemulsification to complete the entire cut along the tunnel made in former steps using a puncture knife [65].

Pseudoexfoliation is related to both glaucoma and cataract. Particularly, these patients have a tendency to achieve a poor pupil dilation; in addition to weak zonules, iridodonesis, phacodonesis or lens subluxation [75, 76]. In addition, patients with PXF may have higher pressures in the postoperative phase [76].

Toric IOLs might also not be successful in patients with an unstable capsular bag, or pseudoexfoliation and/or weak zonules, as the lens and bag may rotate or tilt once implanted, altering the patients' vision. There is a potential error if a toric IOL is implanted at the same time a glaucoma procedure is done, since a glaucoma surgery might induce keratometric changes depending on sutures and their tension, and further changes may occur if those sutures are removed or lysed, negating any benefit from the toric implant [77].

5.5. Multifocal IOLs

Multifocal intraocular lenses platforms are indeed valid options for glaucoma patients; however some considerations should be noted regarding its selection. Several lenses affect the monitoring of visual fields, recent reports by Inoue et al., revealed that multifocal IOLs can reduce contrast sensitivity and may alter raw values, gray scale and mean deviation values. Further, increased glare may reduce the sensitivity [77]. In addition, multifocal IOL implants cause significant nonspecific reduction in mean deviation (MD) values in automated perimetry in healthy eyes with multifocal compared to monofocal intraocular lens (IOL) implants on Humphrey Visual Field 10-2 testing that does not improve with time or neuroadaptation [77, 78]. Multifocal IOL implants may be inadvisable in patients where central visual field reduction may not be tolerated, such as macular degeneration, retinal pigment epithelium changes and glaucoma.

Long-term medical therapy used for several glaucoma patients can induce some degree of pupil rigidity, and in these cases, it is advisable to avoid multifocal IOLs if pupil diameter is less than 3.5 mm. Nevertheless, diffractive multifocal IOLs, which are not pupil-size dependent, can be considered for these patients. Irregular-shaped pupils, however, may increase the photopic symptoms and glare [77–79].

It is important to emphasize that multifocal platforms can be safely used in glaucoma suspects and ocular hypertensive patients with no disk or visual field damage who have been stable. In addition, glaucoma patients with early or mild visual field damage that has been controlled and stable, as well as glaucoma patients with a level of glaucoma in the fellow eye that is similar, and not severe, advanced or progressive.

Large trials providing scientific evidence-based data on the impact of multifocal IOL's in glaucoma patients, decisions regarding the implantation in a glaucoma patient should be individualized, taking into account patients' motivation and the rate of progression of glaucoma.

6. Conclusions

Cataract surgery is one of the most performed surgeries in the developed world. In addition to its significant impact on visual acuity, it has a proven potential effect on IOP decrease, but does not reduce IOP peaks [55]. More than 20 million Americans over 40 have cataract symptoms and more than 3 million cataract surgeries are performed in this country each year [80]. On the other hand, cataracts and glaucoma are the main causes of blindness in the world (51 and 8%, respectively). Glaucoma is the second cause of irreversible blindness, which increases with age [56]. Having both the same trend factor (age), they often coexist. Cataract has an overall prevalence of 15.5%, which increases to 45.9% in subjects older than 75 years and is estimated to be doubling by 2020 [58].

Does cataract and glaucoma coexistence represent a natural key to the management to both conditions? The answer to this question is under discussion, but it is important to note that 30% of patients who underwent cataract surgeries in the United States in the Medicare program had concomitant glaucoma [80, 81]. In addition, another study revealed that 9.1% of patients diagnosed with cataract coexist with the diagnosis of glaucoma [82].

Combined surgery seems to be the most understandable approach in the management of these two conditions. Cataract surgery in conjunction with conventional filtering procedures, such as trabeculectomy and valve implants, is indicated in patients with moderate to severe damage, although there is not real consensus [83, 84].

An important aspect of combined surgery is IOP peaks reduction. Traditional combined surgery produces a significant reduction on IOP, but with a higher risk of complications.

It is at this point that MIGS represents a revolution in combined surgery for glaucoma patients, certainly the IOP reduction is moderate (20%), but the complications number is reduced, it is an additional option to mild glaucoma or topical drug intolerance.

With the advent of these devices, a new vision is established in the glaucoma management, in earlier stages, leaving behind the traditional concept of glaucoma surgery in moderate or severe damage, even more the combination of these procedures with phacoemulsification, defines a new paradigm not only in the IOP control, also in a more audacious and timely visual rehabilitation, inclusive some cases premium lens implant.

On the other hand, the implementation of these novel techniques, require a prominent knowledge of the angular anatomy and be a surgeon experienced in glaucoma surgery, moreover, provides the opportunity to experts in phacoemulsification, to perform minimally invasive techniques and to do appropriate management in glaucomatous patients with mild damage. Cataract surgery with MIGS is an alternative in scrupulously selected patients (mild and moderate). There is insufficient evidence of the long-term intraocular pressure with these devices and techniques (MIGS) may become the most popular surgery in the glaucoma management and with a greater cost-benefit compared to topical treatment; however, there is not enough evidence on this, so it is advisable to consult it constantly and be cautious in the patient selection. Moreover, it is essential to recognize the inherent benefit of the combined procedure and the impact on the visual health and quality of life of our patients.

Author details

Jesús Jiménez-Román[1], Carolina Prado-Larrea[1], Luis Laneri-Pusineri[1] and Roberto Gonzalez-Salinas[2]*

*Address all correspondence to: dr.gonzalezsalinas@gmail.com

1 Glaucoma Department, Asociación para Evitar la Ceguera, Mexico City, Mexico

2 Research Department, Asociación para Evitar la Ceguera, Mexico City, Mexico

References

[1] Martinez de la Casa JM. Cirugía de glaucoma mínimamente invasiva (MIGS): Dónde estamos y hacia dónde caminamos. Archivos de la Sociedad Española de Oftalmología. 2012;**87**(11):351-352

[2] Caprioli J, Kim JH, Friedman DS, Kiang T, Moster MR, Parrish RK, Rorer EM, Samuelson T, Tarver ME, Singh K, Eydelman MB. Special commentary: Supporting innovation for safe and effective minimally invasive glaucoma surgery. Ophthalmology. 2015; **122**(9):1795-1801

[3] Saheb H, Ahmed II. Micro-invasive glaucoma surgery: Current perspectives and future directions. Current Opinion in Ophthalmology. 2012;**23**(2):96-104

[4] Malvankar-Mehta MS, Iordanous Y, Chen YN, Wang WW, Patel SS, Costella J, Hutnik CM. iStent with phacoemulsification versus phacoemulsification alone for patients with glaucoma and cataract: A meta-analysis. PLoS One. 2015;**10**(7):e0131770

[5] Bull H, von Wolff K, Körber N, Tetz M. Three-year canaloplasty outcomes for the treatment of open-angle glaucoma: European study results. Graefe's Archive for Clinical and Experimental Ophthalmology. 2011;**249**(10):1537-1545

[6] Tetz M, Koerber N, Shingleton BJ, von Wolff K, Bull H, Samuelson TW, Lewis RA. Phacoemulsification and intraocular lens implantation before, during, or after canaloplasty in eyes with open-angle glaucoma: 3-year results. Journal of Glaucoma. 2015;**24**(3):187-194

[7] Nguyen Q. Combined Cataract Surgery and MIGS: Which Procedures will Be a Match Made in Heaven? March/April: Glaucoma Today; 2013

[8] Fea AM. Phacoemulsification versus phacoemulsification with micro-bypass stent implantation in primary open-angle glaucoma: Randomized double-masked clinical trial. Journal of Cataract & Refractive Surgery. 2010;**36**(3):407-412

[9] Vold S, Ahmed II, Craven ER, Mattox C, Stamper R, Packer M, Brown RH, Ianchulev T, CyPass Study Group. Two-year COMPASS trial results: Supraciliary microstenting with phacoemulsification in patients with open-angle glaucoma and cataracts. Ophthalmology. 2016;**123**(10):2103-2112

[10] García-Feijoo J, Rau M, Grisanti S, Grisanti S, Höh H, Erb C, Guguchkova P, Ahmed I, Grabner G, Reitsamer H, Shaarawy T. Supraciliary micro-stent implantation for open-angle glaucoma failing topical therapy: 1-year results of a multicenter study. American Journal of Ophthalmology. 2015;**159**(6):1075-1081

[11] Hoeh H, Vold SD, Ahmed IK, Anton A, Rau M, Singh K, Chang DF, Shingleton BJ, Ianchulev T. Initial clinical experience with the CyPass micro-stent: Safety and surgical outcomes of a novel supraciliary microstent. Journal of Glaucoma. 2016;**25**(1):106-112

[12] Francis BA, Berke SJ, Dustin L, Noecker R. Endoscopic cyclophotocoagulation combined with phacoemulsification versus phacoemulsification alone in medically controlled glaucoma. Journal of Cataract & Refractive Surgery. 2014;**40**(8):1313-1321

[13] Siegel MJ, Boling WS, Faridi OS, Gupta CK, Kim C, Boling RC, Citron ME, Siegel MJ, Siegel LI. Combined endoscopic cyclophotocoagulation and phacoemulsification versus phacoemulsification alone in the treatment of mild to moderate glaucoma. Clinical & Experimental Ophthalmology. 2015;**43**(6):531-539

[14] Nyska A, Glovinsky Y, Belkin M, Epstein Y. Biocompatibility of the ex-PRESS miniature glaucoma drainage implant. Journal of Glaucoma. 2003;**12**(3):275-280

[15] Dahan E, Carmichael TR. Implantation of a miniature glaucoma device under a scleral flap. Journal of Glaucoma. 2005;**14**(2):98-102

[16] Condon GP, Moster MR. Minimizing the invasiveness of traditional trabeculectomy surgery. Journal of Cataract & Refractive Surgery. 2014;**40**(8):1307-1312

[17] Traverso CE, De Feo F, Messas-Kaplan A, Denis P, Levartovsky S, Sellem E, Badalà F, Zagorski Z, Bron A, Belkin M. Long term effect on IOP of a stainless steel glaucoma drainage implant (Ex-PRESS) in combined surgery with phacoemulsification. British Journal of Ophthalmology. 2005;**89**(4):425-429

[18] Stewart RM, Diamond JG, Ashmore ED, Ayyala RS. Complications following Ex-PRESS glaucoma shunt implantation. American Journal of Ophthalmology. 2005;**140**(2):340-3e1

[19] Tavolato M, Babighian S, Galan A. Spontaneous extrusion of a stainless steel glaucoma drainage implant (Ex-PRESS). European Journal of Ophthalmology. 2006;**16**(5):753-755

[20] Dahan E. Subconjunctival insertion of Ex-PRESS R-50 miniature glaucoma implant. Journal of Cataract & Refractive Surgery. 2008;**34**(5):716

[21] Garg SJ, Kanitkar K, Weichel E, Fischer D. Trauma-induced extrusion of an Ex-PRESS glaucoma shunt presenting as an intraocular foreign body. Archives of Ophthalmology. 2005;**123**(9):1270-1272

[22] Lan J, Sun DP, Wu J, Wang YN, Xie LX. Ex-PRESS implantation with phacoemulsification in POAG versus CPACG. International Journal of Ophthalmology. 2017;**10**(1):51

[23] Huerva V, Soldevila J, Ascaso FJ, Lavilla L, Muniesa MJ, Sánchez MC. Evaluation of the Ex-PRESS® P-50 implant under scleral flap in combined cataract and glaucoma surgery. International Journal of Ophthalmology. 2016;**9**(4):546

[24] Zetterström C, Behndig A, Kugelberg M, Montan P, Lundström M. Changes in intraocular pressure after cataract surgery: Analysis of the Swedish National Cataract Register Data. Journal of Cataract & Refractive Surgery. 2015;**41**(8):1725-1729

[25] Mathalone N, Hyams M, Neiman S, Buckman G, Hod Y, Geyer O. Long-term intraocular pressure control after clear corneal phacoemulsification in glaucoma patients. Journal of Cataract & Refractive Surgery. 2005;**31**(3):479-483

[26] Heijl A, Leske MC, Bengtsson B, Hyman L, Bengtsson B, Hussein M. Reduction of intraocular pressure and glaucoma progression. Archives of Ophthalmology. 2002; **120**(10):1268-1279

[27] Prata TS, Ushida M, Dorairaj S. Cataract surgery alone cannot be considered an IOP-lowering procedure for open-angle glaucoma patients: An evidence-based perspective. Arquivos Brasileiros de Oftalmologia. 2015;**78**(5):V-I

[28] Issa SA, Pacheco J, Mahmood U, Nolan J, Beatty S. A novel index for predicting intraocular pressure reduction following cataract surgery. British Journal of Ophthalmology. 2005;**89**(5):543-546

[29] Yang HS, Lee J, Choi S. Ocular biometric parameters associated with intraocular pressure reduction after cataract surgery in normal eyes. American Journal of Ophthalmology. 2013;**156**(1):89-94

[30] Huang G, Gonzalez E, Lee R, Chen YC, He M, Lin SC. Association of biometric factors with anterior chamber angle widening and intraocular pressure reduction after uneventful phacoemulsification for cataract. Journal of Cataract & Refractive Surgery. 2012;**38**(1):108-116

[31] Elgin U, Şen E, Şimşek T, Tekin K, Yılmazbaş P. Early postoperative effects of cataract surgery on anterior segment parameters in primary open-angle glaucoma and pseudoexfoliation glaucoma. Turkish Journal of Ophthalmology. 2016;**46**(3):95

[32] Shingleton BJ, Pasternack JJ, Hung JW, O'donoghue MW. Three and five year changes in intraocular pressures after clear corneal phacoemulsification in open angle glaucoma patients, glaucoma suspects, and normal patients. Journal of Glaucoma. 2006; **15**(6):494-498

[33] Slabaugh MA, Bojikian KD, Moore DB, Chen PP. The effect of phacoemulsification on intraocular pressure in medically controlled open-angle glaucoma patients. American Journal of Ophthalmology. 2014;**157**(1):26-31

[34] Chen PP, Lin SC, Junk AK, Radhakrishnan S, Singh K, Chen TC. The effect of phacoemulsification on intraocular pressure in glaucoma patients: A report by the American Academy of Ophthalmology. Ophthalmology. 2015;**122**(7):1294-1307

[35] Tham YC, Li X, Wong TY, Quigley HA, Aung T, Cheng CY. Global prevalence of glaucoma and projections of glaucoma burden through 2040: A systematic review and meta-analysis. Ophthalmology. 2014;**121**(11):2081-2090

[36] Sihota R, Lakshmaiah NC, Walia KB, Sharma S, Pailoor J, Agarwal HC. The trabecular meshwork in acute and chronic angle closure glaucoma. Indian Journal of Ophthalmology. 2001;**49**(4):255

[37] Nonaka A, Kondo T, Kikuchi M, Yamashiro K, Fujihara M, Iwawaki T, Yamamoto K, Kurimoto Y. Cataract surgery for residual angle closure after peripheral laser iridotomy. Ophthalmology. 2005;**112**(6):974-979

[38] Özyol P, Özyol E, Sül S, Baldemir E, Çavdar S. Intra-ocular pressure fluctuation after cataract surgery in primary angle-closure glaucoma eyes medically controlled after laser iridotomy. Acta Ophthalmologica. 2016 Nov;**94**(7):e528-e533

[39] Gunning FP, Greve EL. Lens extraction for uncontrolled angle-closure glaucoma: Long-term follow-up. Journal of Cataract & Refractive Surgery. 1998;**24**(10):1347-1356

[40] Azuara-Blanco A, Burr J, Ramsay C, Cooper D, Foster PJ, Friedman DS, Scotland G, Javanbakht M, Cochrane C, Norrie J. EAGLE study group. Effectiveness of early lens extraction for the treatment of primary angle-closure glaucoma (EAGLE): A randomised controlled trial. The Lancet. 2016;**388**(10052):1389-1397

[41] Tham CC, Kwong YY, Leung DY, Lam SW, Li FC, Chiu TY, Chan JC, Chan CH, Poon AS, Yick DW, Chi CC. Phacoemulsification versus combined phacotrabeculectomy in medically controlled chronic angle closure glaucoma with cataract. Ophthalmology. 2008;**115**(12):2167-2173

[42] Tham CC, Kwong YY, Baig N, Leung DY, Li FC, Lam DS. Phacoemulsification versus trabeculectomy in medically uncontrolled chronic angle-closure glaucoma without cataract. Ophthalmology. 2013;**120**(1):62-67

[43] Collaborative Normal Tension Glaucoma Study Group. Comparison of glaucomatous progression between untreated patients with normal-tension glaucoma and patients with therapeutically reduced intraocular pressures. American Journal of Ophthalmology. 1998;**126**(4):487-497

[44] Klink J, Schmitz B, Lieb WE, Klink T, Grein HJ, Sold-Darseff J, Heinold A, Grehn F. Filtering bleb function after clear cornea phacoemulsification: A prospective study. British Journal of Ophthalmology. 2005;**89**(5):597-601

[45] Awai-Kasaoka N, Inoue T, Takihara Y, Kawaguchi A, Inatani M, Ogata-Iwao M, Tanihara H. Impact of phacoemulsification on failure of trabeculectomy with mitomycin-C. Journal of Cataract & Refractive Surgery. 2012;**38**(3):419-424

[46] Jin GJ, Crandall AS, Jones JJ. Phacotrabeculectomy: Assessment of outcomes and surgical improvements. Journal of Cataract & Refractive Surgery. 2007;**33**(7):1201-1208

[47] Chen DZ, Koh V, Sng C, Aquino MC, Chew P. Complications and outcomes of primary phacotrabeculectomy with mitomycin C in a multi-ethnic asian population. PLoS One. 2015;**10**(3):e0118852

[48] Ong C, Nongpiur M, Peter L, Perera SA. Combined approach to phacoemulsification and trabeculectomy results in less ideal refractive outcomes compared with the sequential approach. Journal of Glaucoma. 2016;**25**(10):e873-e878

[49] Woodcock MG, Richards JC, Murray AD. The last 11 years of Molteno implantation at the University of Cape Town. Refining our indications and surgical technique. Eye. 2008;**22**(1):18-25

[50] Chung AN, Aung T, Wang JC, Chew PT. Surgical outcomes of combined phacoemulsification and glaucoma drainage implant surgery for Asian patients with refractory glaucoma with cataract. American Journal of Ophthalmology. 2004;**137**(2):294-300

[51] Valenzuela F, Browne A, Srur M, Nieme C, Zanolli M, López-Solís R, Traipe L. Combined phacoemulsification and Ahmed glaucoma drainage implant surgery for patients with refractory glaucoma and cataract. Journal of Glaucoma. 2016;**25**(2):162-166

[52] Schoenberg ED, Chaudhry AL, Chod R, Zurakowski D, Ayyala RS. Comparison of surgical outcomes between phacocanaloplasty and phacotrabeculectomy at 12 months' follow-up: A longitudinal cohort study. Journal of Glaucoma. 2015;**24**(7):543-549

[53] Funnell CL, Clowes M, Anand N. Combined cataract and glaucoma surgery with mitomycin C: Phacoemulsification-trabeculectomy compared to phacoemulsification-deep sclerectomy. British Journal of Ophthalmology. 2005;**89**(6):694-698

[54] Vinod K, Gedde SJ, Feuer WJ, Panarelli JF, Chang TC, Chen PP, Parrish RK. Practice preferences for glaucoma surgery: A survey of the American Glaucoma Society. Journal of Glaucoma. 2017;**26**(8):687-693

[55] Pascolini D, Mariotti SP. Global estimates of visual impairment: 2010. British Journal of Ophthalmology. 2012;**96**(5):614-618

[56] Budenz DL, Gedde SJ. New options for combined cataract and glaucoma surgery. Current Opinion in Ophthalmology. 2014;**25**(2):141-147

[57] Quigley HA, Broman AT. The number of people with glaucoma worldwide in 2010 and 2020. British Journal of Ophthalmology. 2006;**90**(3):262-267

[58] Asbell PA, Dualan I, Mindel J, Brocks D, Ahmad M, Epstein S. Age-related cataract. The Lancet. 2005;**365**(9459):599-609

[59] Guan H, Mick A, Porco T, Dolan BJ. Preoperative factors associated with IOP reduction after cataract surgery. Optometry and Vision Science. 2013;**90**(2):179-184

[60] Marchini G, Ceruti P, Vizzari G. Berzaghi D, Zampieri A. Management of concomitant cataract and glaucoma. Dev Ophthalmol. 2017;**59**:155-164

[61] Liaska A, Papaconstantinou D, Georgalas I, Koutsandrea C, Theodosiadis P, Chatziste-fanou K. Phaco-trabeculectomy in controlled, advanced, open-angle glaucoma and cataract: Parallel, randomized clinical study of efficacy and safety. Seminars in Ophthalmology. 2014;**29**(4):226-235

[62] Hou JH, Crispim J, Cortina MS, De La Cruz J. Image-guided femtosecond laser–assisted cataract surgery in Peters anomaly type 2. Journal of Cataract & Refractive Surgery. 2015;**41**(11):2353-2357

[63] Chan E, Mahroo OA, Spalton DJ. Complications of cataract surgery. Clinical & Experimental Optometry. 2010;**93**(6):379-389

[64] Nagy ZZ. New technology update: Femtosecond laser in cataract surgery. Clinical ophthalmology (Auckland, NZ). 2014;**8**:1157

[65] Conrad-Hengerer I, Al Juburi M, Schultz T, Hengerer FH, Dick HB. Corneal endothelial cell loss and corneal thickness in conventional compared with femtosecond laser–assisted cataract surgery: Three-month follow-up. Journal of Cataract & Refractive Surgery. 2013;**39**(9):1307-1313

[66] Mastropasqua L, Toto L, Mastropasqua A, Vecchiarino L, Mastropasqua R, Pedrotti E, Di Nicola M. Femtosecond laser versus manual clear corneal incision in cataract surgery. Journal of Refractive Surgery. 2014;**30**(1):27-33

[67] Kerr NM, Abell RG, Vote BJ, Toh TY. Intraocular pressure during femtosecond laser pretreatment of cataract. Journal of Cataract & Refractive Surgery. 2013;**39**(3):339-342

[68] Schultz T, Conrad-Hengerer I, Hengerer FH, Dick HB. Intraocular pressure variation during femtosecond laser-assisted cataract surgery using a fluid-filled interface. Journal of Cataract & Refractive Surgery. 2013;**39**(1):22-27

[69] Darian-Smith E, Howie AR, Abell RG, Kerr N, Allen PL, Vote BJ, Toh TY. Intraocular pressure during femtosecond laser pretreatment: Comparison of glaucomatous eyes and nonglaucomatous eyes. Journal of Cataract & Refractive Surgery. 2015;**41**(2):272-277

[70] Leske MC, Nemesure B, He Q, Wu SY, Hejtmancik JF, Hennis A. Barbados Family Study Group. Patterns of open-angle glaucoma in the Barbados Family Study. Ophthalmology. 2001;**108**(6):1015-1022

[71] Williams AL, Gatla S, Leiby BE, Fahmy I, Biswas A, De Barros DM, Ramakrishnan R, Bhardwaj S, Wright C, Dubey S, Lynch JF. The value of intraocular pressure asymmetry in diagnosing glaucoma. Journal of Glaucoma. 2013;**22**(3):215-218

[72] Ritch R, Prata TS, De Moraes CG, Vessani RM, Costa VP, Konstas AG, Liebmann JM, Schlötzer-Schrehardt U. Association of exfoliation syndrome and central retinal vein occlusion: An ultrastructural analysis. Acta Ophthalmologica. 2010;**88**(1):91-95

[73] Siddiqui Y, Ten Hulzen RD, Cameron JD, Hodge DO, Johnson DH. What is the risk of developing pigmentary glaucoma from pigment dispersion syndrome? American Journal of Ophthalmology. 2003;**135**(6):794-799

[74] Jabbur NS, Tuli S, Barequet IS, O'Brien TP. Outcomes of laser in situ keratomileusis in patients with pigment dispersion syndrome. Journal of Cataract & Refractive Surgery. 2004;**30**(1):110-114

[75] Paciuc M, Velasco CF, Naranjo R. Acute angle-closure glaucoma after hyperopic laser in situ keratomileusis. Journal of Cataract & Refractive Surgery. 2000;**26**(4):620-623

[76] Jimenez-Roman J, Lazcano-Gomez G, Martínez-Baez K, Turati M, Gulías-Cañizo R, Hernández-Zimbrón LF, Ochoa-De la Paz L, Zamora R, Gonzalez-Salinas R. Effect of phacoemulsification on intraocular pressure in patients with primary open angle glaucoma and pseudoexfoliation glaucoma. International Journal of Ophthalmology. 2017;**10**(9):1374

[77] Ichhpujani P, Bhartiya S, Sharma A. Premium IOLs in glaucoma. Journal of Current Glaucoma Practice. 2013;**7**(2):54

[78] Inoue M, Bissen-Miyajima H, Yoshino M, Suzuki T. Wavy horizontal artifacts on optical coherence tomography line-scanning images caused by diffractive multifocal intraocular lenses. Journal of Cataract & Refractive Surgery. 2009;**35**(7):1239-1243

[79] Farid M, Chak G, Garg S, Steinert RF. Reduction in mean deviation values in automated perimetry in eyes with multifocal compared to monofocal intraocular lens implants. American Journal of Ophthalmology. 2014;**158**(2):227-231

[80] Centers for Disease Control and Prevention. U.S. Outpatient Surgeries on the Rise [internet]. Available at: www.cdc.gov/media/pressrel/2009/r090128.htm. [Accessed January 15, 2014]

[81] Cullen KA, Hall MJ, Golosinskiy A. Ambulatory Surgery in the United States, 2006. US Department of Health and Human Services, Centers for Disease Control and Prevention, National Center for Health Statistics; 2009

[82] Tseng VL, Yu F, Lum F, Coleman AL. Risk of fractures following cataract surgery in Medicare beneficiaries. Journal of the American Medical Association. 2012;**308**(5):493-501

[83] Lochhead J, Casson RJ, Salmon JF. Long term effect on intraocular pressure of phacotrabeculectomy compared to trabeculectomy. British Journal of Ophthalmology. 2003; **87**(7):850-852

[84] Ogata-Iwao M, Inatani M, Takihara Y, Inoue T, Iwao K, Tanihara H. A prospective comparison between trabeculectomy with mitomycin C and phacotrabeculectomy with mitomycin C. Acta Ophthalmol. 2013 Sep;**91**(6):e500-e501

8

Presbyopia Correction During Cataract Surgery with Multifocal Intraocular Lenses

Iva Dekaris, Nikica Gabrić, Ante Barišić and
Adis Pašalić

Abstract

Introduction: The first generations of multifocal intraocular lenses (MFIOLs) were designed to provide patients good distance and near vision, but intermediate was not satisfactory. Trifocal, a bifocal of low-add and quadrifocal MFIOLs were invented, offering possibility to correct vision for distance, near, and intermediate tasks. The novel IOL, extended range of vision (EROV), is covering mostly intermediate and distance vision, with lower level of photic phenomena.

Patients and methods: We have evaluated visual results in 4408 eyes implanted with different MFIOLs in 12 years period (2004–2016). Postoperative uncorrected visual acuity for far, intermediate, and near was evaluated. Postoperative satisfaction and complication rate and management of complications are presented.

Results: In the first generation MFIOLs, almost 70% of eyes gained uncorrected distance visual acuity of 1.0. Uncorrected near visual acuity was J1–J2 in 95% of eyes with diffractive IOLs. Modern MFIOL designs enabled improvement of vision at intermediate distance, without compromising vision at far and near.

Conclusion: With the first generations of MFIOLs, good distance and near uncorrected vision was achieved. With novel MFIOLs a very good uncorrected vision was achieved at far, intermediate and near, while with EROV lens, near vision was less satisfactory, but patients had less photic phenomena.

Keywords: multifocal, presbyopia, cataract surgery, refractive lens exchange, bifocal diffractive lens, intraocular lenses, refractive lens, trifocal lens, quadrifocal lens, extended range of vision lens

1. Introduction

The main cause for cataract or opacification of the lens is age, although it can also be a congenital disease or a consequence of ocular and systemic diseases (uveitis and diabetes), systemic medication (steroids), trauma, and inherited abnormalities (Marfan syndrome, Lowe syndrome). According to WHO data, it accounts for 48% of world blindness, and surgical removal of cataract is the only available treatment for a patient with developed cataract. The prevalence of cataract surgery increases with age, from 16% in the 65–69 age group up to 71% in more than 85 years age group [1]. Removal of cataract by phacoemulsification of the lens, followed by intraocular lens implantation, is in fact one of the most common surgical procedures. According to estimates, 20 million cataract surgeries are performed annually worldwide, but despite this impressive statistic, the number of patients visually handicapped by cataract still globally increases every year. Modern cataract surgery had tremendous development during the past 10–15 years. Improved surgical technique and modern materials have enlarged indication profile for cataract surgery. This also created higher postoperative expectations from patients. Although it is often expected that patient will not need spectacle correction after cataract surgery (at least for far vision), more than 50% of operated eyes need spectacles after surgery to achieve optimal vision. This is due to the fact that with the standard monofocal intraocular lenses (IOL), first of which had been implanted in 1950 by Sir Harold Ridley, only a spherical component of the refractive error can be corrected, without taking care of the astigmatism. In order to determine accurate IOL power for each patient's eye, it is essential to determine keratometric values and axial length readings. Based on such readings, a calculation of the spherical power of the monofocal IOL is made with specially designed formulas adapted for each refractive error. Monofocal IOLs are readily available in different optical powers in every operating theater and thus can be implanted during a standard cataract case, correcting patient's spherical error and providing good distance vision. However, full visual recovery in patients with corneal astigmatism and presbyopia will be limited by the fact that both corneal astigmatism and presbyopia were not corrected with the implantation of standard monofocal lens. Every patient with such IOL will lose its ability to focus near objects and will need spectacle correction of approximately +2.5 diopters for near vision. With the increasing patient's expectations regarding their vision after the surgery, newer generations of intraocular lenses had to be provided.

First, IOLs successfully dealing with presbyopia, named multifocal lenses (MFIOLs) or "premium lenses," were launched on the market in the early 1980s and were represented with diffractive and refractive design [2]. They were the first step toward full vision correction after cataract surgery. Bifocal diffractive IOL with +4.00D near addition is designed along the principles of diffractive optics and was available in a silicone or hydrophobic acrylic model. This lens consists of a three-piece or single-piece, square-edged 6.0 mm optic with a prolate anterior surface producing −0.27 spherical aberration. The posterior surface of the optic features a diffractive zone. The near addition is +4.00D translating to +3.00D at the spectacle plane. In the theory, the optical design redistributes incident light, 50% for near and 50% distance, independent of pupil size. Bifocal diffractive IOL with +3.00D near addition is aspheric one-piece hydrophobic IOL with central apodized diffractive structure and peripheral refractive zone. The near addition of +3.00D refers to +2.4D at spectacle plane. These lenses, due to their diffractive design, were able to provide patients with good near vision even without the use of spectacles, thus correcting presbyopia [3]. Refractive IOLs available at that time were multizonal IOLs with different areas for distant and near vision. They are a three-piece refractive acrylic lens with five concentric zones. Three zones, including the central one, are for far vision, and two zones are for near vision. An aspheric transition provides a balanced intermediate vision. The near add-power is +3.50D, translating to +2.50D at the spectacle plane. A unique edge design provides a 360° barrier aimed to offset the incidence of posterior capsular opacification (PCO) and minimizes edge glare. They gave good distant and intermediate visual acuity but poorer near vision with a significant problem with halos in night driving.

Disadvantages of MFIOLs caused by lens design were halo and glare (especially at night) in some patients, loss of contrast sensitivity, and the fact that patients needed some time for their brain to adapt to MFIOLs [4]. Moreover, the first multifocal IOLs were unable to correct vision at intermediate distance, which is mostly important for younger presbyopes who often use computers or other tasks at the distance of 60 cm to 1 m. Later on, newer, modern designs of MFIOLs were invented, trifocal, bifocal, and "low-add" lenses with different add-powers, extended range of vision, and quadrifocal IOLs, successfully correcting vision for all visual needs at distance, intermediate, and near [5–7]. Trifocal IOL is an aspheric, diffractive intraocular lens. The optical zone of trifocal lens had +3.33D near addition and a +1.66D intermediate addition (although different add-powers are also available). It has asymmetrical light distribution of 50, 20, and 30% for far, intermediate, and near foci, respectively. The IOL is fabricated from a hydrophilic acrylic material with a 25% water content and hydrophobic surface. This is a single-piece IOL with 6.0 mm optic diameter. Central 4.34 mm zone includes trifocal optic, and peripheral 1.66 mm zone has bifocal optic. It has a four-haptic design with an angulation of 0° and a 360° square edge to prevent posterior capsule opacification. Quadrifocal IOL is a non-apodized diffractive trifocal IOL with an intermediary 4.5 mm diffractive zone that distributes light to three focal points independent on pupil size. The IOL is a single-piece lens fabricated from a hydrophobic and ultraviolet- and blue light-filtering acrylate/methacrylate copolymer material. This novel diffractive structure has optimized light utilization, transmitting 88% of light at the simulated 3.0 mm pupil size to the retina. The light is split into two, with one half allocated to the distance focus and the other half split evenly between the near and intermediate focuses. The lens design is intended to improve the intermediate vision tasks and increase patient satisfaction, with a third focal point at an optimal intermediate distance of 60 cm, tending to provide more continuous vision. Bifocal diffractive "low-add" IOLs are provided with different add-powers (e.g., +2.75D, +3.25D, +4.00D add), and they have a full diffractive profile on the posterior surface of the optic. The relief height of the diffractive rings is equal in all three models; they have equal light distribution to distance and near regardless of pupil size or add-power. The focal point distance is controlled by the number and spacing of the diffractive rings, and patients have same contrast sensitivity and low-light visual acuity for all add-powers. Extended range of vision IOL delivers a continuous, full-range vision with reduced incidence of halos and glare. It merges two complementary technologies: echelette design which introduces a novel pattern of light diffraction that elongates the focus of the eye, resulting in an extended range of vision, and achromatic technology for the correction of longitudinal chromatic aberration which causes contrast enhancement. It is a diffractive, single-piece, aspheric IOL.

Although MFIOLs were able to fully correct vision in high percentage of patients, especially when modern lens designs are used, they were not applicable in eyes with the astigmatism, since such eyes have an individual need for correction of cylindrical power and axis which is different in each eye. In general population, 35% of eyes have the astigmatism of ≥1.25 diopter (D), 61% having with the rule astigmatism, 25% against the rule astigmatism, and 14% oblique astigmatism. Both the cataract itself and the astigmatism reduce patient's vision and thus the quality of life. The anterior corneal surface shifts from with-the-rule to against-the-rule astigmatism with aging, whereas posterior corneal astigmatism remains as against the rule in most cases. Total corneal astigmatism is calculated from anterior and posterior corneal curvature measurements [8]. The quantity and axis of the astigmatic refractive error are different in each patient's eye and can be corrected by spectacles with cylindrical power. If the eye scheduled for cataract surgery has a significant astigmatism, postoperative vision will be impaired by this refractive error, and patient will need spectacles to obtain adequate distance and near vision. For patients with significant astigmatism, solution was found with the invention of toric IOLs, which were designed for two functions: to restore visual acuity deteriorated by cataract and to correct corneal astigmatism [9–13]. Toric IOLs must be produced individually since each eye with the corneal astigmatism has a unique combination of spherical and astigmatic correction (regarding both the amount and the axis of astigmatism). Moreover, in a proper calculation of toric intraocular lens power, one should evaluate total corneal astigmatism as a better predictor than keratometric astigmatism [8, 14]. Since the prevalence of against-the-rule astigmatism significantly increases with age, such astigmatism should be treated more aggressively during cataract surgery [15]. The most recent advancement in IOL technology is a combination of multifocal and toric design, resulting in multifocal toric design of the lens which provides a complete visual recovery for patients with astigmatism and presbyopia [9, 16, 17].

Based on the positive visual outcome with the implantation of newer generation of lenses in a cataract surgery, modern IOLs have become treatment of choice for many patients with presbyopia and astigmatism even when their natural lens is still clear and has no cataract [18–20]. Namely, refractive errors such as hyperopia and myopia combined with presbyopia, and also plano-presbyopia, cannot be fully treated with refractive surgery on the cornea. Laser corneal ablation is highly effective in correction of refractive errors and may be the best option for younger population [21]. However, for patients aged 45 or more, only distance vision can be corrected by laser ablation, but the problem of presbyopia remains. With the surgery on the lens, called refractive lens exchange, and implantation of MFIOL full vision can be restored: distance, intermediate, and near vision. If MF toric IOL design is used, also the preexisting astigmatism can be fully corrected [9, 16, 17].

In this chapter, we have analyzed postoperative visual results in our patients operated for cataract and refractive lens exchange with implantation of different types of MFIOLs, used in our setting throughout the last 12 years.

2. Patients and methods

A total of 4408 eyes were implanted with different presbyopia-correcting intraocular lenses in our hospital throughout a period of 12 years (2004–2016). Exclusion criteria for MFIOL implantation were corneal disease, retinal or optic nerve disease, or sever dry eye syndrome. Preoperative assessment included precise biometry and IOL calculation (IOL Master 500, Zeiss, Germany), corneal topography (Pentacam, Oculus, USA), aberrometry (Wavefront Aberrometer, USA), pupillometry, endothelial cell analysis (Noncontact Specular Microscope, Topcon, USA), optical coherence tomography (OCT, Zeiss, Germany), ultrasound, and careful examination of the retinal status. Patient's selection and preoperative counseling were made by experienced cataract surgeons.

The first group of eyes included 2546 eyes implanted with bifocal diffractive MFIOLs (ReSTOR 4+, ReSTOR 3+, Tecnis, Acrylisa) and refractive design (ReZoom) MFIOLs, with a follow-up of 5 years. Most of the patients were implanted with same lens design in both eyes, while in 440 eyes, a technique so-called "mix and match" was used to enhance intermediate vision. In "mix and match" approach, a refractive IOL (ReZoom) was implanted in dominant eye and diffractive IOL (Tecnis or ReSTOR) in non-dominant eye. The second group of eyes included 1862 eyes implanted with MFIOLs of the following designs: (a) trifocal (Zeiss AT LISA tri), (b) quadrifocal (AcrySof IQ PanOptix), (c) combination of "low-add" bifocals with different add-powers (Tecnis ZKBOO +2.75D in dominant and Tecnis ZLBOO +3.25D add in non-dominant eye), and (d) extended range of vision (Symfony ZXR00) (see **Table 1**). Follow-up was at least 6 months (range 6–144 months). All eyes were operated under topical anesthesia, as a conventional phacoemulsification procedure on two phaco machines (Whitestar Signature, Abbott Medical Optics and Infinity Vision System, Alcon, USA). Special attention was made during the following surgical steps: small incision preferably on the steep axis, continuous curvilinear manual capsulorhexis with 5 mm diameter, careful polishing of the posterior and anterior capsule, and viscoelastic removal behind the IOL. Same MFIOL was implanted in both eyes simultaneously, except in case of "low-add" lenses where "low-add" with addition of +2.75 was implanted in dominant and "low-add" of +3.25 add in a non-dominant eye. Postoperative uncorrected visual acuity (UCVA) for far, intermediate, and near vision was evaluated for different types of MFIOL. For MF toric IOL implantation, the axis of astigmatism was marked on a patient's eye during preoperative preparation, in a seated position on a slit lamp, and toric IOL was aligned with this mark during the surgery. The amount of corrected astigmatism was evaluated. Postoperative satisfaction rate, complication rate, and management of complications are presented for all MFIOLs.

Type of multifocal IOL	Number of eyes
Diffractive +4.00 bifocal	1160
Diffractive +3.00 bifocal	826
Refractive	560
Trifocal	649
Low-add	550
Extended range of vision	663
Quadrifocal	30

Table 1. Number of eyes implanted with different types of multifocal intraocular lenses throughout a 12-year period.

3. Results

The number of eyes implanted with different types of multifocal intraocular lenses throughout a 12-year period in our hospital is represented in **Table 1**. In the first 5 years of MFIOL use, mainly lenses of diffractive bifocal and refractive design were implanted, while later on newer generations of MFIOL like trifocal, "low-add" combination, extended range of vision, and quadrifocal lenses were used.

Visual outcome after implantation of first-generation MFIOLs of diffractive and refractive design is represented in **Figure 1**. Close to 70% of eyes gained uncorrected distance visual acuity (UDVA) of 1.0, while <10% of eyes had UDVA of less than 0.8. Uncorrected near visual acuity (UNVA) was J1–J2 in 95% of eyes with diffractive IOLs and in 84% of eyes with refractive lens design. Overall, close to 90% of eyes was spectacle independent. "Mix and match" technique did not change visual outcome for distance vision and had slightly negative impact on near vision; however, it did increase percentage of spectacle-free time since it improved intermediate vision.

With the first generation of lenses, the optical design could not provide good vision at intermediate distance. Therefore, we have started to implant the first lenses designed to improve intermediate vision—lenses of trifocal design and compared the outcome of these lenses with bifocal ones (**Figure 2**). With trifocal design very good UDVA and UNVA were preserved, and there was a significant improvement in uncorrected intermediate vision (UIVA), with mean visual acuity of 0.8 for intermediate tasks. With even newer design of trifocal lens—so-called quadrifocal IOL—more continuous vision at intermediate distance was obtained due to superior visual outcome at 60 cm (arm length). Novel technology of extended range of vision (EROV) lenses became available, and a combination of two different add-on powers in "low-add" bifocal lenses aimed to improve intermediate vision of our patients. Visual outcome of UDVA, UIVA, and UNVA in patients implanted with four modern lens designs compared to older lens designs are represented in **Figure 3**. As shown, modern MFIOL designs enabled a significant improvement of vision at distance of 60–100 cm (intermediate) as compared to diffractive and refractive MFIOLs, without compromising very good visual results at far and near. Satisfaction rate after MFIOL implantation according to preoperative refractive error is presented in **Table 2**. In patients with the astigmatism of >1D, multifocal toric lenses were implanted to correct the astigmatic part of the refractive error. The axis of toric MFIOL implantation was always marked in a sitting position, to avoid misplacement of the lens due to cyclotorsion while the patient is lying down. After toric MFIOL implantation, the mean preoperative astigmatism of 2.25 D was reduced to a mean of 0.32 D (**Figure 4**). The appearance of a bilaterally implanted trifocal toric IOLs, in a primary position (left) and with a dilated pupil (right), correcting patient's vision in both eyes to 100% distance, intermediate, and near vision without any spectacles, is shown in **Figure 5**.

Complications related to MFIOL design like halo and glare were determined among our patients: 15% of patients with refractive lenses reported halos and glare during night driving. Due to

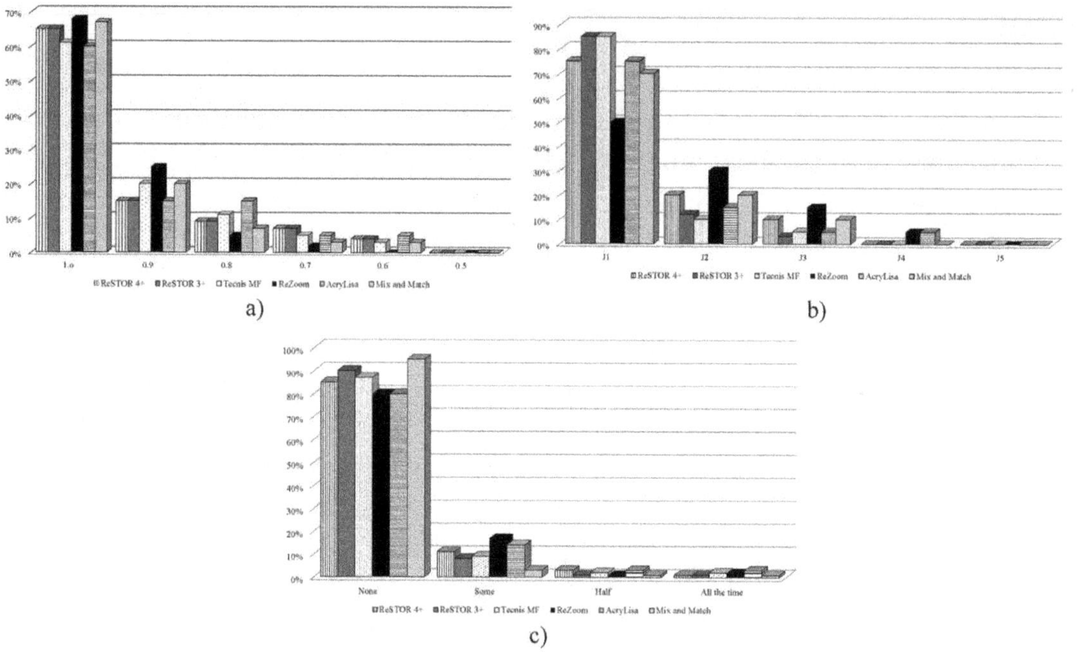

Figure 1. Percentage of eyes achieving (a) uncorrected distance visual acuity of >0.5, (b) uncorrected near visual acuity of >J5, and (c) a portion of time wearing glasses in eyes implanted with different types of multifocal intraocular lenses, in a 5-year follow-up.

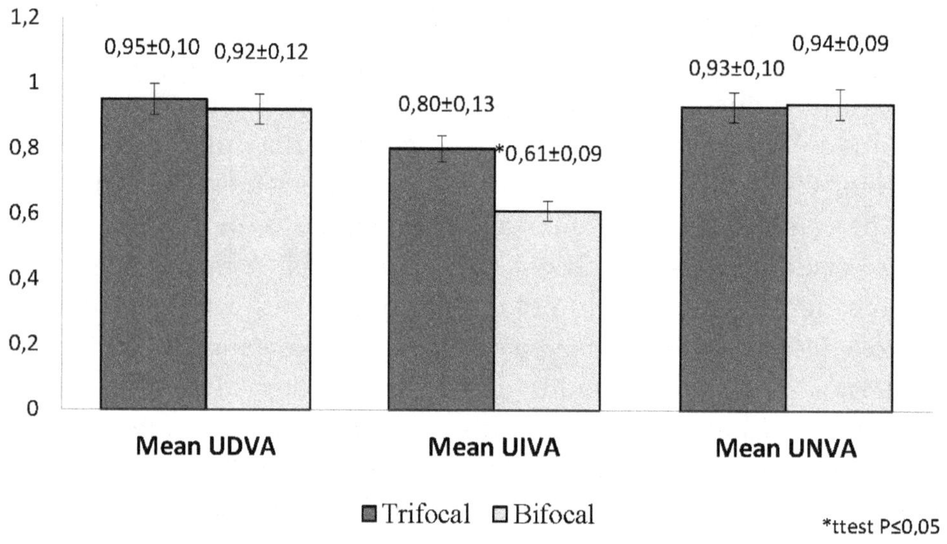

Figure 2. Comparison of mean uncorrected distance visual acuity (UDVA), uncorrected intermediate visual acuity (UIVA), and uncorrected near visual acuity (UNVA) between eyes implanted with trifocal and bifocal multifocal intraocular lenses (expressed in decimal values).

severe halo and glare, we had to explant 12 out of 560 (2.1%) refractive IOLs and replace them with bifocal diffractive IOLs. In modern lens designs, the percentage of halo and glare ranged from 4 to 9%, being lowest in EROV IOL (**Table 3**). Postoperative residual refractive errors were solved with laser refractive surgery. Laser surgery was needed in 6.1% of patients with diffractive bifocal IOLs, while in another groups, enhancement rate was between 1 and 3% (**Table 3**).

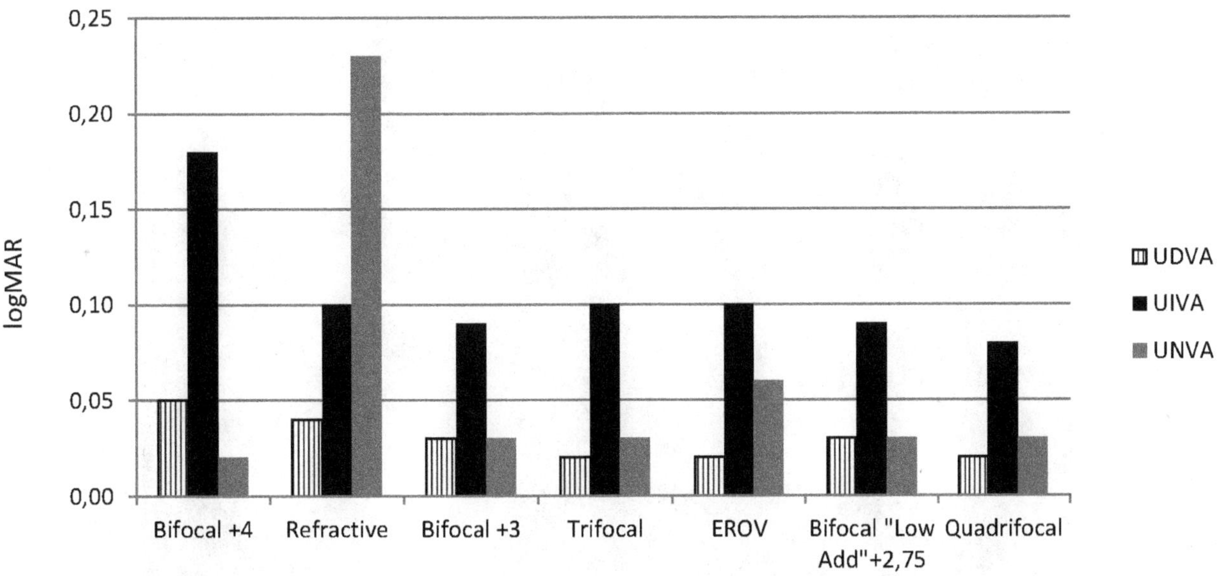

Figure 3. Comparison of uncorrected distance visual acuity (UDVA), uncorrected intermediate visual acuity (UIVA), and uncorrected near visual acuity (UNVA) between eyes implanted with diffractive (bifocal +4 and bifocal +3), refractive, trifocal, extended range of vision (EROV), "low-add," and quadrifocal multifocal intraocular lenses.

Patient refraction	Satisfaction after surgery; average mark [1–10]
High hyperopia	9.6
Low hyperopia	9.1
Plano-presbyopia	8.7
High myopia	8.2
Low myopia	8.1

Table 2. Satisfaction rate after bilateral multifocal intraocular lens implantation, according to preoperative refractive error.

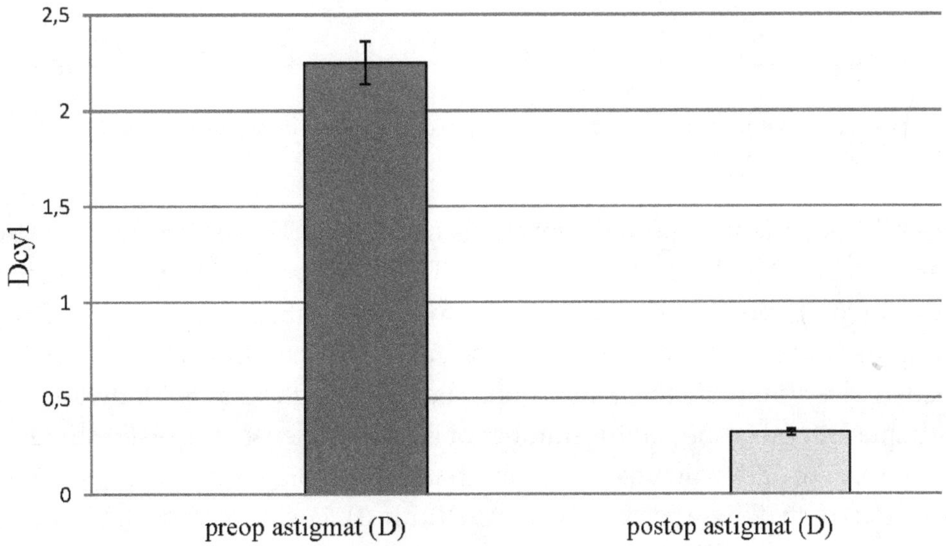

Figure 4. Change in the amount of astigmatism in eyes implanted with toric multifocal intraocular lens.

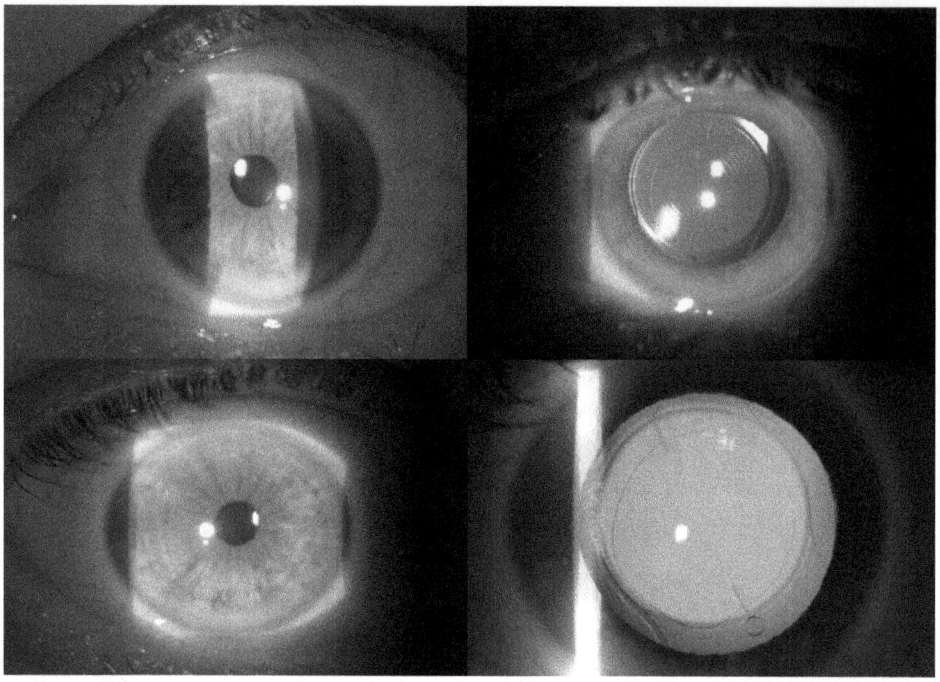

Figure 5. Patient aged 56, after bilaterally implanted trifocal toric IOLs, in a primary position (left) and with a dilated pupil (right). Visual acuity in both eyes is 100% for distance, intermediate (80 cm), and near, without any spectacles.

Lens design/complication rate (%)	Halo and glare	Laser enhancement for residual refractive error	Need for spectacle wear
Bifocal diffractive (Tecnis)	7.7	6.1	5.5
Bifocal diffractive (ReSTOR)	7.2	1.3	4
Refractive (ReZoom)	15	2.6	25.2
Trifocal	9	1.6	1.2
Extended range of vision	4	1.76	4.42
"Low-add" bifocal	8.6	2	1.3
Quadrifocal	5	0	1

Table 3. Complication rate after implantation of different types of multifocal intraocular lenses.

Almost one-third of patients reported symptoms of dry eye. Those patients were treated with artificial tears and punctal plugs when necessary. The need for spectacles was highest in refractive IOL group (25%), mostly for near reading. In bifocal diffractive group, 4–5% of patients had to wear glasses, mostly for computer or tasks at 60–100 cm. In EROV IOL group, 4.22% of patients needed glasses mainly for near vision. The best spectacle independence is achieved in patients with quadrifocal (although the number of implanted lenses is greatly smaller compared to other groups, so the data will most probably change with bigger numbers), trifocal, and bifocal diffractive IOL with "low-add" combination (**Table 3**). Posterior capsular opacification rate was very hard to compare because of a different follow-up (range 3–6%), but trifocal lens did have higher PCO rate compared to others, possibly due to hydrophilic material.

4. Discussion

Nowadays, cataract surgery is becoming a more and more refractive surgery at the same time. Patient's expectations are growing; but thanks to development of new technologies, surgery techniques, and intraocular lens designs, ophthalmologist can fulfill those demands. The aim of modern cataract surgery is to achieve good unaided vision at all distances together with high quality of vision in a safe manner and with a fast recovery. Presbyopia-correcting intraocular lenses are currently the most efficient and permanent treatment for presbyopia. First, IOLs successfully dealing with presbyopia, named multifocal intraocular lenses (MFIOLs), were launched on the market in the early 1980s. They were designed to have several foci in order to provide full vision correction after cataract surgery. These lenses, due to their design, were able to provide patients with good distance and near vision even without the use of spectacles [22]. However, due to their design, MFIOLs have also some disadvantages caused by the presence of several foci. Halo and glare (especially at night) are produced by defocused image and scattered light. Higher near additions at IOL optics increase halo and glare. Moreover, patients need some time for their brain to adapt to MFIOL (so-called neuroadaptation). Very often with neuroadaptation, symptoms of halo and glare tend to decrease. Another characteristic of MFIOL is loss of contrast sensitivity caused by separation of the light entering to the eye in two or three foci. Patients record this as slightly washed out or grayish image, especially in low-light conditions. MFIOLs are also very dependent on eventual residual refractive error, dryness of the eye, IOL centration, posterior capsule opacification, pupil size, and presence of vitreal opacities.

In eye hospital "Svjetlost," MFIOLs are in use since 2004, and currently around one-third of all implanted lenses are MFIOLs. For the first 5 years, we have used MFIOLs available at that time: bifocal diffractive lenses with +4.00D addition (later on also with +3.00D addition) and refractive IOLs. Bifocal diffractive IOLs enabled very good uncorrected far vision and near vision at 30–40 cm, with very good satisfaction rate among patients who did not perform many tasks at intermediate distance (60–100 cm). Refractive IOLs performed somewhat better at intermediate distance range, but near vision was significantly worse as compared to diffractive design. Visual outcome after implantation of the first diffractive and refractive lenses recorded among our patients was similar to other published data [23, 24]. However, lack of good intermediate vision was unacceptable for younger presbyopes performing many tasks at a distance of 60–100 cm. In an attempt to enhance intermediate vision, a technique called "mix and match" was invented aiming to ensure uncorrected vision at all distances. Refractive IOL was implanted in dominant eye (for far and intermediate) vision and diffractive IOL in non-dominant eye (for far and near). It worked well in majority of patients; however, in our hands around 25% of patients were complaining at different images in two eyes (because we used two different technologies) and/or photic phenomena. Some authors have reported very high satisfaction rate with "mix and match" approach, despite the fact that in a presented group of their patients also high percentage of halo and glare was reported [25]. These data show that despite some objective photic phenomena many patients still remain happy with the surgical outcome since they have gained spectacle independence. However, from physician's point of view, we were not satisfied enough with the outcome of "mix and match" method, so we stopped using this technique and switched to newer generations of lens designs emerging on the market: trifocal, combination of "low-add" bifocals with different add-powers, and extended range of vision (EROV) technology [25–27].

In our hands, all types of new-generation or "premium" MFIOLs (trifocal, quadrifocal, "low-add" combination, and EROV) provided similar and very good UDVA. The main improvement of modern lens designs is the quality of uncorrected intermediate vision, which is very satisfying with all lenses. Trifocal lenses provided excellent far, intermediate, and near vision, which seems to be more "continuous" with quadrifocal design mainly for tasks at 60 cm distance. The EROV provided excellent distance and intermediate vision, performing slightly worse at near if emmetropia was aimed in both eyes. Thus, to improve near vision with EROV lens, we are now implanting many patients with a planned myopic shift of −0.5% in a non-dominant eye ("mini-monovision"), and in this manner, better near vision was achieved. The advantage of EROV IOL is that it maintains a very similar level of visual quality as monofocal IOL, less visual disturbances compared to bi- and trifocals, and we have successfully implanted this lens also in amblyopic patients and those with the previous refractive surgery on the cornea. To conclude, both EROV and trifocal IOLs are good options for patients with intermediate distance requirements, while in patients having numerous near-vision tasks, EROV IOL should be aimed slightly myopic in a non-dominant eye, or trifocal/quadrifocal technology may be used. Comparing to other lens designs, PCO occurrence was higher in trifocal lens, but subsequent YAG capsulotomy did not affect long-term visual outcome. Implantation of two "low-add" lenses with different near add-powers provided good near, intermediate, and distance vision, comparable to the outcome with EROV and trifocal/quadrifocal IOLs.

In our patients with the astigmatism >1D, multifocal toric IOLs were implanted. These lenses are capable of correcting both presbyopia and astigmatism. Invention of multifocal toric IOLs was based on very good results in astigmatic correction with monofocal toric IOLs, which showed to be safe and effective in correcting astigmatism and improving vision even in cataract patients with very high astigmatism such as topographically stable keratoconus, pellucid marginal degeneration, and post-penetrating keratoplasty astigmatism [28–30]. The systematic literature review shows that spectacle independence for patients treated with four brands of monofocal toric IOLs increased from 15 to 85% of those who never wore spectacles [1]. There are several specific requirements for the IOLs aimed to treat the astigmatism; the lens has to be easy to manipulate in the capsular bag in order to achieve good alignment and needs good long-term positional stability, as low as possible induction of capsular shrinkage and posterior capsule opacification. Namely, toric IOL which has to be produced for each individual case is marked on its surface for proper alignment in the capsular bag. Axis of astigmatism has to be determined and marked in a seating position due to cyclotorsional movements of the eye while the patient is lying down for the surgery. Proper alignment of toric IOL during surgery is crucial since misalignment of only 10° leads to a loss of one-third of the astigmatic correction. Moreover, even a small decentration of IOL of less than 1 mm will induce aberrations and poorer visual result [31]. Shrinkage of the capsular bag may also lead to decentration of the lens and thus have negative impact on its proper alignment. Misaligned toric intraocular lens has to be repositioned into its proper position by surgical revision. If surgical correction is needed, the intervention should be performed as soon as possible after the primary surgery to avoid manipulation in the capsular bag with abundant fibrosis. Although it is recommended to re-center the lens in the first months after primary surgery, it has been reported that lens can be safely repositioned even 15 months after its implantation [32]. According to our results, with properly calculated and implanted toric MFIOL, both spherical and cylindrical errors can be successfully corrected.

In recent years, special medical equipment and centering systems were invented to minimize potential sources of errors during each step of the surgery (e.g., Verion Image Guided System or Zeiss Callisto). Both systems may improve precision, and size of the incisions enables perfect shape and size of the capsulorhexis and more precise alignment of the toric IOL or multifocal IOL along the optical axis. Such a computer-assisted cataract surgery will make premium IOL surgery even more precise, but it will take some time till all the cataract surgery units embrace this technology. All the results presented in this chapter are obtained without the use of advanced computerized systems. Therefore, the outcome and performance of different MFIOL designs implanted in our hospital in the last 12 years are in fact more objective to compare, since the methodology of surgery did not change significantly throughout this period. Once we add sophisticated computer-controlled systems into standard equipment used during cataract surgery with MFIOL implantation, the results should improve further.

Finally, very important or maybe the most important issue when we discuss about MFIOL use is the issue which cannot be presented by pure scientific data—preoperative counseling. Spectrum of lens design available nowadays on the market is quite large, and only careful discussion over patient lifestyle, everyday activities, job, and expectations may provide to write answer on which lens design to use. Patients who are looking for guaranties, "perfect" vision, or 100% spectacle independence are not good candidates for MFIOLs. The first step toward good results is that the surgeon working with MFIOL understand that there is no perfect lens for every patient, and then to transfer in a proper way this information to a patient. Looking at the preoperative refractive errors, hyperopic patients are the best candidates for such surgery. It is very wise to under-promise how it is going to be with implanted MFIOLs and then hopefully over-deliver. With such a proper preoperative counseling, and subsequent choice of the MFIOL best suited to individual patient needs, all currently available MFIOLs will provide a high level of both spectacle independence and patient satisfaction.

Author details

Iva Dekaris*, Nikica Gabrić, Ante Barišić and Adis Pašalić

*Address all correspondence to: iva.svjetlost@gmail.com

Department of Ophthalmology, Specialty Eye Hospital 'Svjetlost', University of Rijeka, Zagreb, Croatia

References

[1] Agresta B, Knorz MC, et al. Visual acuity improvements after implantation of toric intraocular lenses in cataract patients with astigmatism: A systematic review. BMC Ophthalmology. 2012;**15**:41. DOI: 10.1186/1471-2415-12-41

[2] Auffarth GU, Dick HB. Multifocal intraocular lenses: A systematic review. Der Ophthalmologe. 2001;**98**(2):127-137

[3] Artigas JM, Menezo JL, et al. Image quality with multifocal intraocular lenses and the effect of pupil size: comparison of refractive and hybrid refractive-diffractive designs. Journal of Cataract & Refractive Surgery. 2007;**33**(12):2111-2117

[4] Pieh S, Weghaupt H, et al. Contrast sensitivity and glare disability with diffractive and refractive multifocal intraocular lenses. Journal of Cataract and Refractive Surgery. 1998; **24**(5):659-662

[5] Gatinel D, Loicq J. Clinically relevant optical properties of bifocal, trifocal, and extended depth of focus intraocular lenses. Journal of Cataract and Refractive Surgery. 2016;**32**(4):273-280. DOI: 10.3928/1081597X-20160121-07

[6] Pedrotti E, Bruni E, et al. Comparative analysis of the clinical outcomes with a Monofocal and an extended range of vision intraocular lens. Journal of Cataract and Refractive Surgery. 2016;**32**(7):436-442. DOI: 10.3928/1081597X-20160428-06

[7] Ganesh S, Brar S, et al. Long-term visual outcomes and patient satisfaction following bilateral implantation of trifocal intraocular lenses. Clinical Ophthalmology. 2017;**11**:1453-1459. DOI: 10.2147/OPTH.S125921 ECollection 2017

[8] Ueno Y, Hiraoka T, et al. Age-related changes in anterior, posterior, and total corneal astigmatism. Journal of Refractive Surgery. 2014;**30**(3):192-197. DOI: 10.3928/1081597X-20140218-01

[9] Visser N, Nuijts RM, et al. Visual outcomes and patient satisfaction after cataract surgery with toric multifocal intraocular lens implantation. Journal of Cataract and Refractive Surgery. 2011;**37**(11):2034-2042. DOI: 10.1016/j.jcrs.2011.05.041. Epub 2011 Sep 22

[10] Visser N, Bauer NJ, et al. Toric intraocular lenses: Historical overview, patient selection, IOL calculation, surgical techniques, clinical outcomes, and complications. Journal of Cataract and Refractive Surgery. 2013;**39**(4):624-637. DOI: 10.1016/j.jcrs.2013.02.020

[11] Pérez-Vives C, Ferrer-Blasco T, et al. Optical quality comparison between spherical and aspheric toric intraocular lenses. European Journal of Ophthalmology. 2014;**24**(5):699-706 DOI: 10.5301/ejo.5000440

[12] Carones F, all KMC e. Influence of co-payment levels on patient and surgeon acceptance of advanced technology intraocular lenses. Journal of Refractive Surgery. 2014;**30**(4):278-281. DOI: 10.3928/1081597X-20140320-07

[13] Sheppard AL, Wolffsohn JS, et al. Clinical outcomes after implantation of a new hydrophobic acrylic toric IOL during routine cataract surgery. Journal of Cataract and Refractive Surgery. 2013;**39**(1):41-47. DOI: 10.1016/j.jcrs.2012.08.055

[14] Vojniković B, Gabrić N, et al. Curvature analyses of the corneal front and back surface. Collegium Antropologicum. 2013;**37**:93-96

[15] Lyall DA, Srinivasan S, et al. Changes in corneal astigmatism among patients with visually significant cataract. Canadian Journal of Ophthalmology. 2014;**49**(3):297-303. DOI: 10.1016/j.jcjo.2014.02.001

[16] Belluci R, Bauer NJ, et al. Visual acuity and refraction with a diffractive multifocal toric intraocular lens. Journal of Cataract and Refractive Surgery. 2013;**39**(10):1507-1518. DOI: 10.1016/j.jcrs.2013.04.036

[17] Alfonso JF, Knorz M, et al. Clinical outcomes after bilateral implantation of an apodized +3.0 D toric diffractive multifocal intraocular lens. Journal of Cataract and Refractive Surgery. 2014;**40**(1):51-59. DOI: 10.1016/j.jcrs.2013.06.026

[18] Goes FJ. Refractive lens exchange with the diffractive multifocal Tecnis ZM900 intraocular lens. Journal of Refractive Surgery. 2008;**24**(3):243-250

[19] Liekfeld A, Torun N, et al. A new toric diffractive multifocal lens for refractive surgery. Ophthalmologe. 2010;**107**(3):256, 258-61. DOI: 10.1007/s00347-009-2000-7

[20] Barišić A, Gabrić N, et al. Comparison of different presbyopia treatments: Refractive lens exchange with multifocal intraocular lens implantation versus LASIK Monovision. Collegium Antropologicum. 2010;**34**(2):95-98

[21] Mozayan E, Lee JK. Update on astigmatism management. Current Opinion in Ophthalmology. 2014;**25**(4):286-290. DOI: 10.1097/ICU.0000000000000068

[22] Barišić A, Dekaris I, et al. Comparison of diffractive and refractive multifocal intraocular lenses in presbyopia treatment. Collegium Antropologicum. 2008;**32**(2):27-31

[23] Cochener B, Lafuma A, et al. Comparison of outcomes with multifocal intraocular lenses: A meta-analysis. Clinical Ophthalmology. 2011;**5**:45-56. DOI: 10.2147/OPTH.S14325

[24] Alió JL, Grabner G, et al. Postoperative bilateral reading performance with 4 intraocular lens models: Six-month results. Journal of Cataract and Refractive Surgery. 2011;**37**(5): 842-852. DOI: 10.1016/j.jcrs.2010.11.039

[25] Lubinski W, Podboraczynska-Jodko K, et al. Visual outcomes three and six months after implantation of diffractive and refractive multifocal IOL combinations. Klinika Oczna. 2011;**113**(7-9):209-215

[26] Goes FJ. Visual results following implantation of a refractive multifocal IOL in one eye and a diffractive multifocal IOL in the contralateral eye. Journal of Refractive Surgery. 2008;**24**(3):300-305

[27] Yoon SY, Song IS, et al. Bilateral mix-and-match versus unilateral multifocal intraocular lens implantation: Long-term comparison. Journal of Cataract & Refractive Surgery. 2013;**39**(11):1682-1690

[28] Parikakis EA, Chatziralli IP, et al. Toric intraocular lens implantation for correction of astigmatism in cataract patients with corneal ectasia. Case Reports in Ophthalmology. 2013;**4**(3):219-228. DOI: 10.1159/000356532

[29] Zvornicanin J, Cabric E, et al. Use of the toric intraocular lens for keratoconus treatment. Acta Informatica Medica. 2014;**22**(2):139-141. DOI: 10.5455/aim.2014.22.139-141

[30] Wade M, Steinert RF, et al. Results of toric intraocular lenses for post-penetrating keratoplasty astigmatism. Ophthalmology. 2014;**121**(3):771-777. DOI: 10.1016/j.ophtha.2013.10.011

[31] Pérez-Vives C, Ferrer-Blasco T, et al. Optical quality of aspheric toric intraocular lenses at different degrees of decentering. Graefe's Archive for Clinical and Experimental Ophthalmology. 2014;**252**(6):969-975. DOI: 10.1007/s00417-014-2629-z

[32] Brandlhuber U, Haritoglou C, et al. Reposition of a misaligned Zeiss AT TORBI 709M® intraocular lens 15 months after implantation. European Journal of Ophthalmology. 2014;**24**(5):800-802. DOI: 10.5301/ejo.5000453

9

Cataract Surgery in Patients with Uveitis: Preoperative and Surgical Considerations

Alejandro Rodriguez-Garcia and C. Stephen Foster

Abstract

Cataract is one of the most frequent visual impairment complications of uveitis, accounting for up to 40% of the visual loss seen in these patients. In general, uveitis patients differ from the general cataract population in that they are younger and have a higher rate of comorbidities, however the rates of inflammatory sequelae vary markedly among uveitic entities. Cataract development may be influenced by the cause and duration of uveitis, the degree of inflammation control, and the use of corticosteroid therapy. Cataract surgery in patients with uveitis represents a serious challenge due to pre-existing ocular comorbidities that may limit the visual outcome and difficult the surgical procedure; the need for preoperative control of inflammation; and the efficacy of postoperative management to avoid immediate and late ocular complications. A detailed ophthalmologic exam prior to surgery is essential to know the status of pre-existing pathologic changes, adjust the medical therapy to achieve absolute control of inflammation, establish a surgical plan, and deliver an objective visual prognosis to the patient or the relatives. The key point to surgical success is the absolute control of inflammation, meaning no cells in the anterior chamber for at least 3 months prior to surgery. Today, minimally invasive phacoemulsification with acrylic foldable intraocular lens implantation is the standard of care for most patients with uveitis. It must be taken into consideration that higher rates of intraoperative and postoperative complications may occur. Vision-limiting pathology related to pre-existing uveitis complications are the major contributing factors for limited postoperative visual outcome.

Keywords: uveitis, cataract, phacoemulsification, intraocular lens, steroids, macular edema, glaucoma

1. Introduction

Cataract represents a significant burden in the management and visual outcome of uveitis patients. Up to 40% of the visual loss seen in these patients is either solely or largely due to cataract [1]. Lens opacification is caused by repeated episodes or sustained intraocular inflammation characterized by the release of free oxygen radicals, lysosomal enzymes, immune complex deposition on the lens capsule, hypoxia, and altered composition of the aqueous humor [2]. The development of cataract depends on the type of uveitis, the degree and duration of the inflammatory process, and on the prolonged and excessive use of corticosteroids [3–5].

Cataract surgery in patients with uveitis represents a serious challenge for the anterior segment surgeon [6, 7]. Nowadays, clear cornea phacoemulsification with intraocular lens (IOL) implantation is the standard of care for most patients with uveitis [8, 9]. However, despite remarkable progress on surgical techniques and IOL materials, certain specific considerations should be taken into account regarding patient selection, preoperative preparation, as well as perioperative and postoperative management for successful long-term results [10, 11]. Nearly one-third of all uveitic eyes have small pupils, which represent a surgical technical difficulty [2]. In such cases, higher rates of additional intraoperative maneuvers are required to obtain proper visualization and phacoemulsification of the cataract [4, 12, 13]. And, while surgery is associated with an improvement in best corrected visual acuity (BCVA), higher rates of both, intraoperative and postoperative complications have been reported [14, 15]. Moreover, it has been shown that the final BCVA in uveitic eyes is worse than in non-uveitic ones [14]. Therefore, identifying the cause of uveitis and pre-existing pathologic changes that affect the visual outcome, achieving absolute control of inflammation before surgery, careful surgical planning, and solving intraoperative and postoperative complications are crucial to obtain a successful result (BCVA ≥ 20/40).

2. Epidemiology

Cataract is the most common ocular complication in children with chronic uveitis with an estimated rate from 35 to 52.0% [16]. In juvenile idiopathic arthritis (JIA)-associated uveitis, the prevalence varies from 40 to 60% and the incidence of new-onset cataract formation has been estimated as 0.04/eye-year [17, 18]. On the other hand, in adult patients it is one of the most frequent complications of uveitis with a prevalence rate as high as 50% as seen in Fuchs uveitis [6, 14, 19, 20]. In HLA-B27-associated anterior uveitis, the most common cause of uveitis in adults, cataract formation is the third most frequent complication with an estimated prevalence of 14%, and an incidence rate of 0.091 during follow-up time (**Table 1**) [21]. Cataract prevalence varies among different causes of uveitis and depends on multiple factors including etiology, localization of the inflammatory process, time elapsed between the onset and diagnosis of uveitis, the degree of inflammation, the clinical course, and the use of corticosteroids [1, 18, 22, 23].

Cause of uveitis	Cataract prevalence range (median)	Successful outcome BCVA ≥ 20/40 (Snellen)	Frequent complications	References
Fuchs uveitis	15–75% (50%)	83%	Intraoperative AC hemorrhage (3.6–76%) Hyphema Ocular hypertension (glaucoma) (3–35%) PCO (14.6%) Progressive vitreous opacification	[20, 27, 48, 49]
Herpetic uveitis	15–75% (24%)	72.2%	Viral reactivation Iris posterior synechiae Secondary glaucoma	[63, 151–153]
Juvenile idiopathic arthritis-associated uveitis	40–60% (50%)	60–70% (67%)	Exuberant postoperative inflammation Iris posterior synechiae Secondary glaucoma (25%) CME Cyclitic membrane Hypotony (Phthisis bulbi)	[4, 17, 18, 25, 26, 81, 95, 97–99, 101, 110]
HLA-B27 associated uveitis	9.2–20.1%	NA	Recurrent uveitis CME Iris synechiae	[21]
Pars planitis	36–42% (40%)	50–83%	Persistent vitritis (haze) CME (50%) Glaucoma (10%) PCO (10%) IOL Cocooning (29%) ERM Optic nerve atrophy	[23, 28, 140, 154]
Adamantiades-Behcet disease	21–26% (38.5%)	72.5% (42.4%)	Exuberant inflammation (12.5%) Iris posterior synechiae (17.5%) CME (12.5%) ERM (7.5%) Papillitis (optic nerve atrophy) (5%) PCO (37.5% most common)	[148, 155, 156]
Vogt-Koyanagi-Harada disease	10–35%	68%	Exuberant inflammation Iris anterior and posterior synechiae Pupillary membrane PCO (76%) Macular scarring	[135, 157]

Cause of uveitis	Cataract prevalence range (median)	Successful outcome BCVA ≥ 20/40 (Snellen)	Frequent complications	References
Sympathetic ophthalmia	31.8%	67.79% (72.2%)	PCO (77.7%) Glaucoma	[158]
Sarcoidosis	21%	61%	PCO (57.1%) Recurrent uveitis CME Glaucoma	[159]

AC = anterior chamber; PCO = posterior capsule opacification; CME = cystoid macular edema; ERM = epiretinal membrane.

Table 1. Prevalence, visual outcome, and complications of cataract surgery in uveitis.

3. Clinical characteristics of diverse forms of uveitis

In general, the uveitic population differs from the general population suffering from cataract in that they are younger and have a higher rate of comorbidities [15]. However, the rates of inflammatory sequelae vary markedly among uveitic entities [7, 24]. For this reason, each uveitis syndrome must be analyzed separately with respect to ocular complications and visual outcome [6, 14] (**Table 1**). While Fuchs uveitis regularly has the best visual prognosis and the least postoperative complications, JIA-associated uveitis has one of the most fear prognosis due to frequent pre-existing pathology, difficulties in reaching absolute control of inflammation, and multiple intraoperative and postoperative complications [4, 25–27].

4. Preoperative evaluation

A correct classification and etiologic diagnosis of the uveitic entity is very helpful to establish the appropriate surgical strategy and to determine the prognosis [8]. Moreover, a complete preoperative ophthalmologic examination is essential since pre-existing pathology will have significant therapeutic and prognostic visual implications [16, 28]. For instance, corneal opacity, vitreous haze, macular edema, and optic nerve atrophy usually result in a poor visual outcome [6, 19]. Therefore, it is very important that the patient and/or their relatives have an objective report on the status of the eye to be operated in order to have a realistic expectation of the final visual result. Ancillary diagnostic tests are always necessary to detect pre-existing pathologic changes that will allow us to render a more accurate visual prognosis. In most cases, it is helpful to perform a macular function test. Several methods are available for this purpose including the potential acuity meter (PAM), the laser interferometer (LI), and the focal electroretinogram (fERG) [29, 30]. The PAM test has proven an accuracy of 84% in patients with poor visual acuity (<20/40) [30]. On the other hand, LI has shown a lower accuracy (65%) and a tendency for over-predicting vision compared to the PAM in these patients [29, 30]. Focal cone ERG is very sensitive for detecting macular pathology, showing 91% accuracy in eyes with poor visual acuity [30].

Linear A-B ultrasound is necessary to identify vitreous hemorrhage and opacity, as well as posterior segment changes like, retinal detachment, optic nerve swelling, and sclerochoroidal thickness [31]. Another very useful device is high-frequency ultrabiomicroscopy (UBM), which generates high-resolution images at an almost histological level. *In vivo* image sections may be obtained up to 3–6 mm in depth, permitting visualization of anterior segment structures [32]. Frequent indications for UBM in uveitis include uveitis-glaucoma-hyphema syndrome (UGH), sclerouveitis, herpetic anterior uveitis, pars planitis, pseudophakic uveitis, hypotony, peripheral toxocariasis, and ciliary body pathology [32, 33].

Retina fluorescein angiography (FA) allows the detection of many different forms of posterior segment inflammatory changes. It is used to evaluate the activity and extent of chorioretinitis and optic nerve involvement; identify macular edema and choroidal neovascularization; diagnose certain posterior uveitic entities with typical features; evaluate retinal vascular involvement and neovascularization; and to monitor the therapeutic response [34]. However, many inflammatory changes occur in the peripheral retina where visualization may be difficult with conventional angiography. Wide field scanning laser ophthalmoscopy performs ultra-wide angle FA allowing clear identification of peripheral lesions and accurate documentation of disease progression [35]. This recently new image technology has replaced conventional angiography for the diagnosis and monitoring of intermediate and many forms of posterior uveitis [35].

Indocyanine green angiography (ICGA) allows the detection of choroidal inflammation. Two patterns of choroidal vasculitis have been described: primary inflammatory choriocapillaropathy and stromal inflammatory vasculopathy [36]. The first pattern is characterized by non-perfusion of the choriocapillaris found in entities like, multiple evanescent white dot syndrome, acute posterior multifocal placoid pigment epitheliopathy, multifocal choroiditis, and serpiginous choroidopathy [36]. The choroidal stromal inflammatory vasculopathy pattern is seen in active Vogt-Koyanagi-Harada disease (VKH), ocular sarcoidosis, tuberculosis, and birdshot chorioretinopathy [37]. In Behcet's disease, as in other forms of uveitis, both ICGA vascular patterns may be seen at different stages of inflammation [38].

Today, the most frequently used imaging technique to detect and monitor macular inflammatory changes is optical coherence tomography (OCT). With an axial resolution in the 5–7 μm range, it provides close to an *in-vivo* histologic view of the retina [39]. There are several types of OCT available for clinical purposes. The spectral-domain OCT is the most used method [40]. It allows high-speed, accurate images of the retina, particularly macular pathology like, cystoid and diffuse macular edema, subretinal fluid accumulation, epiretinal membrane formation, macular holes, and choroidal neovascularization [41]. Longer wavelength OCT systems, including the swept-source technology and en-face imaging, enhance the detection of subtle microstructural changes in chorioretinal disorders by improving imaging of the choroid [42–44]. A technique that produces high-resolution cross-sectional images of the entire choroid called enhanced depth imaging technique (EDI-OCT) has identified increased subfoveal choroidal thickness in patients with active Behcet [45] and VKH disease, as well as loss of focal hyperreflectivity of the inner choroid in the acute and convalescent phases of VKH [46].

Once the preoperative evaluation is completed, a postoperative visual prognosis may be assumed, therapeutic adjustments may be applied, and a surgical plan is prepared based on pre-existing pathologic findings.

5. Preoperative preparation and therapeutic strategies

The key to surgical success in patients with uveitic cataract is the absolute control of inflammation, meaning no cells in the anterior chamber for at least 3 months prior to surgery [7]. This requisite is crucial to obtain an optimal surgical result and to minimize postoperative complications [7, 24]. Active uveitis at the time of cataract surgery has been associated with worse visual outcomes [15, 47]. Moreover, postoperative cystoid macular edema (CME) is more likely to develop in eyes with active inflammation within a 3-month period before surgery (relative risk 6.19) than those under control [41]. However, this general consensus of no cells in the anterior chamber prior to surgery has its exemptions [2]. In Fuchs uveitis, minimal but persistent anterior chamber cells and flare are frequently found despite intensive and sustained treatment with topical corticosteroids [48]. Hence, anti-inflammatory treatment is not indicated for the low-grade anterior chamber reaction seen in Fuchs uveitis and only occasionally, a short-course of corticosteroids is indicated for symptomatic exacerbations [49]. Other exemptions are related to the necessity for prompt surgical intervention in cases like, lens-induced uveitis, cyclitic membrane formation with hypotony, persistent vitreous opacity or hemorrhage, and retinal detachment [50, 51].

Preoperative management depends specifically on the type and etiology of uveitis. For inactive idiopathic anterior non-granulomatous uveitis as for Fuchs uveitis, topical administration of prednisolone acetate 1% four times a day, starting 3–7 days before surgery may be sufficient to avoid an outburst of postoperative inflammation [24]. On the contrary, patients with JIA-associated uveitis, anterior granulomatous uveitis, intermediate, posterior, and panuveitis also require oral prednisone (1.0 mg/kg/day) starting 3 days before surgery and continued for a week after cataract removal and then tapered slowly according to the inflammatory status [52, 53]. Preoperative oral steroids have been shown to be effective in reducing the risk of CME [41]. If patients are on immunosuppressive chemotherapy and/or biologics, they should be continued at current dosage [11]. In case that systemic corticosteroids are contraindicated (e.g., diabetes mellitus, metabolic disease, acid-peptic disease, obesity, or osteoporosis), periocular administration (transseptal or sub-Tenon's) of triamcinolone acetonide (40 mg/ml) should be considered [54, 55]. Alternative immunosuppressive agents like, cyclosporin-A, tacrolimus, or anti-metabolites may be administered to these patients considering that most of these medications require a longer period of time (usually 4–6 weeks) to reach an optimal therapeutic effect [56].

The use of topical non-steroidal anti-inflammatory drugs (NSAIDs) like, ketorolac 0.4%, nepafenac 0.15%, or bromfenac 0.09%, have become a standard of care practice for the perioperative management of inflammation, pain, surgical-induced miosis, and cystoid macular edema in uneventful and also in uveitic cataract surgery [57–59]. A systematic review found high-quality evidence that topical NSAIDs are more effective than topical steroids in preventing the short-term pseudophakic CME in non-uveitic cataract surgery [60]. On the other hand, a recent evidence-based review conducted by the American Academy of Ophthalmology found that the claimed made about the synergistic effect of combined topical steroids and NSAIDs remains unproven [61]. In addition, NSAIDs have only a short-term therapeutic effect on prompt visual recovery and reduction of established CME, but no effect on the long-term visual outcome [57, 58, 61]. There is good collective clinical evidence and rationale that the application of a topical NSAID 3 days before surgery reduces CME and improves vision in the short-term [61]. Because the COX-2 enzyme is inducible and mostly responsible for the inflammatory process, the selective inhibitory effect of nepafenac and bromfenac makes them more suitable for this purpose [62]. Nepafenac has shown the shortest time to reach maximal concentration and the greatest aqueous humor peak concentration compared to ketorolac and bromfenac in eyes having cataract surgery [62]. After the surgical procedure, topical NSAIDs use is usually extended for 4–6 weeks [1, 10].

There are other special conditions in uveitis in which certain specific actions should be taken before cataract extraction is performed. Such is the case of herpetic uveitis in which prophylactic anti-viral therapy with acyclovir or valacyclovir should be administered at least 1 week before surgery in order to avoid recurrent viral infection [63, 64]. Other special consideration is the preoperative management of prominent band keratopathy interfering with cataract visualization which may be treated with EDTA 1–2% calcium chelation, or Excimer laser PTK before cataract surgery [65, 66].

Cataract and glaucoma frequently coexist as uveitis complications, and a combined surgical procedure may be associated with an increased risk of glaucoma surgery failure [67, 68]. In such cases, it may result better to perform a clear cornea small-incision cataract extraction first, followed later on by filtration surgery or a valve implantation with anti-metabolites [69, 70]. One must consider that uveitic glaucoma eyes operated for trabeculectomy with mitomycin-C which had previous cataract surgery or granulomatous uveitis, have a higher risk of surgical failure (RR = 2.957, P = 0.0344, and RR = 3.805, P = 0.0106, respectively) [71]. A higher risk of glaucoma surgical failure has also been associated with idiopathic, intermediate, and Fuchs uveitis; active intraocular inflammation at the time of surgery; and relapse of uveitis [72]. Moreover, the success rate of filtration surgery in uveitic eyes is significantly lower than that of non-uveitic, and many patients with successful intraocular pressure (IOP) control still require anti-glaucoma therapy to maintain adequate IOP levels in the postoperative period [72].

Posterior vitrectomy and cataract extraction may be an alternative for patients with prominent posterior segment pathology including vitreous opacity, hemorrhage, cystoid macular edema, and tractional retinal detachment [73]. There is reasonable evidence that cataract phacoemulsification combined with posterior vitrectomy has a favorable visual outcome for some patients with refractory inflammation, particularly those with significant vitreous opacity and chronic macular edema [13, 74]. In children, this combined surgical approach has been used for JIA-associated uveitis, pars planitis, and other forms of posterior uveitis [75].

However, this technique is not exempt of serious postoperative complications like, glaucoma, macular edema, and exuberant inflammation [75, 76]. For specific cases with various ocular complications, multiple combined surgical strategies have been postulated including phacoemulsification with IOL implantation, posterior vitrectomy, intravitreal sustained-release corticosteroid injection, and glaucoma tube implantation with promising results [77].

6. Surgical technique and intraoperative maneuvers

Nowadays, small clear corneal incision phacoemulsification surgery is preferred over extracapsular cataract extraction (ECCE) and lensectomy for most patients with uveitis [78, 79]. Since cataract surgery in these patients is frequently complicated by corneal opacification, iris synechiae, pupillary and cyclitic membranes, among others, the surgical technique should be minimally invasive with precise and delicate maneuvers [10, 24] (**Figure 1**). Most studies report a higher rate of additional maneuvers, notably iris and pupillary manipulation within a range between 19 and 67% of eyes [4–6, 25].

Dealing with unexpected intraoperative complications like, corneal stromal edema; anterior chamber hemorrhage; pigment dispersion; posterior capsule rupture with vitreous exposure is key to achieve the best surgical outcome possible [6, 19, 75]. The first challenge that the surgeon faces is an adequate exposure and visualization of the cataract. Iris synechiolysis, pupillary membrane removal, and pupil distension with iris hooks or iris stretch devices are frequently required for proper cataract visualization [80, 81]. There is no general consensus on what is the best way to deal with the pathologic changes of the anterior segment encountered in uveitic eyes. However, it is generally agreed that

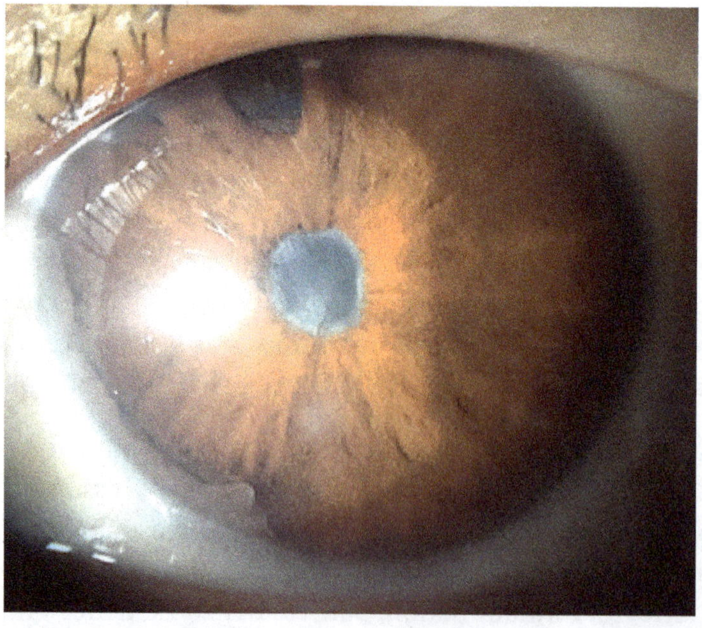

Figure 1. Anterior segment appearance of a patient with Vogt-Koyanagi-Harada disease showing extensive peripheral anterior and posterior synechiae, shallow anterior chamber and a pupillary membrane in front of a secondary cataract.

attempts should be made to minimize surgical maneuvers in order to lessen tissue manipulation and trauma as possible [6, 24, 26].

The capsulorhexis should measure between 5 and 6 mm in diameter because smaller apertures are frequently associated with capsular phimosis and posterior iris synechiae to the anterior capsule remnant [82–84] (**Figure 2**). On the other hand, larger diameter capsulorhexis may affect the IOL centration and stability [83]. The phacoemulsification technique may vary depending on the density and zonular status of the cataract, but an effort should be made to use the less ultrasound power and time possible, to perform vigorous cortical and posterior capsule cleaning, and to avoid posterior capsule rupture [11, 19]. Avoiding the latter is crucial to obtain a good postoperative result, especially in chronic and recurrent uveitis like, herpetic uveitis, pars planitis, VKH disease, toxoplasmosis, among others [6, 24, 85]. In these cases, posterior capsule rupture with vitreous exposure may be a contraindication for IOL implantation due to a high probability of postoperative excessive and persistent inflammation [12, 86]. In uveitic eyes with encapsulated and subluxated IOLs with extensive fibrosis, IOL removal may be necessary at some point of the postoperative period to control severe inflammation and reduce its consequences [87–89]. For eyes with extensive membrane formation in the anterior vitreous, vitrectomy after performing a posterior central capsulorhexis must be considered [90].

Decision making regarding the type of IOL to be used; anterior or posterior chamber IOL implantation; possible IOL sulcus fixation; combined filtration surgery, MIGS, or valve implantation; central posterior capsulorhexis after PC-IOL implantation with anterior vitrectomy; lensectomy, as well as posterior vitrectomy with or without retinal surgery are frequently met during uveitic cataract surgery, and the surgeon must be prepared to make the best decision for the particular case [91–94]. The implantation of a foldable IOL "in the bag" is ideal for most cases of uveitis with certain exceptions [4, 95]. Until now, it is not clear how to proceed in children with uveitic cataract, and randomized controlled trials (RCT) are necessary to elucidate

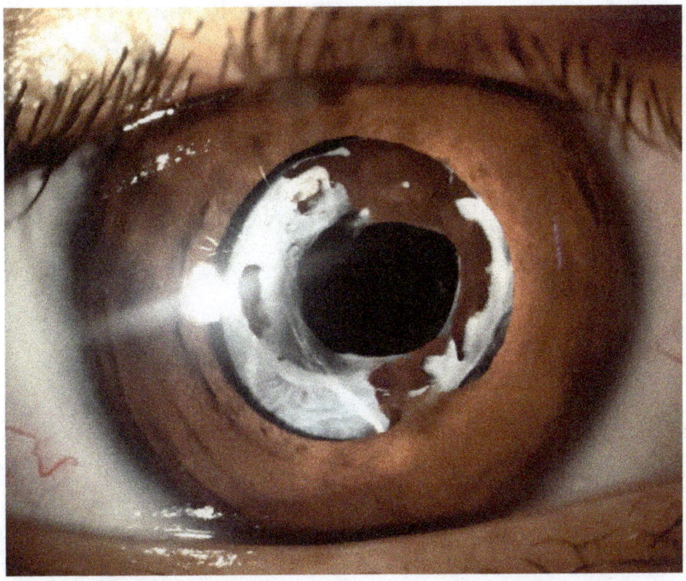

Figure 2. Patient with ankylosing spondylitis and HLA-B27-associated uveitis after cataract surgery showing capsular phimosis and partial adherence of the pigmentary epithelium of the iris to the anterior capsule remnant.

this matter [4, 25, 26, 81]. Historically, uveitic cataract surgery during childhood has been associated with a higher rate of surgical complications, particularly excessive postoperative inflammation [6, 10]. In the past, this situation made that the preferred surgical techniques for cataract extraction in this group including ECCE with posterior pars plana vitrectomy or lensectomy [4, 95]. However, recent evidence favors the implantation of foldable PC-IOLs in children with uveitis, including patients with JIA-associated iridocyclitis [25, 26, 96–101].

Intraocular corticosteroids can be administered during surgery. Intracameral dexamethasone phosphate (400 μg/0.1 ml) or intravitreal triamcinolone (4 mg/0.1 ml) injection (IVTA) may be administered intraoperatively, except in advanced secondary glaucoma or known steroid-responsive patients [4, 102]. A prospective and comparative RCT between oral corticosteroids and preservative-free IVTA injection showed no differences in postoperative anterior chamber reaction, IOP levels, and central macular thickness (CMT) [103]. Another study found a better effect of IVTA versus orbital floor TA on macular edema and postoperative inflammation after cataract surgery in patients with uveitis [55]. However, IVTA injections have a temporary effect therefore, may require repeated injections which are not exempt of serious ocular complications like, elevated IOP (30–43% eyes), bacterial endophthalmitis, vitreous hemorrhage, and retinal detachment [104]. For those eyes at higher risk for intravitreal injection, sub-Tenon's or transseptal TA can be administered at the end of surgery [19].

Intravitreal steroid sustained-release devices containing fluocinolone acetonide 0.59 mg or dexamethasone phosphate 0.7 mg have proven to be beneficial for the control of inflammation, prevention of CME, or reduction of CMT if applied a few days to weeks before or during cataract surgery [105]. Although no general consensus exists on the appropriate surgical time, it seems reasonable to perform the cataract surgery within 4–6 weeks from the last steroid implantation [105–107]. The most fear complication of sustained-release steroid devices is ocular hypertension (OHT). A meta-analysis found that 66% of eyes develop OHT after the implantation of the 0.59 mg fluocinolone acetonide device, compared to 32% following 4 mg IVTA, and only 15% with the 0.7 mg dexamethasone implant [108]. Risk factors for developing OHT include, pre-existing glaucoma, higher baseline IOP, younger age, OHT following previous injection, uveitis, higher steroid dosage, and fluocinolone implant [108]. A new sustained-release implant containing 0.19 mg fluocinolone acetonide has shown promising results improving visual acuity and reducing CMT with a significant reduction of IOP compared to the dexamethasone implant and IVTA [109].

7. Considerations for intraocular lenses

The general consensus regarding cataract surgery in patients with uveitis is that implantation of IOLs may be safely performed when ocular inflammation is completely abolished for a minimum period of 3 months [4, 7]. However, a debate still exists if an IOL should be implanted in specific circumstances like, lens-induced uveitis, JIA-associated iridocyclitis, young children with posterior or panuveitis, and intraoperative rupture of the posterior capsule with vitreous exposure [25, 26, 91, 110]. The implantation of an IOL triggers different intraocular responses including inflammation and foreign body reaction, as well as activation of the complement and coagulation cascades [83, 111–113]. These reactions along with the breakdown of the blood-aqueous barrier induced by surgery may increase cellular adhesion and lens epithelial cell (LEC) proliferation on the anterior surface of the IOL, resulting in anterior capsule phimosis, fibrosis, and posterior capsule opacification (PCO) [114]. With the advent of technologic development, many advances have been made to reduce IOL-induced reactions and to improve their biocompatibility [115]. The inflammatory response induced by IOLs is inversely related to its biocompatibility, so the higher the biocompatibility, the lower the inflammatory response [15, 83, 115]. Even though they were considered biologically inert, the first IOLs made of polymethyl-methacrylate (PMMA) were capable of producing foreign body reaction, as well as activate the complement and coagulation cascades [113, 116].

Different strategies have been used to reduce the host response, including the modification of the IOL surface by making it hydrophilic, like in heparin-coated PMMA IOLs, or hydrophobic such as surface passivated [83]. Heparin surface-modified IOLs have improved biocompatibility compared with unmodified PMMA IOLs in eyes at risk for severe postoperative inflammation, including those with uveitis [117, 118].

Foldable IOLs may be hydrophobic, including silicone IOLs or hydrophilic, and both surfaces have demonstrated to be relatively inert [114, 119]. Hydrophobic surfaces resist cell adhesion while hydrophilic ones reduce electrostatic forces and cellular adhesion, preventing the attraction of inflammatory cells and their activation, as well as adherence of fibroblasts to the IOL surface [120, 121].

Anterior capsule phimosis has been related to the degree of fibrotic reaction produced by pro-inflammatory cytokines released by residual LEC [122, 123]. Careful vacuuming the undersurface of the anterior capsule helps to reduce the number of LEC [82, 124]. Capsular phimosis has been reported more frequently with hydrogel (poly-HEMA) than acrylic, and silicone IOLs [83, 125]. Foreign body giant cell precipitates are less frequently seen in hydrophilic than on hydrophobic IOL surfaces and heparin-coated PMMA IOLs [115, 126]. The frequency of posterior capsule opacification (PCO) is highest with PMMA IOLs, less with silicone and minimal with acrylic IOLs [124, 127].

Few studies have evaluated the visual outcome following cataract surgery in uveitis with silicone IOL implantation. Overall, only 30% of eyes have achieved 20/40 of better vision with silicone IOLs, fewer than any other type of IOL [15]. Silicone was the first material available for foldable IOLs, but its use has declined particularly because it cannot be used for a monobloc open-loop designed, the preferred choice for preloaded injectors that allow implantation through small corneal incisions [128].

With the advent of acrylic foldable IOLs, the biocompatibility issue has become a minor concern, but controversy still exists of which material, hydrophilic or hydrophobic is best suitable for patients with uveitis [120, 126, 129]. Since the lens is surrounded by aqueous humor, it was thought that hydrophilic materials were more biocompatible than hydrophobic for patients with uveitis [89, 92]. However, there is insufficient evidence to determine the effects of different types of IOL materials, including hydrophobic and hydrophilic acrylic IOLs in patients with uveitis [129]. Results from the largest RCT provide only preliminary evidence that acrylic IOLs may perform better than silicone IOLs in terms of improving vision and reducing the chances of postoperative inflammation and complications [129, 130]. A large multicenter RCT with standardized outcome measurements is necessary to properly address the surgical outcome of patients with uveitic cataract.

8. Immediate postoperative management

The postoperative management is as important as the preoperative preparation and the surgical procedure itself. Since the first postoperative moments, intense topical corticosteroids (1% prednisolone acetate hourly), topical NSAIDs (anti-COX-2 selective), topical wide spectrum antibiotics (fourth generation fluoroquinolones), overnight steroid ointment, as well as mydriatic-cycloplegic combinations (e.g., 1% tropicamide + 5% phenylephrine every 6-hours × 5–7 days) should be administered [11, 24, 131]. Topical corticosteroids are wined down according to the grade of anterior chamber inflammatory reaction, the presence of glaucoma, or OHT in steroid-responders [54]. In case the patient was given systemic corticosteroids, they should be maintained at immunosuppressive levels (1 mg/kg/day) for 7–10 days before reducing them slowly to a minimum dose of 7.5 mg/day [56]. In case the patient is on immunosuppressive chemotherapy or biologic therapy, it should be continued at maintenance dose [19, 131]. Systemic anti-virals used for herpetic uveitis should be kept at therapeutic dose for 7–14 days postoperative, and then reduced to prophylactic levels (acyclovir, 600–800 mg/day and valacyclovir 500–1000 mg/day) for several weeks to months before stopping them [63, 64, 132].

9. Postoperative complications and their management

Postoperative complications after cataract surgery in patients with uveitis are relatively frequent [8]. The reported prevalence of complications is higher in ECCE than in phacoemulsification [78, 79, 133]. The risk for postoperative complications also depends on the type of uveitis and the degree of ocular involvement [8, 12, 85] (**Table 1**). Despite all preventive measurements taken before and during surgery, the most frequent and fear postoperative complication is the outburst of inflammation out of expected proportions [5]. Significant inflammation characterized by >2+ anterior chamber cells, extensive protein exudation with fibrin and plasmoid bodies formation, as well as fibrinoid membranes covering the pupil, and hypopyon may be seen [7, 19, 24, 134]. This aggressive inflammatory response is commonly associated with early postoperative iris synechiae formation and pupillary inflammatory membranes, particularly in disorders like JIA-associated uveitis, and VKH, among others [4, 6, 131, 135]. The best way to deal with this unexpected postoperative inflammatory response consists on avoiding it by previous absolute control of inflammation and the implementation of perioperative measurements discussed before. Nevertheless, in those cases in which a significant inflammatory reaction occurs, an adjustment to the systemic prednisone dose and the administration of atropine 1% will help to control the inflammation [52–54].

Other immediate postoperative complications that may be seen are hyphema and significant pigment dispersion throughout the anterior segment [19, 24]. Pigment dispersion is related to a variety of factors including, surgical trauma, small pupil, and age [24, 83, 91]. In both cases, regular tonometry is mandatory for opportune detection of severe OHT related to clogging of the trabecular meshwork by ghost cells or pigment, respectively [6]. If anti-glaucoma therapy is required, prostaglandin analogs as well as alpha-adrenergic drugs should be avoided as possible because they may exacerbate the inflammatory process [69]. In some patients with corneal stromal edema and Descemet folds due to high IOP, oral carbonic anhydrase inhibitors (e.g., acetazolamide 250 mg, 3–4 times a day) may be administered [69]. If the IOP becomes uncontrollable with medical therapy, filtration surgery or valve implantation should be considered to avoid further optic nerve damage [69, 136]. Finally, an excessive postoperative inflammatory process may produce significant vitreous opacity and membrane formation [5]. Once acute infectious endophthalmitis has been ruled out in such cases, aggressive anti-inflammatory therapy with systemic, periocular, and even intravitreal corticosteroids should be administered [52, 54, 55, 106]. If vitreous condensation and organization persist, a pars plana vitrectomy with or without intravitreal corticosteroid injection should be performed [13, 73, 75, 137].

In the late postoperative period, ocular complications are usually related with recurrent intraocular inflammation occurring from 8.3 to 53% of cases [8, 12, 85, 133]. Recurrent postoperative uveitis may produce anterior and/or posterior iris synechiae which may cause an angle or pupillary block glaucoma, respectively [69].

Certainly one of the most frequent ocular complications observed in this late period is posterior capsule opacification seen in up to 58% of cases [82, 83, 85, 124, 133]. Nd-Yag laser capsulotomy usually resolves this problem, but in some cases retrolental hyaloid-vitreous opacification or significant deposition of pigment and inflammatory debris on the IOL surface may occur therefore, recurrent low-energy Nd-Yag laser and other operative procedures may be needed for polishing the IOL [82, 138]. It must be considered that Nd-Yag laser capsulotomy in patients with uveitis is associated with a higher risk for vision-threatening complications, including OHT, CME, IOL damage or luxation, as well as retinal detachment [40, 139].

Another very important visual-threatening postoperative complication is macular edema occurring from 33 to 56% after ECCE and from 12 to 59% after phacoemulsification [12, 85, 133, 140]. The appearance of CME depends on multiple factors including the cause of uveitis and the type of surgical procedure performed [41]. Treatment of uveitic macular edema (UME) includes the administration of periocular injections of depot corticosteroids [54, 141]. However, as stated before, IVTA has shown to be superior to orbital floor injection for the treatment of UME [55, 142]. OHT is a potential complication of both types of steroid administration and should always be considered, particularly after repeated intravitreal injections [55, 108, 143]. Sustained-delivery corticosteroid devices may also be administered for this purpose [105, 106, 144]. In patients with bilateral UME, steroid-responders or those who do not accept periocular or intravitreal corticosteroid injections, oral prednisone along with oral carbonic anhydrase inhibitor (e.g., acetazolamide 250 mg every 12 hours) may be administered [54]. Epiretinal membrane formation is more commonly seen in patients with chronic

UME with a prevalence ranging from 15 to 56% [12, 145, 146]. Treatment consists of pars plana vitrectomy and internal limiting membrane delamination [73, 146, 147].

Other less common, but serious complications is retinal detachment and hypotony [5, 26]. Hypotony may be related to the retinal detachment per se, or to a low aqueous humor production due to inflammation of the ciliary process, or tractional detachment of the ciliary body due to cyclitic membrane formation [26]. Postoperative hypotony may evolve to pthisis bulbi [10, 88]. Both complications should be attended immediately by retinopexy, and/or posterior vitrectomy with cyclitic membrane and sometimes intraocular lens removal, as well as peri- or intraocular corticosteroid administration [87, 88].

10. Prognosis and visual outcome

The outcome of cataract surgery in patients with uveitis is less predictable than in other causes of cataract. Many factors may contribute to this uncertainty including, pre-existing pathologic changes, intraoperative technical challenges, the impact of postoperative exuberant inflammation, and the reversibility of postoperative complications derived from it [14]. Vision-limiting pathology related to pre-existing uveitis complications, especially macular edema and optic neuropathy are probably the major contributing factors for limited postoperative visual outcome [8, 15, 85].

Different studies suggest that visual prognosis varies according to uveitis subtypes [5, 15, 26]. For instance, the proportion of eyes achieving 20/40 or better vision is better in Fuchs uveitis and worse in Behcet's disease, VKH disease, or sympathetic ophthalmia [20, 27, 47, 148]. In general, diseases that spare the posterior segment have a better prognosis than those affecting it, particularly macular and optic nerve involvement [5, 6, 8, 85]. In addition, acute uveitic entities tend to be associated with better outcome than chronic ones [12].

Uveitic cataract surgery has been associated with worse postoperative visual acuity, higher IOP, and more than double prevalence of UME when compared with non-uveitic cataract surgery [14]. Moreover, the visual outcome following uveitic cataract extraction is not as good as that of age-related cataract surgery with the exception of Fuchs uveitis [27, 149]. Systematic reviews found a successful visual outcome (20/40 or better) in 96% of eyes with age-related cataract surgery compared to 70% in uveitic eyes undergoing either phacoemulsification or ECCE [15, 149]. ECCE and phacoemulsification seem to have similar visual outcomes compared to half less successful rate after pars plana lensectomy [15]. With respect to the comparable visual results reported between ECCE and phacoemulsification, it must be taken into account that most ECCE trials have more exclusion criteria than phacoemulsification studies, favoring better visual outcomes [15, 85, 150].

Finally, regarding IOL implantation, more eyes (71%) undergoing cataract surgery with IOL implantation than eyes left aphakic (52%) achieved a BCVA ≥ 20/40 vision postoperatively [14]. Eyes receiving acrylic IOLs or heparin surface-modified PMMA had better visual outcomes than those receiving non-heparin-PMMA or silicone IOLs [14, 15, 83, 94].

Author details

Alejandro Rodriguez-Garcia[1*] and C. Stephen Foster[2,3,4]

*Address all correspondence to: immuneye@gmail.com

1 Tecnológico de Monterrey, Escuela de Medicina y Ciencias de la Salud, Institute of Ophthalmology and Visual Sciences, Ocular Immunology and Uveitis Service, Monterrey, Mexico

2 Massachusetts Eye Research and Surgery Institute, Waltham, MA, USA

3 Ocular Immunology and Uveitis Foundation, Weston, MA, USA

4 Department of Ophthalmology, Harvard Medical School, Boston, MA, USA

References

[1] Durrani OM. Degree, duration, and causes of visual loss in uveitis. The British Journal of Ophthalmology. 2004;**88**:1159-1162

[2] Hooper PL, Rao NA, Smith RE. Cataract extraction in uveitis patients. Survey of Oph_ thalmology. 1990

[3] Urban RC, Cotlier E. Corticosteroid-induced cataracts. Survey of Ophthalmology. 1986; **31**:102-110

[4] Foster CS, Barrett FR. Cataract development and cataract surgery in patients with juvenile rheumatoid arthritis-associated iridocyclitis. Ophthalmology. 1993;**100**:809-817

[5] Elgohary MA, McCluskey PJ, Towler H, Okhravi N, Singh RP, Obikpo R, Lightman SS. Outcome of phacoemulsification in patients with uveitis. The British Journal of Ophthalmology. 2007;**91**:916-921

[6] Agrawal R, Murthy S, Ganesh SK, Phaik CS, Sangwan V, Biswas J. Cataract surgery in uveitis. International Journal of Inflammation. 2012;**2012**:1-16

[7] Foster CS, Fong LP, Singh G. Cataract surgery and intraocular lens implantation in patients with uveitis. Ophthalmlogy. 1989;**96**:281-288

[8] Yoeruek E, Deuter C, Gieselmann S, Saygili O, Spitzer MS, Tatar O, Bartz-Schmidt KU, Szurman P. Long-term visual acuity and its predictors after cataract surgery in patients with uveitis. European Journal of Ophthalmology. 2010;**20**:694-701

[9] Pershing S, Kumar A. Phacoemulsification versus extracapsular cataract extraction: Where do we stand? Current Opinion in Ophthalmology. 2011;**22**:37-42

[10] Jancevski M, Foster CS. Cataracts and uveitis. Current Opinion in Ophthalmology. 2010;**21**:10-14

[11] Foster CS, Rashid S. Management of coincident cataract and uveitis. Current Opinion in Ophthalmology. 2003;**14**:1-6

[12] Estafanous MF, Lowder CY, Meisler DM, Chauhan R. Phacoemulsification cataract extraction and posterior chamber lens implantation in patients with uveitis. American Journal of Ophthalmology. 2001;**131**:620-625

[13] Walker J, Rao NA, Ober RR, Liggett PE, Smith REA. Combined anterior and posterior approach to cataract surgery in patients with chronic uveitis. International Ophthalmology. 1993;**17**:63-69

[14] Chu CJ, Dick AD, Johnston RL, Yang YC, Denniston AK. Cataract surgery in uveitis: A multicentre database study. The British Journal of Ophthalmology. 2017;**101**:1132-1137

[15] Mehta S, Linton MM, Kempen JH. Outcomes of cataract surgery in patients with uveitis: A systematic review and meta-analysis. American Journal of Ophthalmology. 2014; **158**:676-692

[16] Rosenberg KD, Feuer WJ, Davis JL. Ocular complications of pediatric uveitis. Ophthalmology. 2004;**111**:2299-2306

[17] Thorne JE, Woreta F, Kedhar SR, Dunn JP, Jabs DA. Juvenile idiopathic arthritis-associated uveitis: Incidence of ocular complications and visual acuity loss. American Journal of Ophthalmology. 2007;**143**:840-846

[18] Thorne JE, Woreta FA, Dunn JP, Jabs DA. Risk of cataract development among children with juvenile idiopathic arthritis-related uveitis treated with topical corticosteroids. Ophthalmology. 2010;**117**:1436-1441

[19] Rojas B, Zafirakis P, Foster SC. Cataract surgery in patients with uveitis. Current Opinion in Ophthalmology. 1997;**8**:6-12

[20] Jones NP. Cataract surgery in Fuchs' heterochromic uveitis: Past, present, and future. Journal of Cataract & Refractive Surgery. 1996;**22**:261-268

[21] Loh AR, Acharya NR. Incidence rates and risk factors for ocular complications and vision loss in HLA-B27-associated uveitis. American Journal of Ophthalmology. 2010; **150**:534-542

[22] Tomkins-Netzer O, Talat L, Bar A, Lula A, Taylor SR, Joshi L, Lightman S. Long-term clinical outcome and causes of vision loss in patients with uveitis. Ophthalmology. 2014; **121**:2387-2392

[23] Niederer RL, Sharief L, Bar A, Lightman SL, Tomkins-Netzer O. Predictors of long-term visual outcome in intermediate uveitis. Ophthalmology. 2017;**124**:393-398

[24] Meier FM, Tuft SJ, Pavésio CE. Cataract surgery in uveitis. Ophthalmology Clinics of North America. 2002;**15**:365

[25] Terrada C, Julian K, Cassoux N, Prieur AM, Debre M, Quartier P, LeHoang P, Bodaghi B. Cataract surgery with primary intraocular lens implantation in children with uveitis: Long-term outcomes. Journal of Cataract & Refractive Surgery. 2011;**37**:1977-1983

[26] Quiñones K, Cervantes-Castañeda RA, Hynes AY, Daoud YJ, Foster CS. Outcomes of cataract surgery in children with chronic uveitis. Journal of Cataract & Refractive Surgery. 2009;**35**:725-731

[27] Tejwani S, Murthy S, Sangwan VS. Cataract extraction outcomes in patients with Fuchs heterochromic cyclitis. Journal of Cataract & Refractive Surgery. 2006;**32**:1678-1682

[28] Heinz C, Schoonbrood S, Heiligenhaus A. Intermediate uveitis in children and young adults: Differences in clinical course, associations and visual outcome. The British Journal of Ophthalmology. 2014;**98**:1107-1111

[29] Cuzzani OE, Ellant JP, Young PW, Gimbel HV, Rydz M. Potential acuity meter versus scanning laser ophthalmoscope to predict visual acuity in cataract patients. Journal of Cataract & Refractive Surgery. 1998;**24**:263-269

[30] Fish GE, Birch DG, Fuller DG, Straach RA. Comparison of visual function tests in eyes with maculopathy. Ophthalmology. 1986;**93**:1177-1182

[31] Gupta V, Al-Dhibi HA, Arevalo JF. Retinal imaging in uveitis. Saudi Journal of Ophthalmology. 2014;**28**:95-103

[32] Tran VT, Lehoang P, Herbort CP. Value of high-frequency ultrasound biomicroscopy in uveitis. Eye (Lond). 2001;**15**:23-30

[33] Ciardella AP, Prall FR, Borodoker N, Cunningham ET. Imaging techniques for posterior uveitis. Current Opinion in Ophthalmology. 2004;**15**:519-530

[34] Khairallah M, Jelliti B. Fluorescein angiography in uveitis. Acta Ophthalmologica. 2011; **89**(s248):0-0. DOI: 10.1111/j.1755-3768.2011.4231.x

[35] Kaines A, Tsui I, Sarraf D, Schwartz S. The use of ultra wide field fluorescein angiography in evaluation and management of uveitis. Seminars in Ophthalmology. 2009;**24**:19-24

[36] Bouchenaki N, Cimino L, Auer C, Tao Tran V, Herbort CP. Assessment and classification of choroidal vasculitis in posterior uveitis using indocyanine green angiography. Klinische Monatsblätter für Augenheilkunde. 2002;**219**:243-249

[37] Herbort CP. Fluorescein and indocyanine green angiography for uveitis. Middle East African Journal of Ophthalmology. 2009;**16**:168-187

[38] Klaeger A, Tran TV, Hiroz CA, Morisod L, Herbort CP. Indocyanine green angiography in Behcet's uveitis. Retina. 2000;**20**:309-314

[39] Hassenstein A, Bialasiewicz AA, Richard G. Optical coherence tomography in uveitis patients. American Journal of Ophthalmology. 2000;**130**:669-670

[40] Nazari H, Dustin L, Heussen FM, Sadda S, Rao NA. Morphometric spectral-domain optical coherence tomography features of epiretinal membrane correlate with visual acuity in patients with uveitis. American Journal of Ophthalmology. 2012;**154**:78-86

[41] Bélair ML, Kim SJ, Thorne JE, Dunn JP, Kedhar SR, Brown DM, Jabs DA. Incidence of cystoid macular edema after cataract surgery in patients with and without uveitis using optical coherence tomography. American Journal of Ophthalmology. 2009;**148**:128-135

[42] Copete S, Flores-Moreno I, Montero JA, Duker JS, Ruiz-Moreno JM. Direct comparison of spectral-domain and swept-source OCT in the measurement of choroidal thickness in normal eyes. The British Journal of Ophthalmology. 2014;**98**:334-338

[43] Tan CS, Cheong KX, Lim LW, Sadda SR. Comparison of macular choroidal thicknesses from swept source and spectral domain optical coherence tomography. The British Journal of Ophthalmology. 2016;**100**:995-999

[44] Chee SP, Chan SWN, Jap A. Comparison of enhanced depth imaging and swept source optical coherence tomography in assessment of choroidal thickness in Vogt-Koyanagi-Harada disease. Ocular Immunology and Inflammation. 2016;**2012**:1-5

[45] Kim M, Kim H, Kwon HJ, Kim SS, Koh HJ, Lee SC. Choroidal thickness in Behcet's uveitis: An enhanced depth imaging-optical coherence tomography and its association with angiographic changes. Investigative Ophthalmology & Visual Science. 2013;**54**: 6033-6037

[46] Nakayama M, Keino H, Okada AA, Watanabe T, Taki W, Inoue M, Hirakata A. Enhanced depth imaging optical coherence tomography of the choroid in Vogt-Koyanagi-Harada disease. Retina. 2012;**32**:2061-2069

[47] Lin CP, Yeh PT, Chen PF, Yang CM, Cataract HFR. Extraction surgery in patients with uveitis in Taiwan: Risk factors and outcomes. Journal of the Formosan Medical Association. 2014;**113**:377-384

[48] Ram J, Kaushik S, Brar GS, Gupta A, Gupta A. Phacoemulsification in patients with Fuchs' heterochromic uveitis. Journal of Cataract & Refractive Surgery. 2002;**28**:1372-1378

[49] Bonfioli AA, Curi ALL, Oréfice F. Fuchs' heterochromic cyclitis. Seminars in Ophthalmology. 2005;**20**:143-146

[50] Marak GE. Phacoanaphylactic endophthalmitis. Survey of Ophthalmology. 1992;**36**: 325-339

[51] Kerkhoff FT, Lamberts QJ, van den Biesen PR, Rothova A. Rhegmatogenous retinal detachment and uveitis. Ophthalmology 2003;**110**:427-431

[52] Rodríguez-García A. When should I consider using systemic corticosteroids to treat uveitis? Curbside Consultation in Uveitis: 49 Clinical Questions. In: Curbside Consultation in Ophthalmology Series. C. Stephen Foster (editor). SLACK Incorporated. Thorofare, NJ, USA. 2012:27-30. ISBN: 978-1-55642-998-9

[53] Meacock WR. Steroid prophylaxis in eyes with uveitis undergoing phacoemulsification. The British Journal of Ophthalmology. 2004;**88**:1122-1124

[54] Rothova A. Corticosteroids in uveitis. Ophthalmology Clinics of North America. 2002;**15**: 389-394

[55] Roesel M, Tappeiner C, Heinz C, Koch JM, Heiligenhaus A. Comparison between intravitreal and orbital floor triamcinolone acetonide after phacoemulsification in patients with endogenous uveitis. American Journal of Ophthalmology. 2009;**147**:406-412

[56] Jabs DA, Rosenbaum JT, Foster CS, Holland GN, Jaffe GJ, Louie JS, Nussenblatt RB, Stiehm ER, Tessler H, Russell NVG, Whitcup SM, Yocum D. Guidelines for the use of immunosuppressive drugs in patients with ocular inflammatory disorders: Recommendations of an expert panel. American Journal of Ophthalmology. 2000;**130**:492-513

[57] Donnenfeld ED, Perry HD, Wittpenn JR, Solomon R, Nattis A, Chou T. Preoperative ketorolac tromethamine 0.4% in phacoemulsification outcomes: Pharmacokinetic-response curve. Journal of Cataract & Refractive Surgery. 2006;**32**:1474-1482

[58] Kim SJ, Flach AJ, Jampol LM. Nonsteroidal anti-inflammatory drugs in ophthalmology. Survey of Ophthalmology. 2010;**55**:108-133

[59] Rodríguez-García A, Hernández-Camarena JC, López-Jaime GR, Nava-García JA. Effect of topical nonsteroidal anti-inflammatory drugs on pupillary size during uncomplicated cataract surgery. Journal of Refractive Surgery. 2017;**33**:236-242

[60] Kim SJ, Schoenberger SD, Thorne JE, Ehlers JP, Yeh S, Bakri SJ. Post-cataract prevention of inflammation and macular edema by steroid and nonsteroidal anti-inflammatory eye drops. Ophthalmology. 2014;**121**:1915-1924

[61] Kim SJ, Schoenberger SD, Thorne JE, Ehlers JP, Yeh S, Bakri SJ. Topical nonsteroidal anti-inflammatory drugs and cataract surgery: A report by the American Academy of Ophthalmology. Ophthalmology. 2015;**122**:2159-2168

[62] Walters T, Raizman M, Ernest P, Gayton J, Lehmann R. In vivo pharmacokinetics and in vitro pharmacodynamics of nepafenac, amfenac, ketorolac, and bromfenac. Journal of Cataract & Refractive Surgery. 2007;**33**:1539-1545

[63] Rodriguez A, Power WJ, Neves RA, Foster CS. Recurrence rate of herpetic uveitis in patients on long-term oral acyclovir. Documenta Ophthalmologica. 1995;**90**:331-340

[64] Barron BA, Gee L, Hauck WW, Kurinij N, Dawson CR, Jones DB, Wilhelmus KR, Kaufman HE, Sugar J, Hyndiuk RA, Laibson PR, Stulting D, Asbel PA. Herpetic eye disease study: A controlled trial of oral acyclovir for herpes simplex stromal keratitis. Ophthalmology. 1994;**101**:1871-1882

[65] Najjar DM, Cohen EJ, Rapuano CJ, Laibson PREDTA. Chelation for calcific band keratopathy: Results and long-term follow-up. American Journal of Ophthalmology. 2004;**137**:1056-1064

[66] Stewart OG, Morrell AJ. Management of band keratopathy with excimer phototherapeutic keratectomy: Visual, refractive, and symptomatic outcome. Eye (Lond). 2003; **17**:233-237

[67] Bohnsack BL, Freedman SF. Surgical outcomes in childhood uveitic glaucoma. American Journal of Ophthalmology. 2013;**155**:134-142

[68] Carreño E, Villarón S, Portero A, Herreras JM, Maquet JA, Calonge M. Surgical outcomes of uveitic glaucoma. Journal of Ophthalmic Inflammation and Infection. 2010;**1**:43-53

[69] Siddique SS, Suelves AM, Baheti U, Foster CS. Glaucoma and uveitis. Survey of Ophthalmology. 2013;**58**:1-10

[70] Shimizu A, Maruyama K, Yokoyama Y, Tsuda S, Ryu M, Nakazawa T. Characteristics of uveitic glaucoma and evaluation of its surgical treatment. Clinical Ophthalmology (Auckland, NZ). 2014;**8**:2383

[71] Iwao K, Inatani M, Seto T, Takihara Y, Ogata-Iwao M, Okinami S, Tanihara H. Long-term outcomes and prognostic factors for trabeculectomy with mitomycin C in eyes with uveitic glaucoma: A retrospective cohort study. Journal of Glaucoma. 2014;**23**:88-94

[72] Park UC, Ahn JK, Park KH, Phacotrabeculectomy YHG. With mitomycin C in patients with uveitis. American Journal of Ophthalmology. 2006;**142**:1005-1012

[73] Androudi S, Ahmed M, Fiore T, Brazitikos P, Foster CS. Combined pars plana vitrectomy and phacoemulsification to restore visual acuity in patients with chronic uveitis. Journal of Cataract & Refractive Surgery. 2005;**31**:472-478

[74] Soheilian M, Mirdehghan SA, Peyman GA. Sutureless combined 25-gauge vitrectomy, phacoemulsification, and posterior chamber intraocular lens implantation for management of uveitic cataract associated with posterior segment disease. Retina. 2008;**28**:941-946

[75] Pålsson S, Nyström A, Sjödell L, Jakobsson G, Byhr E, Andersson Grönlund M, Zetterberg M. Combined phacoemulsification, primary intraocular lens implantation, and pars plana vitrectomy in children with uveitis. Ocular Immunology and Inflammation. 2015; **23**:144-151

[76] Shinoda K, O'hira A, Ishida S, et al. Posterior synechia of the iris after combined pars plana vitrectomy, phacoemulsification, and intraocular lens implantation. Japanese Journal of Ophthalmology 2001;**45**:276-280

[77] Ahmad ZM, Hughes BA, Abrams GW, Mahmoud TH. Combined posterior chamber intraocular lens, vitrectomy, Retisert, and pars plana tube in noninfectious uveitis. Archives of Ophthalmology. 2012;**130**:908-913

[78] Chee SP, Ti SE, Sivakumar M, Tan D. Postoperative inflammation: Extracapsular cataract extraction versus phacoemulsication. Journal of Cataract & Refractive Surgery. 1999; **25**:1280-1285

[79] Oshika T, Yoshimura K, Miyata N. Postsurgical inflammation after phacoemulsication and extracapsular extraction with soft or conventional intraocular lens implantation. Journal of Cataract & Refractive Surgery. 1992;**18**:356-361

[80] Oetting TA, Omphroy LC. Modified technique using flexible iris retractors in clear corneal surgery. Journal of Cataract & Refractive Surgery. 2002;**28**:596-598

[81] Lam LA, Lowder CY, Baerveldt G, Smith SD, Traboulsi EI. Surgical management of cataracts in children with juvenile rheumatoid arthritis-associated uveitis. American Journal of Ophthalmology. 2003;**135**:772-778

[82] Dana MR, Chatzistefanou K, Schaumberg DA, Foster CS. Posterior capsule opacification after cataract surgery in patients with uveitis. Ophthalmology. 1997;**104**:1387-1394

[83] Rauz S, Stavrou P, Murray PI. Evaluation of foldable intraocular lenses in patients with uveitis. Ophthalmology. 2000;**107**:909-919

[84] Rahman I, Jones NP. Long-term results of cataract extraction with intraocular lens implantation in patients with uveitis. Eye (Lond). 2004;**19**:191-197

[85] Okhravi N. Assessment of visual outcome after cataract surgery in patients with uveitis. Ophthalmology. 1999;**106**:710-722

[86] Ram J, Gupta A, Kumar S, Kaushik S, Gupta N, Severia S. Phacoemulsification with intraocular lens implantation in patients with uveitis. Journal of Cataract & Refractive Surgery. 2010;**36**:1283-1288

[87] Adán A, Gris O, Pelegrín L, Torras J, Corretger X. Explantation of intraocular lenses in children with juvenile idiopathic arthritis-associated uveitis. Journal of Cataract & Refractive Surgery. 2009;**35**:603-605

[88] Foster CS, Stavrou P, Zafirakis P, Rojas B, Tesavibul N, Baltatzis S. Intraocular lens removal from [corrected] patients with uveitis. American Journal of Ophthalmology. 1999;**128**:31-37

[89] Abela-Formanek C, Amon M, Schild G, Schauersberger J, Kolodjaschna J, Barisani-Asenbaum T, Kruger A. Inflammation after implantation of hydrophilic acrylic, hydrophobic acrylic, or silicone intraocular lenses in eyes with cataract and uveitis: Comparison to a control group. Journal of Cataract & Refractive Surgery. 2002;**28**:1153-1159

[90] Lam DS, Law RW, Wong AK. Phacoemulsification, primary posterior capsulorhexis, and capsular intraocular lens implantation for uveitic cataract. Journal of Cataract & Refractive Surgery. 1998;**24**:1111-1118

[91] Holland GN, Van Horn SD, Margolis TP. Cataract surgery with ciliary sulcus fixation of intraocular lenses in patients with uveitis. American Journal of Ophthalmology. 1999;**128**:21-30

[92] Papaliodis GN, Nguyen QD, Samson CM, Foster CS. Intraocular lens tolerance in surgery for cataracta complicata: Assessment of four implant materials. Seminars in Ophthalmology. 2002;**17**:120-123

[93] Diamond JG, Kaplan HJ. Uveitis: Effect of vitrectomy combined with lensectomy. Ophthalmology. 1979;**86**:1320-1327

[94] Tomlins PJ, Sivaraj RR, Rauz S, Denniston AK, Murray PI. Long-term biocompatibility and visual outcomes of a hydrophilic acrylic intraocular lens in patients with uveitis. Journal of Cataract & Refractive Surgery. 2014;**40**:618-625

[95] Magli A, Forte R, Rombetto L, Alessio M. Cataract management in juvenile idiopathic arthritis: Simultaneous versus secondary intraocular lens implantation. Ocular Immunology and Inflammation. 2014;**22**:133-137

[96] Nemet AY, Raz J, Sachs D, Friling R, Neuman R, Kramer M, Suresh K, Oandi MD, Vidushi S, Assia EI. Primary intraocular lens implantation in pediatric uveitis: A comparison of 2 populations. Archives of Ophthalmology. 2007;**125**:354-360

[97] Ganesh SK, Sudharshan S. Phacoemulsification with intraocular lens implantation in juvenile idiopathic arthritis. Ophthalmic Surgery, Lasers & Imaging. 2010;**41**:104-108

[98] Kotaniemi K, Penttila H. Intraocular lens implantation in patients with juvenile idiopathic arthritis-associated uveitis. Ophthalmic Research. 2006;**38**:318-323

[99] Probst LE, Holland EJ. Intraocular lens implantation in patients with juvenile rheumatoid arthritis. American Journal of Ophthalmology. 1996;**122**:161-170

[100] Lundvall A, Zetterström C. Cataract extraction and intraocular lens implantation in children with uveitis. The British Journal of Ophthalmology. 2000;**84**:791-793

[101] Grajewski RS, Zurek-Imhoff B, Roesel M, Heinz C, Heiligenhaus A. Favourable outcome after cataract surgery with IOL implantation in uveitis associated with juvenile idiopathic arthritis. Acta Ophthalmologica. 2011;**90**:657-662

[102] Okhravi N, Morris A, Kok HS, Menezo V, Dowler JG, Hykin PG, Lightman S. Intraoperative use of intravitreal triamcinolone in uveitic eyes having cataract surgery: Pilot study. Journal of Cataract & Refractive Surgery. 2007;**33**:1278-1283

[103] Dada T, Dhawan M, Garg S, Nair S, Mandal S. Safety and efficacy of intraoperative intravitreal injection of triamcinolone acetonide after phacoemulsification in cases of uveitic cataract. Journal of Cataract & Refractive Surgery. 2007;**33**:1613-1618

[104] van Kooij B, Rothova A, de Vries P. The pros and cons of intravitreal triamcinolone injections for uveitis and inflammatory cystoid macular edema. Ocular Immunology and Inflammation. 2006;**14**:73-85

[105] Larochelle MB, Smith J, Dacey MS. Dexamethasone intravitreal implant in the treatment of uveitic macular edema in the perioperative cataract setting: A case series. American Journal of Ophthalmology. 1999;**166**:149-153

[106] Chieh JJ, Carlson AN, Jaffe GJ. Combined fluocinolone acetonide intraocular delivery system insertion, phacoemulsification, and intraocular lens implantation for severe uveitis. American Journal of Ophthalmology. 2008;**146**:589-594

[107] Arcinue CA, Cerón OM, Foster CSA. Comparison between the fluocinolone acetonide (Retisert) and dexamethasone (Ozurdex) intravitreal implants in uveitis. Journal of Ocular Pharmacology and Therapeutics. 2013;**29**:501-507

[108] Kiddee W, Trope GE, Sheng L, Beltran-Agullo L, Smith M, Strungaru MH, Baath J, Buys YM. Intraocular pressure monitoring post intravitreal steroids: A systematic review. Survey of Ophthalmology. 2013;**58**:291-310

[109] Shah SP, Yarian DL, Prenner J, Friedman ES, Wheatley ES, Fine HF, Mantopoulos D, Roth DB. One-year results of fluocinolone acetonide intravitreal implant for diabetic macular edema in highly treated eyes. Presented at: American Society of Retina Specialists 35th Annual Meeting, Boston, MA. 11-15 August 2017

[110] Holland GN. Intraocular lens implantation in patients with juvenile rheumatoid arthritis-associated uveitis: An unresolved management issue. American Journal of Ophthalmology. 2014;**122**:255-257

[111] Apple DJ. Influence of intraocular lens material and design on postoperative intracapsular cellular reactivity. Transactions of the American Ophthalmological Society. 2000;**98**:257-283

[112] Mondino BJ, Nagata S, Glovsky MM. Activation of the alternative complement pathway by intraocular lenses. Investigative Ophthalmology & Visual Science. 1985;**26**:905-908

[113] Sievers H, von Domarus D. Foreign-body reaction against intraocular lenses. American Journal of Ophthalmology. 1984;**97**:743-751

[114] Majima K. An evaluation of the biocompatibility of intraocular lenses. Ophthalmic Surgery, Lasers and Imaging. 1996;**27**:946-951

[115] Amon M, Menapace R. In vivo documentation of cellular reactions on lens surfaces for assessing the biocompatibility of different intraocular implants. Eye (Lond). 1994; **8**:649-656

[116] Mondino BJ, Rajacich GM. Comparison of complement activation by silicone intraocular lenses and polymethyl-methacrylate intraocular lenses with polypropylene loops. Archives of Ophthalmology. 1987;**105**:989-990

[117] Stavrou P, Murray PI. Heparin surface modified intraocular lenses in uveitis. Ocular Immunology and Inflammation. 1994;**2**:161-168

[118] Percival P. Use of heparin-modified lenses in high-risk cases for uveitis. Developments in Ophthalmology. 1991;**22**:80-83

[119] Kang S, Kim MJ, Park SH, Joo CK. Comparison of clinical results between heparin surface modified hydrophilic acrylic and hydrophobic acrylic intraocular lens. European Journal of Ophthalmology. 2008;**18**:377-383

[120] Ravalico G, Baccara F, Lovisato A, Tognetto D. Postoperative cellular reaction on various intraocular lens materials. Ophthalmology. 1997;**104**:1084-1091

[121] Umezawa S, Shimizu K. Biocompatibility of surface-modified intraocular lenses. Journal of Cataract & Refractive Surgery. 1993;**19**:371-374

[122] Kurosaka D, Ando I, Kato K, Oshima T, Kurosaka H, Yoshino M, Nagamoto T, Ando N. Capsule contraction syndrome. Journal of Cataract & Refractive Surgery. 1999; **25**:930-935

[123] Nishi O, Nishi K, Imanishi M, Tada Y, Shirasawa E. Effect of the cytokines on the prostaglandin E2 synthesis by lens epithelial cells of human cataracts. The British Journal of Ophthalmology. 1995;**79**:934-938

[124] Hollick EJ, Spalton DJ, Ursell PG, Meacock WR, Barman SA, Boyce JF. Posterior capsular opacification with hydrogel, polymethylmethacrylate, and silicone intraocular lenses: Two-year results of a randomized prospective trial. American Journal of Ophthalmology. 2000;**129**:577-584

[125] Lüke C, Dietlein TS, Jacobi PC, Konen W, Krieglstein GK. Massive anterior capsule shrinkage after plate-haptic silicone lens implantation in uveitis. Journal of Cataract & Refractive Surgery. 2001;**27**:333-336

[126] Hollick EJ, Spalton DJ, Ursell PG, Pande MV. Biocompatibility of poly (methyl-methacrylate), silicone, and AcrySof intraocular lenses: Randomized comparison of the cellular reaction on the anterior lens surface. Journal of Cataract & Refractive Surgery. 1998;**24**:361-366

[127] Hollick EJ, Spalton DJ, Ursell PG, Pande MV, Barman SA, Boyce JF, Tilling K. The effect of polymethylmethacrylate, silicone, and polyacrylic intraocular lenses on posterior capsular opacification 3 years after cataract surgery. Ophthalmology. 1999;**106**:49-55

[128] Bellucci R. An introduction to intraocular lenses: Material, optics, haptics, design and aberration. In: Cataract. ESASO Course Series. Güell JL, editor. Basel, Karger; 2013;**3**:38-55. ISBN: 978-3-318-02410-4 (Print) eISBN: 978-3-318-02411-1 (Online). https://doi.org/10.1159/000350902

[129] Leung TG, Lindsley K, Kuo IC. Types of intraocular lenses for cataract surgery in eyes with uveitis. Cochrane Database of Systematic Reviews. 2014;(3):CD007284. DOI:10.1002/14651858.CD007284.pub2

[130] Alio JL, Chipont E, BenEzra D, Fakhry MA, International Ocular Inflammation Society, Study Group of Uveitic Cataract Surgery. Comparative performance of intraocular lenses in eyes with cataract and uveitis. Journal of Cataract & Refractive Surgery. 2002;**28**:2096-2108

[131] Foster CS, Vitale AT. Cataract surgery in uveitis. Ophthalmology Clinics of North America. 1993;**6**:139-146

[132] Schuster AK, Harder BC, Schlichtenbrede FC, Jarczok MN, Tesarz J. Valacyclovir versus acyclovir for the treatment of herpes zoster ophthalmicus in immunocompetent patients. Cochrane Database of Systematic Reviews. 2016;**11**:CD011503

[133] Krishna R. Long-term follow-up of extracapsular cataract extraction and posterior chamber intraocular lens implantation in patients with uveitis. Ophthalmology. 1998;**105**:1765-1769

[134] Pande MV, Spalton DJ, Kerr-Muir MG, Marshall J. Postoperative inflammatory response to phacoemulsification and extracapsular cataract surgery: Aqueous flare and cells. Journal of Cataract & Refractive Surgery. 1996;**22**(Suppl 1):770-774

[135] Moorthy RS, Rajeev B, Smith RE, Rao NA. Incidence and management of cataracts in Vogt-Koyanagi-Harada syndrome. American Journal of Ophthalmology. 2014;**118**:197-204

[136] Merayo-Lloves J, Power WJ, Rodriguez A, Pedroza-Seres M, Foster CS. Secondary glaucoma in patients with uveitis. Ophthalmologica. 1999;**213**:300-304

[137] Kiryu J, Kita M, Tanabe T, Yamashiro K, Miyamoto N, Ieki Y. Pars plana vitrectomy for cystoid macular edema secondary to sarcoid uveitis. Ophthalmology. 2001;**108**:1140-1144

[138] Liesegang TJ, Bourne WM, Ilstrup DM. Secondary surgical and neodymium-YAG laser discissions. American Journal of Ophthalmology. 1985;**100**:510-519

[139] Steinert RF, Puliafito CA, Kumar SR, Dudak SD, Patel S. Cystoid macular edema, retinal detachment, and glaucoma after Nd:YAG laser posterior capsulotomy. American Journal of Ophthalmology. 1991;**112**:373-380

[140] Ganesh SK, Babu K, Biswas J. Phacoemulsification with intraocular lens implantation in cases of pars planitis. Journal of Cataract & Refractive Surgery. 2004;**30**:2072-2076

[141] Choudhry S, Ghosh S. Intravitreal and posterior subtenon triamcinolone acetonide in idiopathic bilateral uveitic macular oedema. Clinical & Experimental Ophthalmology. 2007;**35**:713-718

[142] Maca SM, Abela-Formanek C, Kiss CG, Sacu SG, Benesch T, Barisani-Asenbauer T. Intravitreal triamcinolone for persistent cystoid macular oedema in eyes with quiescent uveitis. Clinical & Experimental Ophthalmology. 2009;**37**:389-396

[143] Young S, Larkin G, Branley M, Lightman S. Safety and efficacy of intravitreal triamcinolone for cystoid macular oedema in uveitis. Clinical & Experimental Ophthalmology. 2001;**29**:2-6

[144] Cunningham Jr ET, de Smet MD, Yeh S, Albini TA, Zierhut M. Sustained-release corticosteroids for uveitis. Ocular Immunology and Inflammation 2015;**23**:421-424

[145] Gilbert C, Hiscott P, Unger W, Grierson I, McLeod D. Inflammation and the formation of epiretinal membranes. Eye (Lond). 1988;**2**(Suppl 6):144-156

[146] Dev S, Mieler WF, Pulido JS, Mittra RA. Visual outcomes after pars plana vitrectomy for epiretinal membranes associated with pars planitis. Ophthalmology. 1999;**106**:1086-1090

[147] Radetzky S, Walter P, Fauser S, Koizumi K, Kirchhof B, Joussen AM. Visual outcome of patients with macular edema after pars plana vitrectomy and indocyanine green-assisted peeling of the internal limiting membrane. Graefe's Archive for Clinical and Experimental Ophthalmology. 2004;**242**:273-278

[148] Berker N, Soykan E, Elgin U, Ozkan SS. Phacoemulsification cataract extraction and intraocular lens implantation in patients with Behcet's disease. Ophthalmic Surgery, Lasers & Imaging Retina. 2004;**35**:215-218

[149] Powe NR, Schein OD, Gieser SC. Synthesis of the literature on visual acuity and complications following cataract extraction with intraocular lens implantation. Archives of Ophthalmology. 1994;**112**:239-252

[150] Foster RE, Lowder CY, Meisler DM, Zakov ZN. Extracapsular cataract extraction and posterior chamber intraocular lens implantation in uveitis patients. Ophthalmology. 1992;**99**:1234-1241

[151] Tugal-Tutkun I, Ötük-Yasar B, Altinkurt E. Clinical features and prognosis of herpetic anterior uveitis: A retrospective study of 111 cases. International Ophthalmology. 2010;**30**:559-565

[152] Miserocchi E, Waheed NK, Dios E, Christen W, Merayo J, Roque M, Foster CS. Visual outcome in herpes simplex virus and varicella zoster virus uveitis: A clinical evaluation and comparison. Ophthalmology. 2002;**109**:1532-1537

[153] Marsh RJ, Cooper M. Ocular surgery in ophthalmic zoster. Eye (Lond). 1989;**3**:313-317

[154] Kaufman AH, Foster CS. Cataract extraction in patients with pars planitis. Ophthalmology. 1993;**100**:1210-1217

[155] Tugal-Tutkun I, Onal S, Altan-Yaycioglu R, Altunbas HH, Urgancioglu M. Uveitis in Behçet disease: An analysis of 880 patients. Ophthalmology. 2004;**138**:373-380

[156] Kadayifçilar S, Gedik Ş, Eldem B, İrkeç M. Cataract surgery in patients with Behçet's disease. Journal of Cataract & Refractive Surgery. 2002;**28**:316-320

[157] Ganesh SK, Babu K, Biswas J. Cataract surgery in patients with Vogt-Koyanagi-Harada syndrome. Journal of Cataract & Refractive Surgery. 2004;**30**:95-100

[158] Ganesh SK, Sundaram PM, Biswas J, Babu K. Cataract surgery in sympathetic ophthalmia. Journal of Cataract & Refractive Surgery. 2004;**30**:2371-2376

[159] Akova YA, Foster CS. Cataract surgery in patients with sarcoidosis-associated uveitis. Ophthalmology. 1994;**101**:473-479

10

FM Continuous Monitoring of Intraocular Pressure: An Engineering Perspective

Adrian E. Rendon-Nava,

Alejandro Díaz-Méndez and Luis Nino-de-Rivera

Abstract

This chapter discusses the problem of continuously monitoring intraocular pressure (IOP) from an engineering perspective. It is aimed to all public in general although we think that medical staff and engineers may benefit the most from it. Although equations are included for engineers to get a glimpse of how the system works, this chapter does not go into great detail in mathematics and physics to make it understandable to medical staff. It provides though references for engineers who wish to get a better understanding of key subjects tackled in this chapter. The chapter is organized as follows: Section 1 introduces intraocular pressure (IOP) and need for its continuous monitoring. Section 2 describes the most recent efforts to develop a continuous IOP monitoring system. Section 3 shows what medical and engineering considerations must be taken into account to effectively measure IOP. Section 4 deals with health issues due to tissue warming and how to prevent them. Section 5 explains how an implant can be fabricated using either passive electronic components or active ones. Finally, Section 6 explains how the pressure sensor and the electronic circuits can be integrated.

Keywords: biomedical implants, IOP monitoring, magnetic coupling, wireless coupling, wireless power transmission

1. Introduction

Before we can begin to talk about intraocular pressure (IOP) continuous monitoring, let us have a look at some key facts according to the World Health Organization (WHO) [1]:

- There are 285 million people estimated to be visually impaired worldwide, of which 246 million have low vision.
- About 90% of the visually impaired people globally live in low-income environments.
- Eighty per cent of all visual impairment can be prevented or cured.

Among the three major causes globally that cause visual impairment is glaucoma. Glaucoma can be understood as a group of ocular diseases mainly associated with a rise in intraocular pressure. All these groups of diseases have in common the progressive injury to the optic nerve [2]. If glaucoma is left untreated, it can cause total blindness.

The problem with diseases such as glaucoma is that they present no symptoms, so trying to diagnose it without previously measuring the IOP becomes a real challenge. Actual methods for IOP measurement involve the use of medical equipment called tonometers. Tonometers measure IOP over the cornea but in some cases, where the hardness of the cornea is above normal standards, important measurement errors can be produced which do not allow a correct IOP estimation.

There are nowadays other indirect methods that have been under research in the last years such as multifocal electroretinography to know the effects of IOP rising [3]. Nevertheless, with available tonometry and electroretinography techniques, it is not possible to take measurements during normal activities of the patient such as the sleep cycle, stage where IOP can be increased in a significant manner. In order to take an IOP measurement with tonometry or multifocal electroretinography methods, the measurement must be taken by qualified personnel which implies that the patient has to be in the hospital facilities.

The development of sensors with the capacity of measuring IOP inside the eyeball is of paramount importance in order to know with all precision not only intraocular pressure values but also IOP variations in daily activities of the patients.

A new measurement instrument is needed that allows medical staff to study the aetiology of diseases such as glaucoma, that is, to provide with a new tool which will enable to know if there is a cause-effect relationship between daily activities of patients and IOP variations in real time.

Fortunately, we are at a point where technology has evolved in such a way that biomedical implants wirelessly powered are now a reality.

2. State of the art

There have been many efforts in different parts of the world over time to build an IOP monitoring system. In this section, we only present a few researches to give the reader a broad idea of what has been done in terms of IOP monitoring systems but references [4–8] are included in case the reader wants to know more about researches not mentioned in this chapter.

Between the first researches carried out, there is the one done by Tufte et al. when in 1962 in Honeywell, they developed piezoresistive sensors with silicon membranes [9].

In 2000, Mokwa, Schnakenberg and collaborators proposed the design and fabrication of an implantable intraocular system for continuous IOP measurement through OPHTAL project [10]. The system consisted of a pressure sensor connected to the integrated circuits altogether in an artificial contact lens. Three prototypes were fabricated. The last one is shown in **Figure 1**.

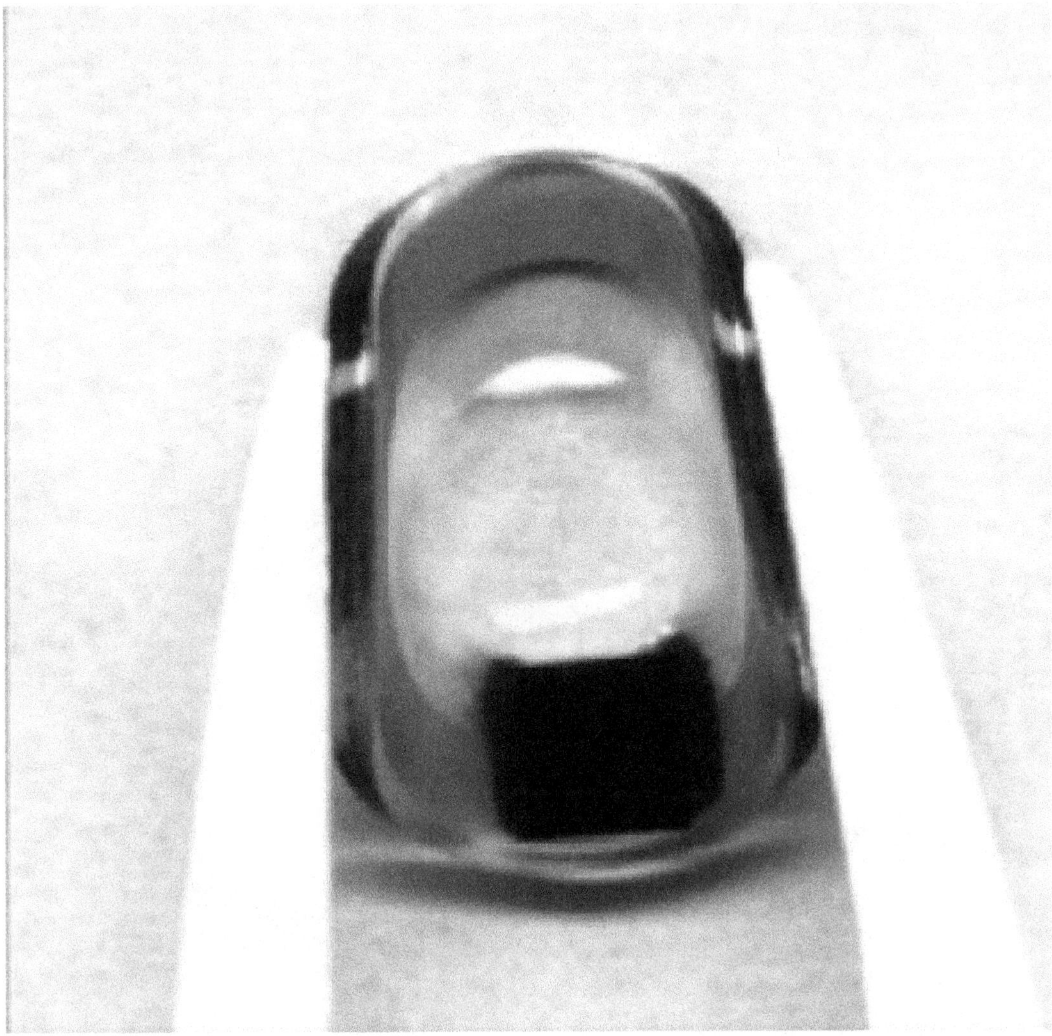

Figure 1. Third pressure sensor prototype.

Humayun and collaborators proposed in 2008 a prototype sensor to measure IOP [11]. Two sensor designs were fabricated, one with a variable capacitor and the other one with a variable capacitor and a variable inductor (**Figure 2**).

The pressure sensor response showed a high sensitivity (>7000 ppm/mmHg) in both designs, confirming a resolution of less than 1 mmHg for biomedical applications. The authors also conducted a 6-month study in animals to verify the implant bio-stability *in vivo* and no surgical or post-operation complications were found.

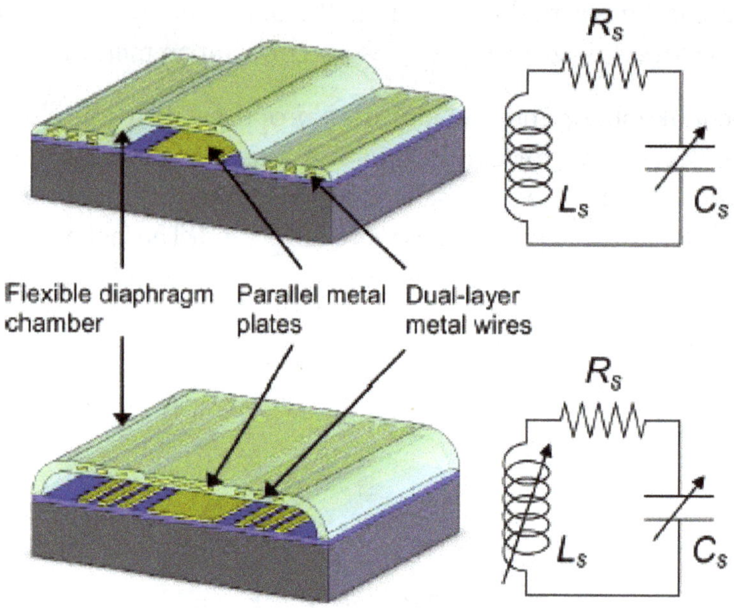

Figure 2. Sensor design variations (cross-sectional view).

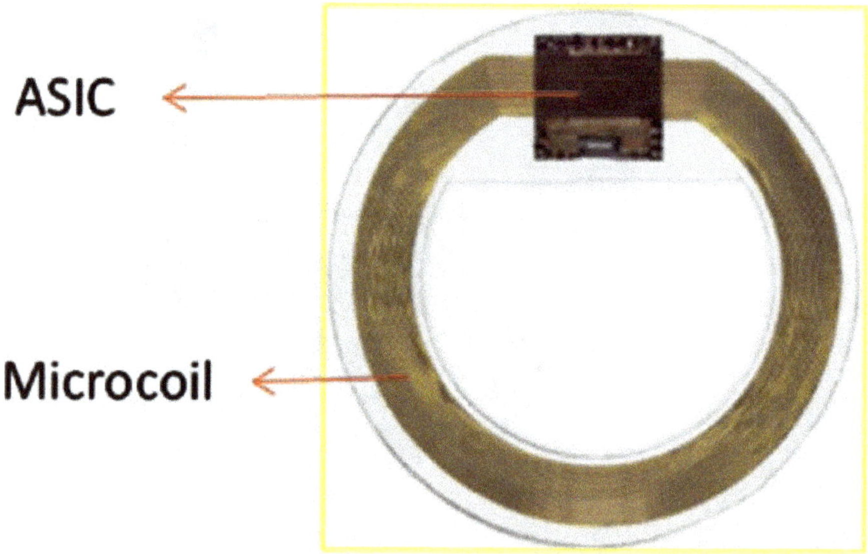

Figure 3. Sensor device.

In 2011, Melki and collaborators published a study with the purpose of determining the biocompatibility of an IOP sensor in rabbits and comparing IOP measurements from the sensor with other IOP sensor devices [12]. **Figure 3** shows the photograph of the sensor encapsulated in a silicon rubber.

The intraocular sensor was implanted in six New Zealand white rabbits. The upper part of the sensor contains the Application-Specific Integrated Circuit (ASIC). The external diameter of the coil was of 11.3 mm, the inner diameter was of 7 mm and the thickness was of 0.9 mm.

The animals were observed and examined in intervals of up to 25 months after surgery. From the obtained results, it was found that the sensor had acceptable tolerance by the eye of the rabbit since no evidence of significant inflammation or scar formation was observed in *in vivo* tests. The measurements made with pneumotonometry, tonometry and with the sensor resulted in standard deviations of 2.70, 3.35 and 0.81 mmHg, respectively.

3. Merging medicine and engineering

As seen in the previous section, all efforts to build a continuous IOP monitoring system proposed a wireless power transmission method. This obeys to the fact that having a battery inside the eye to power the biomedical implant can be both bulky and most importantly health threatening to the patient due to the hazardous chemicals it contains.

If we are to develop a continuous IOP monitoring system, we need to approach the problem with a multidisciplinary focus.

3.1. Medical considerations

The human eyeball measures approximately 2.5 cm in diameter so there is a restriction in terms of the maximum area that the implant can have to be successfully implanted in the patient. Among medical factors that come into play for implanting a continuous IOP monitoring system are the following:

- The location of the implant must not interfere with the vision and movement of the eye.
- Surgery should be as less invasive as possible.
- Implant design must be such that it allows the physician to implant the monitoring system in the shortest time possible.

3.1.1. Electromagnetic radiation

At frequencies between 10 MHz and 30 GHz, organic tissue warming is the major effect in electromagnetic energy absorption and temperature increases of more than 1 or 2°C can have adverse health effects [13].

A great number of physiological effects have been observed in cellular studies and with animals when electromagnetic energy is absorbed in levels that cause an increment in body temperature of more than 1 or 2°C [14]. These effects include alterations in neural and neuromuscular functions, increased permeability of the blood-brain barrier, ocular damage, changes in the immune system associated with stress, haematological changes, reproductive changes and changes in cell morphology.

Experimental data available indicate that human exposition in a resting position to electromagnetic fields for 30 min, which produce a specific absorption rate (SAR) in the whole body of 1–4 W kg^{-1}, will result in an increase of temperature of less than 1°C. Exposition to electromagnetic fields more intense producing SAR values of more than 4 W kg^{-1} may overwhelm the thermoregulatory capacity of the body and produce warming tissue harmful levels. **Table 1** shows basic restrictions for exposure to time-varying electric and magnetic fields for frequencies up to 10 GHz.

Nature of the exposition	Frequency range	Current density for head and trunk (mA·m^{-2}) (rms)	SAR average for the whole body (W·kg^{-1})	Localized SAR (head and trunk) (W·kg^{-1})	Localized SAR (limbs) (W·kg^{-1})
Occupational exposure	Up to 1 Hz	40	---	---	---
	1–4 Hz	40/*f*	---	---	---
	4 Hz to 1 kHz	10	---	---	---
	1–100 kHz	*f*/100	---	---	---
	100 kH to ·10 MHz	*f*/100	0.4	10	20
	10 MHz to 10 GHz	---	0.4	10	20
General public exposure	Up to 1 Hz	8	---	---	---
	1–4 Hz	8/*f*	---	---	---
	4 Hz to 1 kHz	2	---	---	---
	1–100 kHz	*f*/500	---	---	---
	100 kH to ·10 MHz	*f*/500	0.08	2	4
	10 MHz to 10 GHz	---	0.08	2	4

Table 1. Basic restrictions for time-varying electric and magnetic fields exposition for frequencies up to 10 GHz.

3.2. Engineering considerations

Regarding technological restrictions for the localization of the implant, we can find the following:

- The implant must have the maximum area possible.
- The implant should be placed as near as possible from the exterior of the body.

Both of the previous considerations are based on the fact that the implant needs to maximize power transfer and magnetic coupling.

IOP measurement requires the size of the implant not to be so large neither so bulky so it can be implanted into the eye of the patient without causing any discomfort. This is the reason why several IOP monitoring systems are based on radiofrequency identification (RFID) technology [15].

Given that power consumption is a key factor in IOP monitoring system design, we may classify electronic implants based on their power consumption briefly as described below.

3.2.1. *Active electronic implant*

An active electronic implant will have active electronic components such as diodes and transistors. By using active electronic components, there is the drawback of higher power consumption. On the other hand, by using transistors and diodes the electronic implant would have the advantage of having more precise and reliable pressure measurements.

3.2.2. *Passive electronic implant*

The passive option consists of having pure passive electronic components (resistors, capacitors and inductors). The main advantage of this proposal is that power demand would be much lower than its active counterpart so a possible health risk in the patient due to tissue warming is greatly reduced.

Both types of implants will be discussed in more detail in Section 5.

4. Health issues due to tissue warming

A vital requirement when designing electronic implants is to limit temperature increment of the implant in order to prevent damaging organic tissue. In general, temperature variation in a body can be described by a partial differential equation of heat conduction which expresses the variation in the temperature of a body with respect of time, but in order for this equation to be used in human tissue, Pennes incorporated a few extra terms into the partial differential heat conduction equation to describe the warming effect of basal metabolism and the influence of blood in temperature regulation of tissue [16]. Pennes bio-heat equation can be written as follows:

$$C\rho\frac{\partial T}{\partial t} = \nabla\cdot\left(K\nabla T\right) + A - B\left(T - T_b\right) \tag{1}$$

where A is the heat production rate due to metabolic processes per volume unit, B is the perfusion constant and T_b is the blood temperature (it is assumed as a constant at $T_b = 37°C$).

The bio-heat equation may be applied to human tissue without any external sources of heat. For our case of study, however, the temperature increase in human tissue is also caused by power dissipation of the electronic implant and by electromagnetic radiation coming from the external device that will be supplying wireless power to the implant.

4.1. Joule heating

When considering an electronic implant inside the human body, power dissipation by electronic circuitry has to be considered. Assuming that heat dissipation per volume unit of an implant is P_i, this can be incorporated in the bio-heat equation as a source of heat and is expressed as

$$P_i = V_i * I_i \tag{2}$$

where V_i is the biasing voltage of the electronic circuitry and I_i is the total electric current circulating through the implant.

4.2. Electromagnetic energy contribution

If a biological tissue is exposed to electromagnetic radiation, the electric field E and the magnetic field H penetrate the tissue causing it to warm up due to electromagnetic deposit. On the other hand, SAR is the specific absorption rate and it is defined as the differential with respect of time, of the increment of dissipated energy by a material. The SAR is related with the magnitude of the electric field $|E|$ so, once we know the electric field distribution in the tissue, we can obtain the SAR from which we can obtain the generated heat per volume unit per time unit to include the term to the bio-heat equation.

In order to have a complete bio-heat equation, we need to include Joule heating and electromagnetic energy contribution. The complete bio-heat equation can be expressed as

$$C\rho\frac{\partial T}{\partial t} = \nabla\cdot(K\nabla T) + A - B(T - T_b) + \rho SAR + P_i \tag{3}$$

Eq. (3) needs to be solved for each particular case of study to know how many degrees of temperature will the tissue increase caused by the implant. For the graphic shown in **Figure 4**, Eq. (3) was solved using Matlab software. **Figure 4** shows a graphic of how an electronic implant heats the tissue of the sclera when exposed to an electromagnetic energy radiation and joule heating. Details of the implant design and characteristics are shown in **Table 2**.

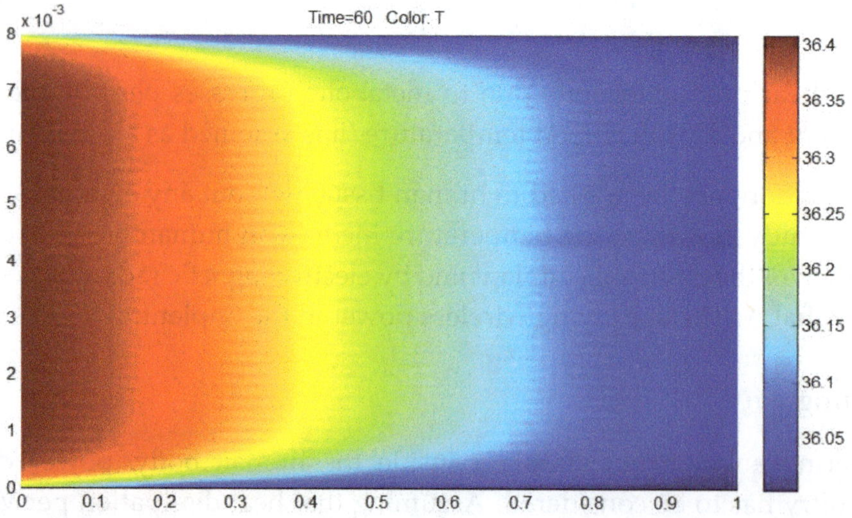

Figure 4. Warming graphic of the sclera. Exposition time: 60 s.

Parameter	Value
Number of turns	18
Metal thickness	0.035 mm
Inner radius	1 mm
Outer radius	10 mm
Width of metal tracks	0.25 mm
Distance between tracks	0.25 mm
Resistance	150 Ω
Inductance	7.84 μH
Quality factor (Q)	3.28

Table 2. Proposed electrical parameters for the simulated reader coil.

5. Implant fabrication with passive and active electronic circuits

As stated in Section 3, we can classify electronic implants based on the nature of their components. Next, we describe both options.

5.1. Passive RLC implant

For this kind of approach, an Resistive Inductive Capacitive (RLC) passive circuit is proposed as an IOP sensor like the one shown in **Figure 5**. The capacitor would be a variable capacitor, sensitive to variations in pressure.

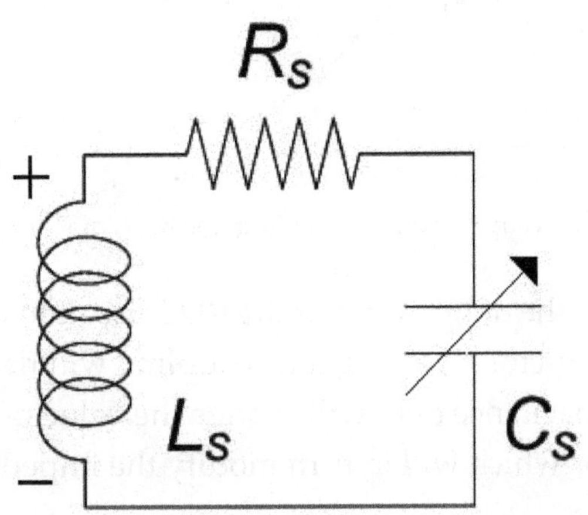

Figure 5. Electric diagram of the circuit proposed as an IOP sensor.

The resonance frequency of the RLC circuit shown in **Figure 5** is given by Eq. (4) where we can note that if the value of capacitance varies, the resonance frequency of the circuit will change too.

$$f = \frac{1}{2\pi\sqrt{L_S C_S}} \tag{4}$$

From electromagnetic theory, we know that if we place two inductors close enough and we make a time-varying electric current circulate through one of the coils, it will induce a voltage in the other coil. This is the principle by which wireless energy transfer is done. **Figure 6** shows a Maxwell-Wien circuit which could act as the external device in charge of both delivering power to the implant and reading data from it.

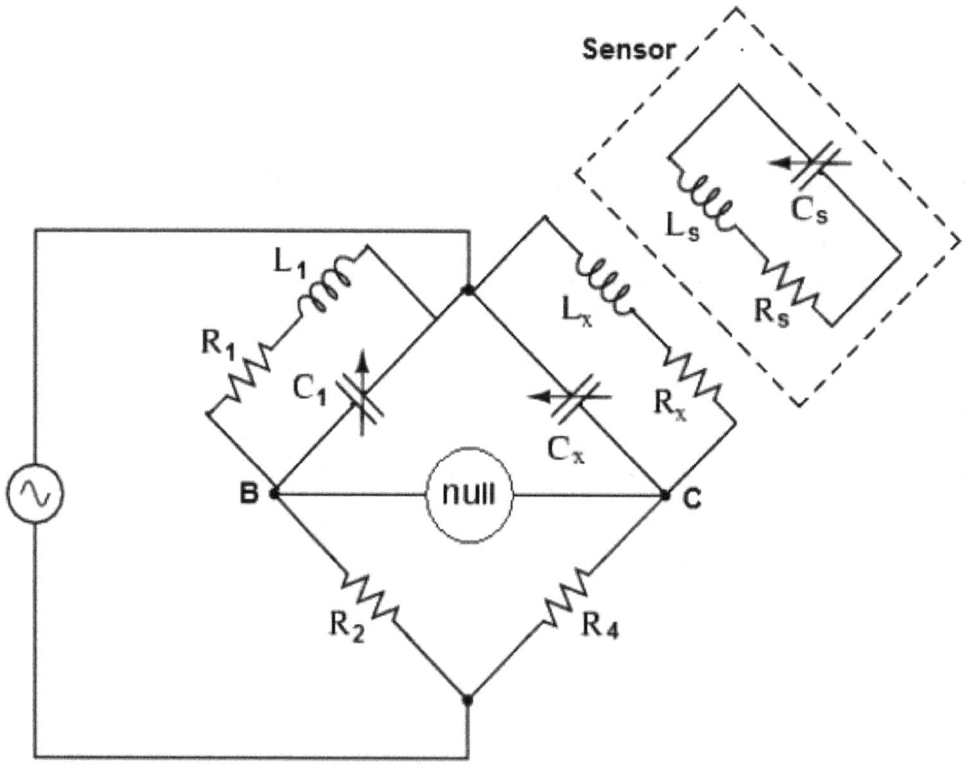

Figure 6. Maxwell-Wien bridge circuit coupled with the coil from the implant.

The implant is shown inside the dotted lines. If the RLC circuit in the implant formed by R_s, L_s and C_s is placed near the inductor L_x, a magnetic coupling will be created. By being L_x and L_s coupled, a change in the capacitance of C_s will change the value of the resonance frequency of the RLC circuit of the sensor which will in turn modify the impedance of L_x coil.

Eq. (5) shows how the impedance of the external device coil will vary by being coupled with the coil of the implant [17]

$$Z_x = j2\pi f L_x \left[1 + k^2 \frac{\left(\frac{f}{f_0}\right)^2}{1 - \left(\frac{f}{f_0}\right)^2 + \frac{1}{Q} j \frac{f}{f_0}} \right] \tag{5}$$

where f is the resonance frequency of the external device, k is the coupling factor between both coils, Q is given by

$$Q = 2\pi f_0 L_s / R_s \tag{6}$$

And f_0 is the resonance frequency of the implant described previously in Eq. (4).

The main disadvantage for this approach is the lack of precision and accuracy in the measurements. If we were to obtain precise and accurate measurements with a very small error, then both coils would have to be at the exact same place each time a measurement is to be taken. We could assume that the implant is always fixed so in order to make this kind of approach to work properly, the system design must be done to ensure that the coils will remain in the same position for each measurement and no misalignment will occur.

Another important issue to be noted is the transmission medium between coils. So far, we have considered air as the transmission medium between coils. Much more realistic calculations and simulations may be performed if organic tissue is considered as the transmission medium [18].

5.2. Electronic implant using transistors

Designing an electronic implant using transistors needs special care since they require a much larger amount of power compared to passive RLC implants. Electronic circuit design must be done in such a way that warming of the tissue does not exceed 1°C to avoid organic tissue damage. Tissue warming is the main disadvantage of designing electronic implants using transistors. On the other hand, they are very precise and accurate since measurements depend only on having enough power available in the implant rather than if the coils are misaligned or not.

The active electronic circuit for the implant can be divided into three sub-modules, which are reviewed below.

5.2.1. Rectifier and regulator circuit

As mentioned in Section 5.1, a time-varying electric current circulating through one coil will induce a time-varying voltage in the other coil. Biasing in electronic circuits, however, requires a direct current (DC) voltage so that is when the rectifier and the regulator circuits come into play.

5.2.1.1. Rectifier circuit

A rectifier circuit changes an alternating current into a direct current. It has a small error though, since at the output the voltage has a little ripple. **Figure 7** shows a full-wave rectifier with P-type metal-oxide semiconductor (PMOS) transistors.

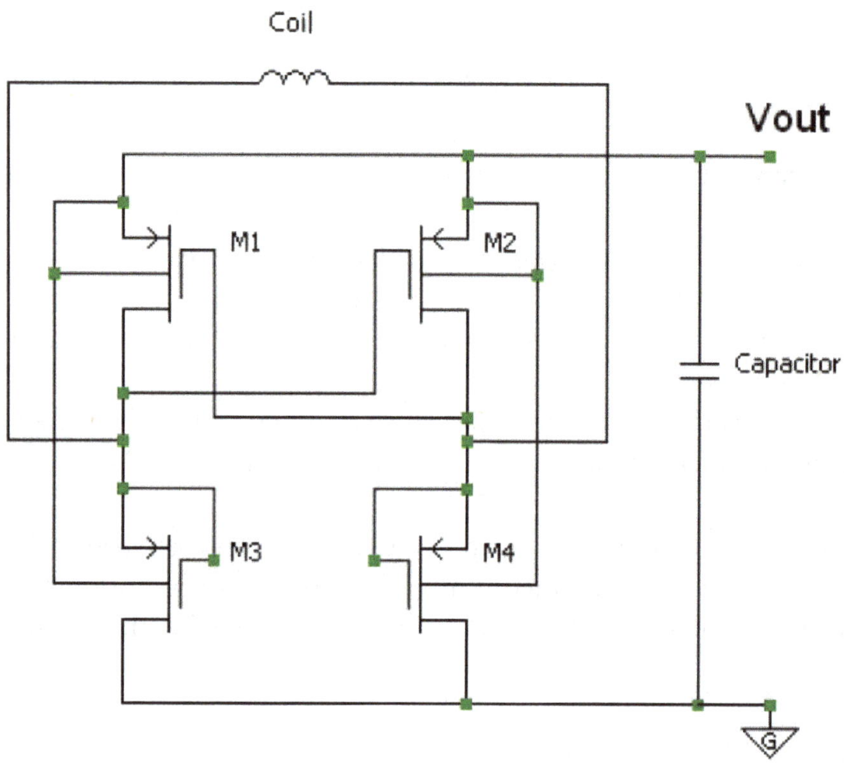

Figure 7. PMOS rectifier circuit.

5.2.1.2. Regulator circuit

To get rid of the small ripple at the output of the rectifier, a regulator circuit is often added.

The aim of the regulator is to deliver a stable power supply voltage for proper operation of the rest of the circuits in the implant. It has a minimum voltage needed at the input below which it will not deliver a constant voltage. If the input voltage is, on the other hand, greater than the minimum, then the regulator will output a constant voltage. This is the circuit responsible for making active electronic implants independent of coils distance. If the distance between coils is enough for the regulator to provide an output, it will provide a steady voltage regardless of how close the coils are. If on the contrary, the distance between coils is not close enough, then the voltage regulator simply will not provide any voltage at all. **Figure 8** depicts a Complementary Metal-Oxide Semiconductor (CMOS) topology for a voltage regulator circuit.

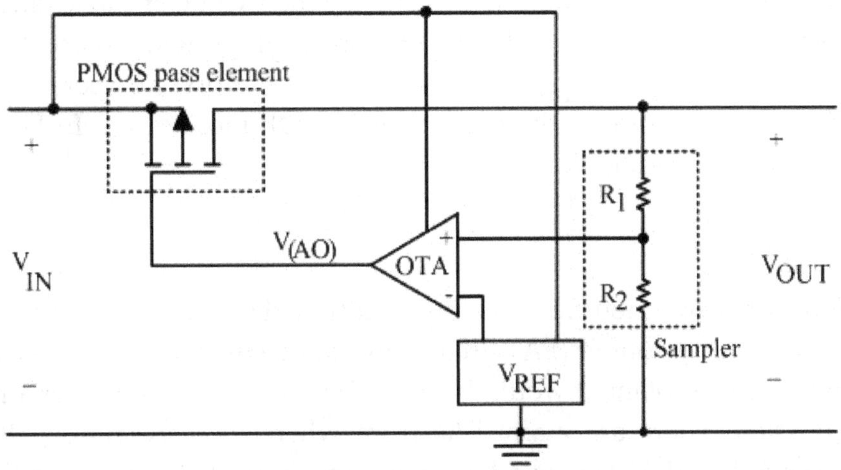

Figure 8. Topology of a voltage regulator. Taken with permission from [19].

5.2.2. Signal-conditioning circuit

Once we have a stable DC voltage, we can move on to the next sub-module of the implant. If the sensor is in charge of transforming an analogue physical signal into an electric variable, the signal-conditioning circuit has the task of taking the analogue electric signal and manipulate it in such a way that it meets the requirements for the next stage in the system. For our case, the next stage would be the transmission circuit.

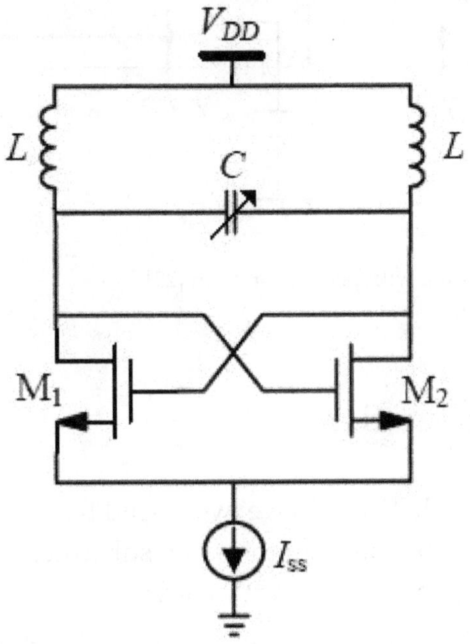

Figure 9. Cross-coupled LC VCO topology.

There are many electric circuit designs that can be used as a signal-conditioning circuit. Here, we take a brief look at a voltage-controlled oscillator (VCO) [20]. As seen in Section 2, most pressure sensors are variable capacitors which change their value of capacitance according to a change in pressure. On the other hand, a VCO is an oscillator with an oscillating frequency that depends on the value of its capacitor. If we connect the pressure sensor with the VCO, then we would have a signal-conditioning circuit for IOP monitoring. In **Figure 9**, a cross-coupled LC VCO topology is shown.

5.2.3. Transmission circuit

The transmission circuit sub-module takes the conditioned signal and transmits it back to the external device. A power amplifier (PA) circuit can achieve the latter. Since we are discussing circuits for an electronic implant, it would be desirable to have a low-power amplifier to deal with the transmission. There are many PAs from where we can choose; there are linear amplifiers (Classes A, B and AB) or switched-mode amplifiers (Classes E and F). In **Figure 10**, a class E PA is shown. Switched-mode amplifiers have a higher efficiency than linear ones (50–70% in the case of linear vs. a theoretical 100% in switched-mode amplifiers). Chapter 5 in [21] has a deeper explanation in power amplifiers for biomedical implants.

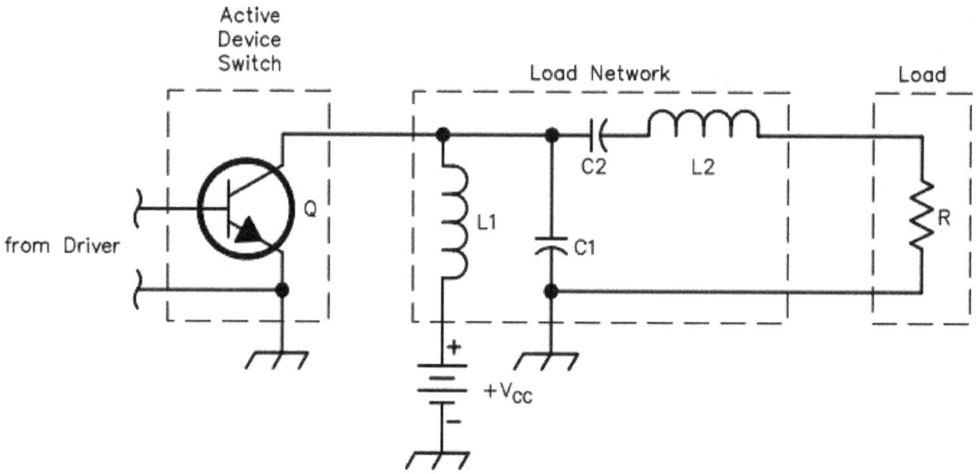

Figure 10. Class E power amplifier. Taken with permission from [22].

6. Sensor and circuit integration

At this point, the reader may ask: Why do we even need this section since at present, sensors and electronic circuits can be fabricated on the same substrate? And the answer is: Because it depends on what type of application we want to develop.

It is true that nowadays it is possible to fabricate sensors and circuits in the same substrate. The inconvenience with actual fabrication processes is that they use a rigid silicon wafer as a substrate. For many applications, this is enough, but for biomedical applications this approach is not useful. That is why in Section 2 all proposals that have active circuits in their designs (such as the one shown in **Figure 3**) tend to divide the fabrication process of the implant. On one hand, they fabricate the coil in a flexible substrate such as parylene, silicone rubber or polyimide so the implant can adapt to the curved surface of the eye. On the other hand, all electronic circuitry and in general all IOP sensors too are fabricated in a rigid silicon wafer. The final step involves connecting the coil with the sensor and the electronic circuits.

The main drawback from this approach is the potential damage that the silicon wafer can cause to the tissue of the eye. Fortunately, there has been a significant advance in terms of electronic circuit fabrication on a flexible substrate. In **Figure 11**, an electronic circuit fabrication process with Carbon Nanotubes (CNT) on a flexible substrate and photographs of the final chip are shown.

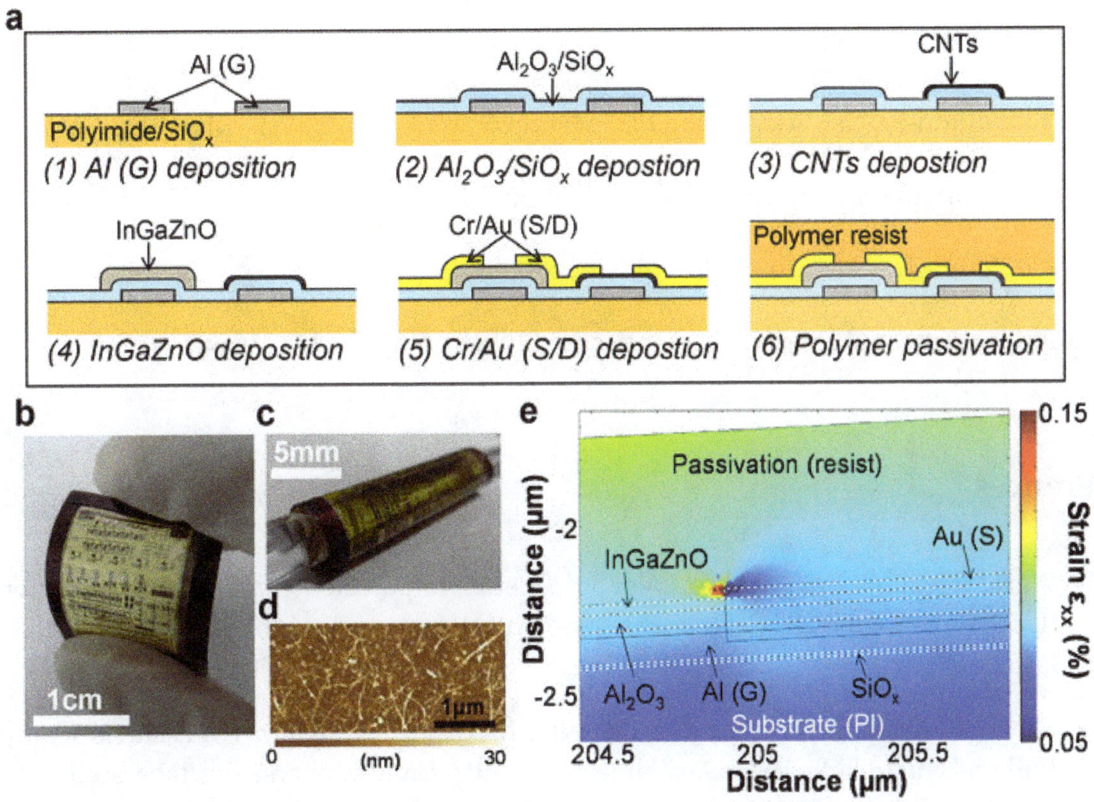

Figure 11. Circuit fabrication process on a flexible substrate. (a) Fabrication process of flexible InGaZnO-CNT CMOS logic circuits. Photographs of flexible CMOS circuits under (b) bending by hand and (c) rolling over a glass bar (~2.6-mm radius). (d) Atomic Force Microscopy (AFM) image of CNT network film for p-type type thin-film Transistors (TFT). (e) FEM simulation plot modelling the strain distribution in the InGaZnO channel region under bending (r = 2.6 mm). Taken with permission from [23].

7. Summary

In this chapter, we presented an overview of how an electronic implant can be designed. We showed what has been done in this area over the years and we pointed to a major medical concern that is tissue warming when it comes to implanting the IOP sensor into a patient.

From an engineering perspective and despite the tremendous advance that has been made in this area, there are still key issues that must be tackled in the years to come such as power efficiency in wireless power transfer. Another aspect, not less important, is the possibility to have electronic circuits fabricated in the same flexible substrate along with the pressure sensor. This is an area of recent creation that has though an immense growth potential. Microelectronic devices fabricated in a flexible substrate can have applications not only in intraocular pressure monitoring but in many other biomedical applications. And these circuits can not only have biomedical applications demand but also in other numerous engineering fields such as energy harvesting, domotics and wearable technology (clothing and accessories).

Author details

Adrian E. Rendon-Nava[1*], Alejandro Díaz-Méndez[2] and Luis Nino-de-Rivera[1]

*Address all correspondence to: adrian_rn78@hotmail.com

1 National Polytechnic Institute, Mexico City, Mexico

2 National Institute of Astrophysics, Optics and Electronics, Puebla, Mexico

References

[1] World Health Organization. WHO | Visual impairment and blindness [Internet]. [Updated: August 2014]. Available from: http://www.who.int/mediacentre/factsheets/fs282/en/ [Accessed: July 5, 2016].

[2] Taber, C. W., editor. Taber's Cyclopedic Medical Dictionary. F. A. Davis Company. Philadelphia, USA; 1993. Available from: http://www.tabers.com/tabersonline/view/Tabers-Dictionary/772170/all/glaucoma [Accessed: December, 2014].

[3] Miguel-Jiménez, J. M., Ortega, S., Boquete, L., Rodríguez-Ascariz, J. M., Blanco, R. Multifocal ERG wavelet packet decomposition applied to glaucoma diagnosis. Biomed. Eng. Online. 2011;10(37):1–13.

[4] Cooper, R. L., Beale, D. Radio telemetry of intraocular pressure in vitro. Invest. Ophthalmol. Visual Sci. 1977;16:168–171.

[5] Rosengren, L., Backlund, Y., Sjostrom, T., Hok, B., Svedbergh, B. A system for wireless intra-ocular pressure measurements using a silicon micromachined sensor. J. Micromech. Microeng. 1992;2:202–204.

[6] Laube, T. et al. Optical energy transfer for intraocular microsystems studied in rabbits. Graefe's Arch. Clin. Exp. Ophthalmol. 2004;242:661–667.

[7] Chow, E. Y., Chlebowski, A. L., Irazoqui, P. P. A miniature-implantable RF-wireless active glaucoma intraocular pressure monitor. IEEE Trans. Biomed. Circ. Syst. 2010;4(6): 340–349. DOI: 10.1109/TBCAS.2010.2081364.

[8] Shin, K. -S., Jang, C. -I., Kim, M. J., Yun, K. -S., Park, K. H., Kang, J. Y., Lee, S. H. Development of novel implantable intraocular pressure sensors to enhance the performance in in vivo tests. J. Microelectromech. Syst. 2015;24(6):1896–1905. DOI: 10.1109/JMEMS.2015.2451214.

[9] Tufte, O. N., Chapman, P. W., Long, D. J. Silicon diffused-element piezoresistive diaphragms. Appl. Phys. 1962;33:3322.

[10] Schnakenberg, U., Mokwa, W., et al. Initial investigations on a system for measuring intraocular pressure. Sensor Actuat. A. 2000;85:287–291.

[11] Chen, P. J., Rodger, D. C., Saati, S., Humayun, M. S. Microfabricated implantable parylene-based wireless passive intraocular pressure sensors. J. Microelectromech. Syst. 2008;17(6):1342–1351.

[12] Todani, A., et al. Intraocular pressure measurement by radio wave telemetry. Invest. Ophthalmol. Vis. Sci. 2011;52:9573–9580.

[13] American Conference of Government Industrial Hygienists, editor. Threshold Limit Values for Chemical Substances and Physical Agents and Biological Exposure Indices. Cincinnati, OH: American Conference of Government Industrial Hygienists; 1996.

[14] Michaelson, S. M., Elson, E. C., Polk, C., Postow, E. Modulated fields and 'window' effects. In: Biological Effects of Electromagnetic Fields. Boca Raton, FL: CRC Press; 1996. p. 435–533.

[15] How Wireless Electricity Transmission Works—Wireless Power Consortium [Internet]. Available from: https://www.wirelesspowerconsortium.com/technology/how-it-works.html [Accessed: 06 July, 2016].

[16] Pennes, H. H. Analysis of tissue and arterial blood temperatures in the resting human forearm. J. App. Physiol. 1948;1(2):93–122.

[17] Fonseca, M., English, J. M., von Arx, M., Allen, M. G. Wireless micromachined ceramic pressure sensor for high-temperature applications. J. Microelectromech. Syst. 2002;11(4):337–343.

[18] Rendon-Nava, A. E., Díaz-Méndez, J. A., Nino-de-Rivera, L., Calleja-Arriaga, W., Gil-Carrasco, F., Díaz-Alonso, D. Study of the effect of distance and misalignment between magnetically coupled coils for wireless power transfer in intraocular pressure measurement. Sci. W. J. 2014;2014:11/692434.

[19] Paulo, C., Luis, F., Tales, P., Robson, M., Leonardo, Z., Edgar, C. (2011). Structural design of CMOS voltage regulator for implantable devices. Current Trends and Challenges in RFID, Prof. Cornel Turcu (Ed.), InTech. DOI:

10.5772/17561. Available from: http://www.intechopen.com/books/current-trends-and-challenges-in-rfid/structural-design-of-cmos-voltage-regulator-for-implantable-devices.

[20] Rendon-Nava, A. E., Nino-de-Rivera, L., Díaz-Méndez, J. A. A 1-V supply voltage controlled oscillator for intraocular pressure measurement. Telecommun. Radio Eng. 2013;72(16):1537–1544.

[21] Siu, C., Iniewski, K. CMOS circuits for wireless medical applications. In: Krzysztof, I., editor. VLSI Circuits for Biomedical Applications. Norwood, MA: Artech House; 2008. p. 111–130.

[22] Sokal, A. D. Class E RF power amplifiers. QEX Mag. 2001;(204):9–20.

[23] Honda, W., Arie, T., Akita, S., Takei, K. Mechanically flexible and high-performance CMOS logic circuits. Sci. Rep. 2015;5:15099. DOI: http://dx.doi.org/10.1038/srep15099.

11

Phacoemulsification Cataract Surgery without Viscoelastic Substance: Bianchi's Method

Germán R. Bianchi

Abstract

Life expectancy of the population increase and cataract development will affect all the people with aging. Cataract surgery, a worldwide performed procedure, evolves and progresses. However, different techniques exist, which could be selected for different cases. Any ideal technique should be safe, simple, fast, and easy to learn with good clinical outcome. This chapter will describe one technique to operate cataracts with those characteristics and to perform phacoemulsification cataract surgery without viscoelastic substance. Some advantages of this technique are related to avoiding viscoelastic potential problems, as postoperative intraocular pressure elevation or anterior chamber inflammation associated with viscoelastic. Moreover, a fundamental factor to remark is the difference between work into the anterior chamber with negative pressure or positive pressure. Because the anterior chamber is maintained by the balanced salt solution with the continuous irrigation without viscoelastic. Performing the capsulorhexis is easier. Other advantages are shorten surgical time, fewer economical cost, and potentially fewer complications. Some limitations are as follows: intraocular lens must be one piece foldable, and principally, patients with corneal endothelial pathology must be excluded. Tips, step-by-step surgery, recommendations, and evolution of the technique will be described, with the wish that many surgeons will try to perform Bianchi's method (bimanual, microincision phacoemulsification cataract surgery without viscoelastic substance) for your next patient.

Keywords: phacoemulsification, cataract surgery, viscoelastic, technique, cataract surgery complications

1. Introduction

The life expectancy is increasing every decade, and the lens of the eye decreases their optical quality over the years [1]. If we could live the number of years what is expected, everybody will have cataracts and will need a cataract surgery. That is a fact. Cataracts are still a leading cause of moderate to severe visual impairment, even blindness worldwide [2–4]. Visual impairment caused by cataract leads to not only an economic loss but also the impaired quality of life [5]. However, cataract is easily treatable by surgery [6]. On the other hand, there are different studies trying to find how cataracts could be prevented [7–9]. In the future, cataractogenesis could be totally elucidated, and maybe cataract surgery will not be necessary. However, until today, the only way to resolve this problem is by a surgical procedure.

Science and technology improve ophthalmology performance to protect the sight. Today, a cataract surgery takes only a few minutes, with topical anesthesia, with sutureless, and with a very fast visual recovery. Moreover, cataract surgery research in this field progresses continuously. And it always is possible to improve for tomorrow what we are doing now. The chapter which I want to share with you is exactly about that: how we could improve cataract surgery technique, with the same surgical equipment usually employed.

I have begun performing cataract surgery since 22 years ago. When I learned to operate cataracts, extracapsular was the surgical technique of choice, without the aid of viscoelastic substance. Their use at those years was not extended widely. And surgeries went well. After that, phacoemulsification technology produces a revolution, improving surgical outcome. At the same time, the intraocular lens (IOL) industry grew up, as well as viscoelastic substances spread worldwide and were included as one necessary medical supply for the surgery. Viscoelastic substance appears to resolve a lot of problems, which could arise when the anterior chamber is opened [10, 11].

The anterior chamber space preservation is relevant to avoid endothelial complications [12]. If anterior chamber space is flattened, the iris could be damaged, the corneal endothelium could suffer, and all of the work inside the eye are riskier. New surgeon generation from developed countries learns to operate cataracts with phacoemulsification equipment using viscoelastic substance as the gold standard technique. And today, femtosecond laser technology is growing and possibly in a close future takes the place of phacoemulsification technique completely. However, more machines, more devices, and more medical supplies are increasing their final cost and not necessarily increasing their visual and refractive results over other techniques. Moreover, there are many surgeons around the world, in developing countries, where that sophisticated technology is not accessible. They help people without an expensive medical device and without viscoelastic substance and still perform cataract surgery by extracapsular technique [13]. The Blumenthal technique of manual small-incision cataract surgery (MSICS), with the help of anterior chamber maintainer, has been proven safe and effective, preventing endothelial cell loss during surgery [14, 15].

Why have I developed this technique to perform phacoemulsification cataract surgery without the aid of viscoelastic substance? After one scientific meeting in Vienna, Austria (European Society of Ophthalmology 2015), I was thinking about the way to decrease my surgery time, simplify the technique without increasing risk, and if possible improve my personal surgery outcome. There are published descriptions to avoid the use of viscoelastic substance during IOL implantation [16, 17] with good results. First, I began doing that and it was fine. However, I want to avoid the use of viscoelastic substance at all. Could capsulorhexis and hydrodissection have been performed without viscoelastic substance safely during phacoemulsification technique? The answer is yes, and also, avoiding completely the use of viscoelastic substance, it could have relevant advantages, as I will describe in this chapter. I propose to myself to perform and develop phacoemulsification cataract surgery without viscoelastic substance. I will share my experience, my technique tips, indications, contraindications, and why today this is my first choice technique to perform cataract surgery.

2. Viscoelastic substance: advantages and problems

Since the 1970s, viscoelastic substance begins to progress, and today they are popular and indispensable for integral parts of intraocular surgery [18]. The main purpose for using viscoelastic substance in cataract surgery is to maintain a stable anterior chamber depth and protect the corneal endothelial cells from being damaged [11]. That decreases surgical complications and makes challenging cases easier. For example, there are cases called "intraoperative floppy iris syndrome," which was associated with tamsulosin, a systemic α-1 blocker used to treat benign prostatic hypertrophy [19]. The clinical intraoperative triad of the syndrome consists of fluttering and billowing of the iris stroma caused by ordinary intraocular fluid currents, a propensity for iris prolapse through the phacoemulsification and/or side-port incisions, and progressive constriction of the pupil during surgery [19]. Also, viscoelastic substance is sometimes helpful to tamponade a posterior capsule rupture for subsequent IOL implantation [20] or to inject viscoelastic substance through a pars plana incision to elevate the nuclear pieces into the anterior chamber [21].

However, there are studies which describe problems related with viscoelastic substance. The IOP elevation by viscoelastic substances is caused by a reduction of aqueous outflow due to blockage of the trabecular meshwork where the fluids exit the eye, which was first published in 1990 [18] and later confirmed by other authors in vivo and in vitro [10, 22, 23]. Therefore, complete removal of viscoelastic substance is recommended after IOL implantation. The IOP elevation is usually transient, peaking at 4–7 h postoperatively and returning to baseline within several days, but the maximum IOP may exceed 30 mmHg. Therefore, careful monitoring of IOP and IOP-lowering therapy may be necessary, especially in patients with glaucoma who have a compromised outflow facility.

Flare or Tyndall effect could be postoperatively detected after cataract surgery, which in part is frequent, but in excess that could be the manifestation of "toxic anterior segment syndrome" (TASS) after cataract surgery, and viscoelastic substance could be associated with this [23, 24]. Also, an extra surgery time is necessary to introduce viscoelastic substance and to completely remove them from the anterior chamber, trying to avoid the problems previously described. Moreover, viscoelastic substance increases the final cost of the surgery. In conclusion, viscoelastic substances could help to perform a more secure surgery, especially in some cases, but also could be the cause of other problems, sometimes serious. Because of that, this work emphasizes and proposes a special technique to perform phacoemulsification cataract surgery without viscoelastic substance.

3. Bianchi's method: patient selection

As any surgical technique, specific indications and contraindications (inclusion/exclusion criteria) will be described, to choose the appropriate case or to exclude patients with high risk:

1. Include patients with cataracts classified as NO1–NC1 to NO4–NC4 according to the LOCS III classification (avoid NO5–NC5, NO6–NC6).
2. Exclude patients with less than 2000 endothelial cell count preoperative. Endothelial cells count evaluation is necessary to be included as a standard preoperative test, and it is advisable to perform as postoperative standard follow-up test.
3. Exclude patients with endothelial defects, *pseudoexfoliation*, posttraumatic cataracts, pupil synechiae or small pupil, uveitis, and/or previous vitreoretinal surgeries.
4. Include only patients programmed to implant foldable one-piece intraocular lens (IOL) models with injector.
5. Exclude patients when three-piece IOL models are programmed to implant. I do not recommend those kinds of IOLs for this procedure because their haptics are hard and the capsule could be broken.

4. Bianchi's method: technique description step by step

When a new surgical technique is presented, there are many questions to be answered. I will try to describe all of the details because I hope many surgeons worldwide probe it with success. One first question: will it be necessary to acquire new equipment, devices, and/or machines? The answer is no. The technique could be correctly performed with different standard phacoemulsification equipment, and any surgeon who perform phacoemulsification with viscoelastic technique could perform the Bianchi's method without viscoelastic substance. Hand positions and movements are similar to "microincision cataract surgery" (MICS). It is just necessary to get a micro-capsulorhexis forceps of 1.1 mm diameter, which must have the same diameter of the irrigation cannula. From standard surgical instruments usually employed to perform phacoemulsification, you will only need the irrigation cannula, but the aspiration cannula is not necessary. **Figure 1** shows the specific surgical tools.

Topical anesthesia must be performed as usual *and then*:

1. Two clear corneal incisions of 1.1 mm were performed with v-lance near the limbus. The first was at "2" o'clock and the second at "10" o'clock.
2. Immediately after the first incision was performed, the irrigation cannula (1.1 mm diameter) was introduced, the second incision was performed, and the micro-capsulorhexis forceps of 1.1 mm diameter was introduced. The size of the v-lance and the irrigation cannula must be the same to avoid leakage through the corneal incision.

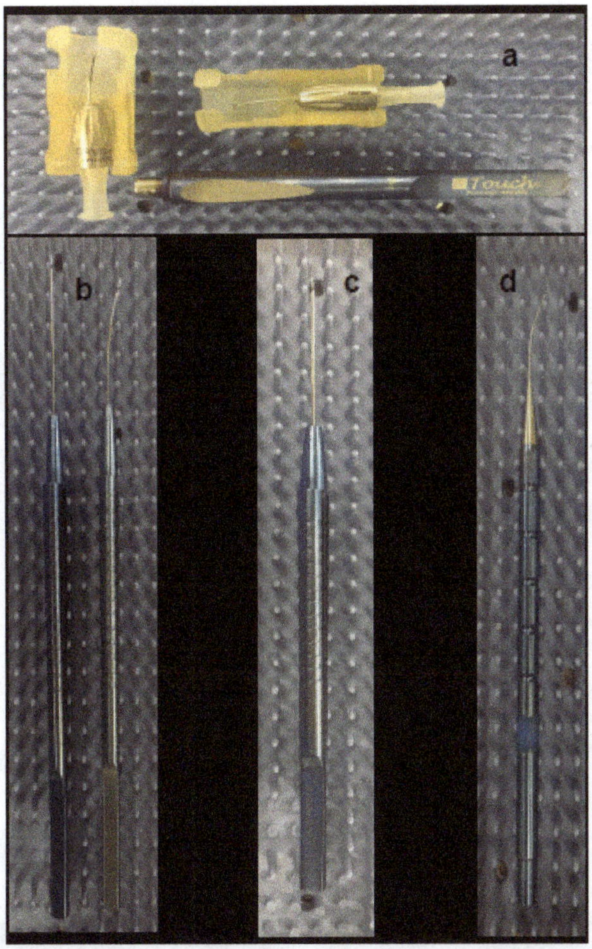

Figure 1. Surgical instruments necessary to perform Bianchi's method. (a) MST Touch Handle and 23g Micro-Holding Forceps for capsulorrhexis; (b) Curve and straight Micro-Scissors; (c) capsulorrhexis micro-forceps and (d) I/A irrigation cannula.

3. The irrigation bottle with balanced salt solution (BSS) must be elevated usually at 80–100 cm above the patient's head level, under continuous irrigation (no more, to avoid IOP increase), to obtain a deep and stable space in the anterior chamber. The irrigation cannula has two lateral vents, which let the BSS leave and move in a centripetal way, toward the equator. That means the liquid circulation is not against the endothelium; therefore, the endothelium is protected. For the learning curve, in the first case, it is recommended to put in the automatic or continuous way the irrigation mode of the phaco. This lets to maintain stable the anterior chamber automatically. With more experience, the surgeon can manage them with the phaco pedal.

   This bimanual technique is suitable for right- or left-handed surgeons. The previous description is for right-handed surgeons. For left-handed surgeons, "2" o'clock incision is for micro-capsulorhexis and the cannula must be located at "10" o'clock incision.

4. Capsulorhexis was performed (**Figure 2**), while the liquid (BSS) circulation in the anterior chamber produces a positive pressure, which determines a stable and safe space to work. This is one of the most important points of the technique. It is easier to perform the

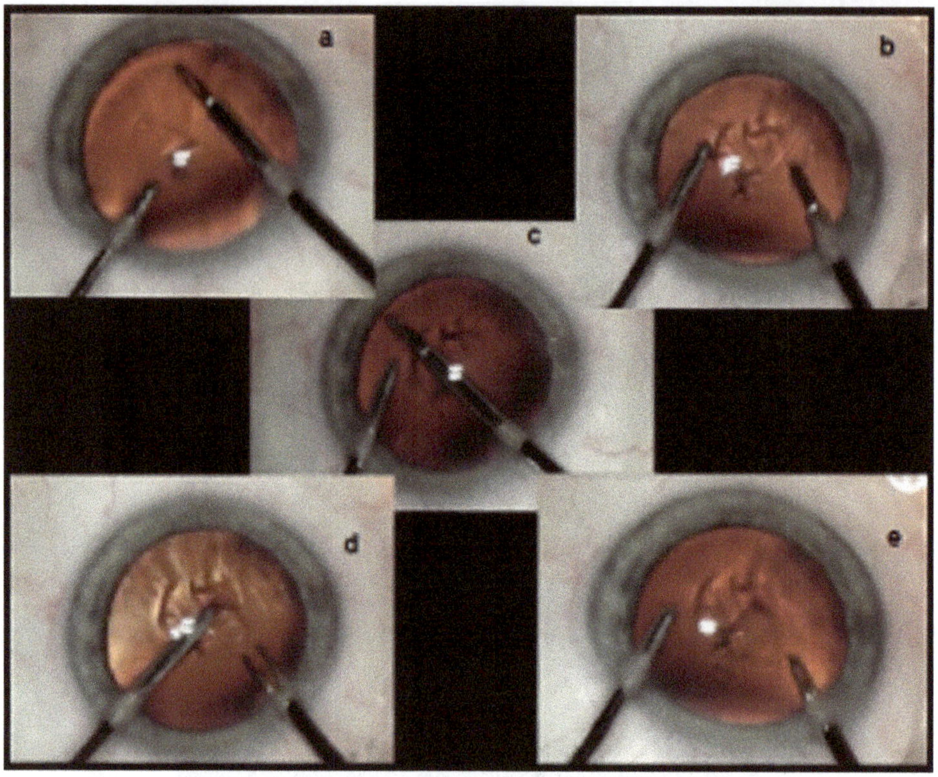

Figure 2. This figure shows from "a" to "e" the capsulorhexis procedure with continuous liquid circulation into the anterior chamber.

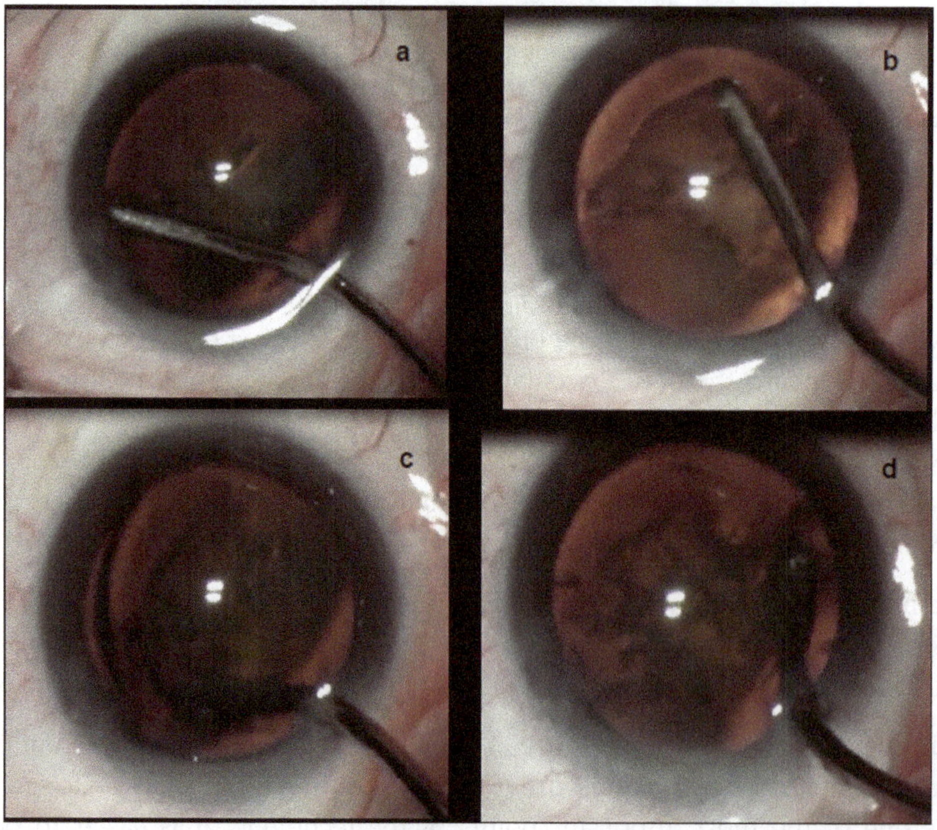

Figure 3. Hydrodissection step performed with the irrigation cannula and from "a" to "d" is possible to see the nucleus rotation.

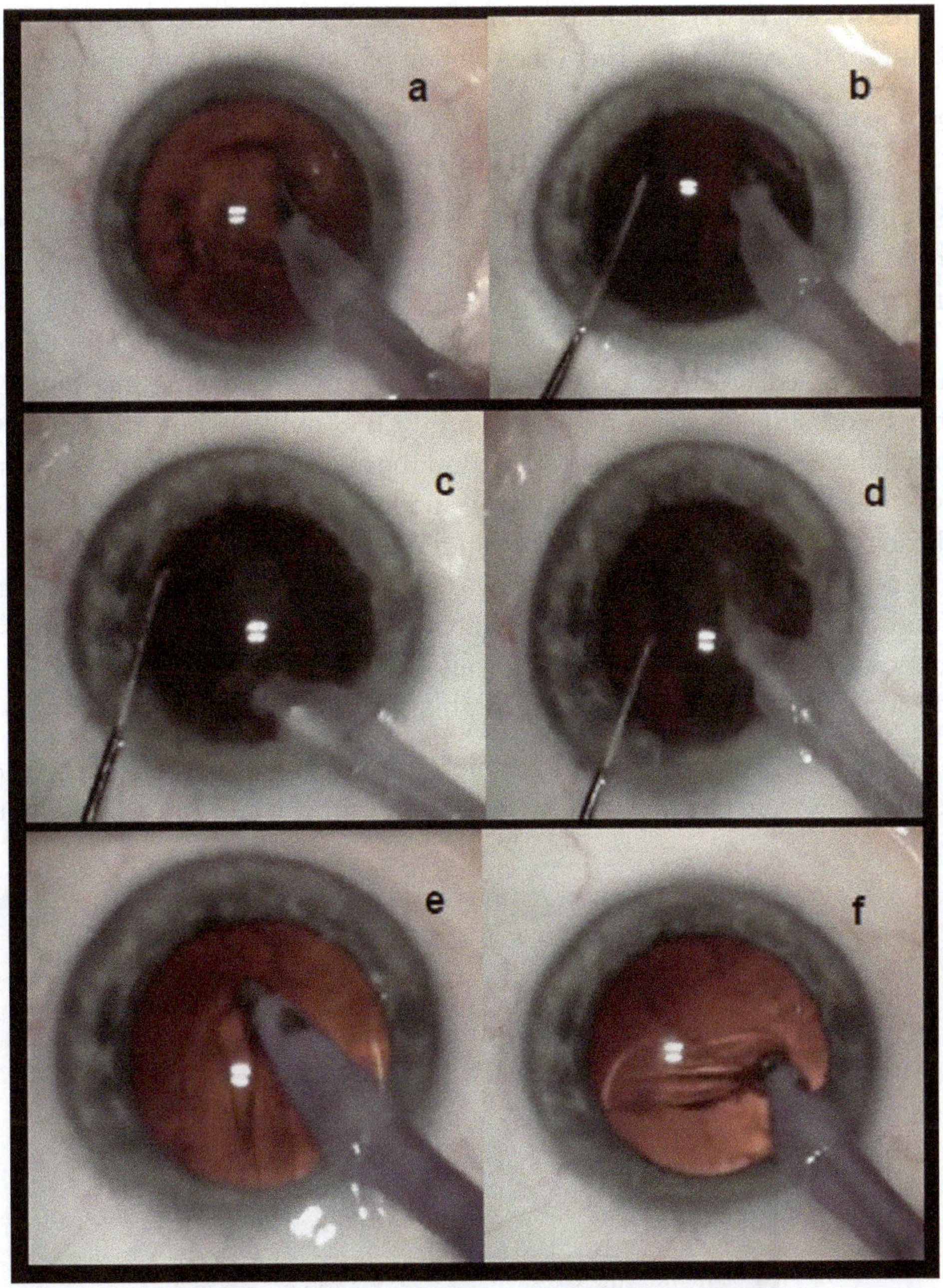

Figure 4. Phacoemulsification, aspiration, and mass extraction were performed as usual.

capsulorhexis under positive pressure than under negative pressure (as what happens with viscoelastic substance), because continuous irrigation flattens the anterior face of the lens. When you are working under positive pressure into the anterior chamber, it is very rare to have the problem of capsulorhexis rupture. In my experience, capsulorhexis failure was more frequent with viscoelastic substance than those cases performed without viscoelastic substance.

5. After that, hydrodissection was performed with the same irrigation cannula until a complete rotation of the nucleus was observed (**Figure 3**). Perform this step carefully, because if you push too much the nucleus, the zonnula could be broken. However, it is not difficult to perform the hydrodissection: simply, let the irrigation cannula position below capsulorhexis, and the liquid diffuses around the nucleus to release it. Or sometimes, a

circular movement of the cannula could be performed to facilitate that the nucleus will be released from the epinucleus. Then, the rotation of the nucleus will easily occur.

6. Phacoemulsification, aspiration, and mass extractions: it will be performed without any difference from a standard procedure (**Figure 4**).

7. Next step: without removing the cannula, the second corneal incision must be increased (**Figure 5**) according to the phaco tip, for the IOL implantation (1.8 mm, 2.2 mm up to 2.8 mm or what the surgeon need) (**Figure 6**). Only foldable one-piece IOL models with injector could be used. Three pieces IOL models are not recommended for this procedure. When the intraocular lens cartridge was introduced through the incision, the anterior chamber could suffer a space reduction due to BSS outflow, but immediately after the IOL injection begins, liquid leakage stops, and the anterior chamber space is restored. The positive pressure expands the capsular bag, and then the IOL is placed with the cannula to help during the unfolding process to obtain the correct IOL position. Also, this procedure let the toric IOLs be easily rotated, if it was necessary. This is another advantage of this technique against standard technique with viscoelastic substance, because sometimes, after removing viscoelastics, toric IOLs could be displaced and are necessary to correct their position again, to obtain the exact location for astigmatism correction.

Finally, I usually inject an intracameral antibiotic (cefuroxime) and the surgery concludes. Most of the surgeries were performed between 4 and 5 min or 6 and 7 min for harder cataracts.

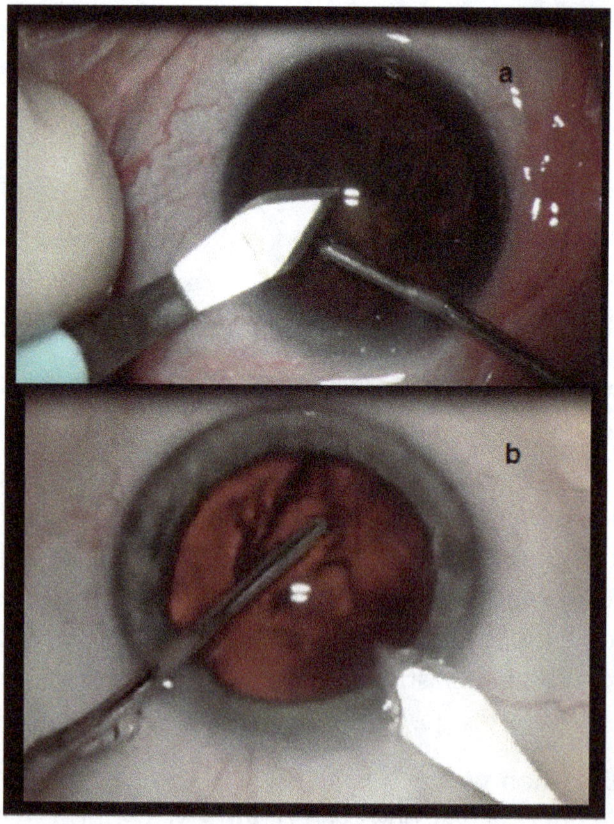

Figure 5. This figure shows the second corneal incision enlargement.

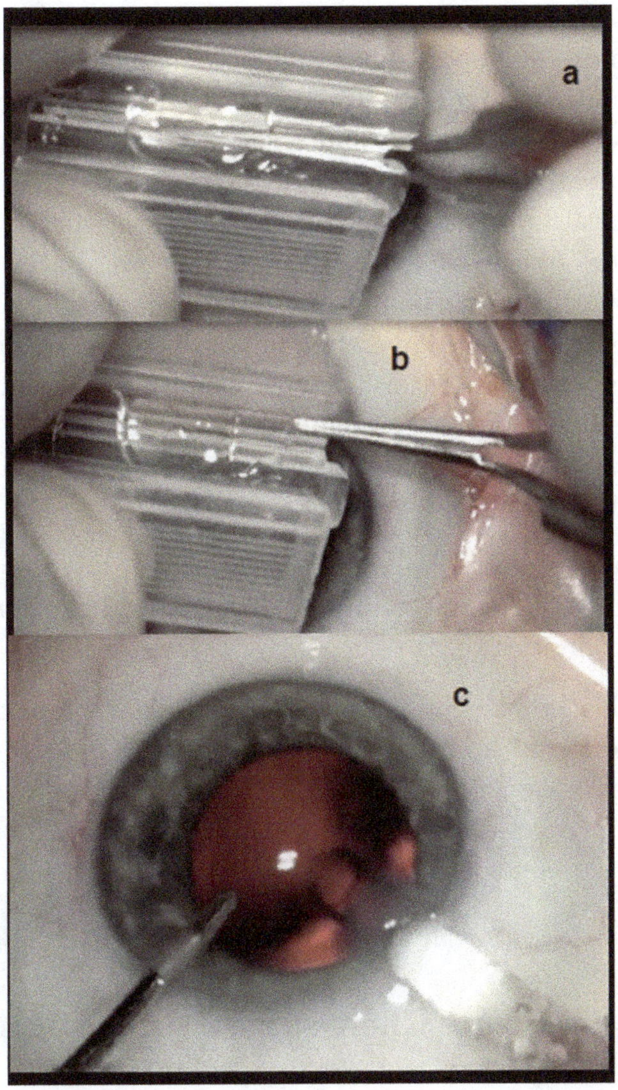

Figure 6. One-piece intraocular lens is placed in an injected.

5. Is this technique secure?

Performing cataract surgery without viscoelastic substances seems to be dangerous for the corneal endothelial tissue. However, with the surgical steps previously described, it is true? To evaluate and control this matter, since my beginning with this technique (July 2015) and after 1500 operated cases, all of the patients are still followed with endothelial cell count and central corneal thickness evaluation (always at the preoperative time and, then, at least 6 months post-op with endothelial cell count follow-up).

A prospective comparative study is ongoing, to evaluate clinical outcomes and complications between both techniques: phacoemulsification with and without viscoelastic substance by Bianchi's method. I can advance some data from this study, as a brief preliminary report. The patient's age was 45–91 years old; none of them has suffered intraoperative or postoperative complications as capsular bag rupture, IOL implantation problems, expulsive hemorrhage, IOP elevation, TASS, and/or endophthalmitis. All of the patients improve their visual acuity. Endothelial cell count and central corneal thickness were compared between patients operated with and without viscoelastic substance, and nonstatistical significant difference was found between both groups. The surgical time with Bianchi's method is between 4 and 5 min (7 min maximum) and for standard phacoemulsification with viscoelastic is 8–10 min (for this study, the surgeon was *German Bianchi MD* for all of the procedures). Why is the surgical time shorter? Because an extra time is needed to insert and completely remove the injected viscoelastic substance. Besides a prolonged operation time, which per se increases overall operation risks and complications, viscoelastic substance removal can immediately affect safety issues. Also, an increased irrigation-aspiration time might also be responsible for endothelial cell loss due to the aspiration trauma. The use of a viscoelastic substance can have side effects and may cause endothelial damage as well.

Even though it is an ongoing study, preliminary data plus the experience of 2 years doing this technique with good outcomes let me confirm that it is secure, fast, and simple. Now, it is my first choice to perform cataract surgery.

I have started to teach this technique to the ophthalmic residents of the clinic where I work, and they told me "it is not difficult" and also the learning curve is fast. However, some colleagues previously told me: "well, is easy for you… but not for everybody!." No, today I can confirm that the Bianchi's method to perform cataract surgery without viscoelastic substances is easy, for any ophthalmic surgeon who used to perform phacoemulsification technique or MICS.

6. Is there another experience where surgeons try to avoid the use of viscoelastic substance?

Schulze et al. [25] avoid their use, only during IOL implantation, without finding difference in endothelial cell loss. Oksuz et al. [26] described a technique without VS to perform capsulorhexis, but they use it after hydrodissection and for the IOL implantation. Finally, they aspirated it from the anterior chamber.

In the past, Wright et al. [13] compare their results of small-incision extracapsular cataract surgery using the anterior chamber maintainer without viscoelastic substance, and they finally show that the magnitude and range of the endothelial cell losses associated with this technique are significantly greater than those described following phacoemulsification. Because of that, these authors finally recommend the use of VS for this extracapsular procedure.

But in 2008, Sallet [27] described a phacoemulsification cataract surgery technique completely performed without VS, where he found no difference in their clinical outcome comparing it with 50 patients operated with VS. However, Galan [28] previously performed a similar technique with 1.6 mm corneal incision and enlargement to 3.0 mm for IOL implantation with less success rate than Sallet G, which Sallet considered could be due to the narrower incisions performed by him of 1.2 and 2.6 mm for IOL implantation. The technique described in this work proposes two corneal microincision, which is 1.1 wide and the enlargement of one of those to 2.2–2.8 mm according to the phacoemulsification tip (Sallet G open 2.6 mm). Small corneal incisions could be in part the key to obtain better surgical results. Another difference with the technique described by Sallet G is about hydrodissection: in the present technique, it is performed by the irrigation cannula.

7. Economical surgery cost

This new technique is not more expensive. In fact, it is more economic, because it is not necessary to buy viscoelastic substances. In the country where I live, the final cost of the surgery increases US$75 per procedure when viscoelastic substance (I use DisCoVisc®) is necessary.

However, as in this chapter was described, there are many patients where viscoelastic substances are not necessary: not only because it increases the surgery cost but moreover because they could be a potential problem, which disrupts the surgical outcome.

8. Final recommendations

As it was mentioned at the beginning of this chapter, lifetime expectancy increases as well as ocular tissues grow older. Our eyes are not prepared for the last years that we are living. Cataracts appear and the possibility to replace them with an IOL let many people stay able to keep their sight and quality of life. Moreover, the improvements in the surgical techniques, device, equipment, and tools let today to resolve high orders of refractive problems with the IOL implantation (with or without removing the lens). The procedure to implant an IOL into the eye is short, simple, and secure. But it is always possible to improve and adequate techniques to different environments.

The technique described in this work was presented in the XXXV Congress of the European Society of Cataract & Refractive Surgeons (ESCRS Lisbon 2017) at the Video Awards Session. There is a mini-review published in September 2017 [29]. Also, the video of the technique could be showed in https://vimeo.com/212631783. If you are a cataract ophthalmic surgeon, try this technique, and you will decrease complications, surgery time, and surgery cost with a better postoperative recovery. Remember the indication and contraindication, choose the right patient, and go ahead.

Below is the list of advantages and limitation.

Advantages:

1. Avoid complications related with viscoelastic (IOP elevation, TASS) and corneal endothelial damage during the viscoelastic substance aspiration.
2. Perform a fast surgery (4–5 min usually, 6–7 min at maximum).
3. Work all the time under positive pressure in the anterior chamber; this let the capsulorhexis becomes easily performed.

4. Short learning curve: usually new cataract surgeons only learn to operate phacoemulsification cataract surgery with viscoelastic substances. I'm not against viscoelastic substance, which is really useful for some cases, although, for other cases, it could be possible to perform a safe procedure without viscoelastic substance, moreover, with "extra" advantages!
5. Surgery cost: the final cost of the surgery decreases for the patient, because you do not need an extra medical supply (you do not need to buy viscoelastic substance for each surgery). And as my scrub nurses happily told me, they also prefer it. Why? Micro-capsulorhexis forceps cleaning and maintenance are more easy when I use BSS than viscoelastic substances. And also, that increases the lifespan of my surgical tool. For all of those reasons, it decreases the total surgical economical cost.
6. One more advantage: you do not need a third-hand incision.

What are the limitations or contraindications?

1. Avoid "hard" cataracts.
2. Avoid three-piece IOL.
3. The technique is not recommended for patients with endothelial corneal pathology, pseudoexfoliation syndrome, traumatic cataracts, and/or history of previous vitreoretinal surgery. However, in those cases, the standard phacoemulsification procedure will also increase the surgical risk. Endothelial corneal transplantation or complete perforated corneal transplant could be necessary at the end because of bullous pseudophakic keratopathy and the consequent corneal edema.
4. Endothelial cell count is a mandatory preoperative study, and I recommend follow-up 6 months after surgery. I know that some places do not have an endothelial cell counter analyzer, but it is a study which I think is relevant to perform not only the Bianchi's method, moreover, for every patient who will need a cataract surgery. Today the people have great expectative about their refractive surgical outcome after cataract surgery, and if a patient has an endothelial problem and if it was possible to have an objective data about it, the surgeon could decrease patient's expectative and explain to him which could be his specific surgical risk, before performing the surgery. I emphasize this point. It is a really important issue to prevent legal problems.
5. If capsulorhexis goes wrong, always convert to viscoelastic standard technique.
6. Hydrodissection must be performed without pressing over the posterior capsule to avoid rupture.
7. Doing the IOL implantation should be obtained in a well expanded anterior chamber, but if not, use viscoelastic substance.

In summary, a bimanual phacoemulsification microincision cataract surgery could be performed without the aid of viscoelastic substance, decreasing their economical cost during 5–7 min. The technique is easy to learn and potentially with fewer complications, which must be scientifically demonstrated in a prospective study (which is an ongoing study), and even better in a multicentric study to confirm that this technique is efficient and reproducible for different ophthalmic surgeons.

And finally, to end this chapter, I want to share with you a little story.

My professor was Dr. Hugo Dionisio Nano, one of the most important ophthalmologists in Argentina, with international recognition around the world. Dr. Nano, with his age of 88 years old, usually goes to his clinics, goes to scientific meetings, and still is an active "ophthalmology teacher" for many colleagues. In 2016, he needed a cataract surgery and chose me as his surgeon, a great honor and a great challenge for me. For his first eye, I have performed the standard phacoemulsification cataract surgery, with viscoelastic substance. Surgery went fine with no complications. However, he had a moderate postoperative inflammation and intraocular pressure rise, which resolved a few days later. One week after, I chose to operate his second eye without viscoelastic substance (Bianchi's method), and he did not have any postoperative problem. This is one anecdote I know, but I hope with this chapter, I could give you enough scientific information and technical tips to encourage you and try "Bianchi's method" in your next cataract surgery.

Acknowledgements

To my wife Carolina and my children, Lucía, Sofía, Manuel, and Giulietta, thanks for all of your patience and for the time you give me to perform my profession.

To my surgical team: thanks for your professionalism and continuous dedication.

To my mother, who encouraged me every day to study, and to my father, who always guided me from the sky, thank you.

I would like to thank Dr. Rodrigo M. Torres, for his motivation and scientific advice to perform medical studies.

Author details

Germán R. Bianchi

Address all correspondence to: germansinio69@gmail.com

Clínica de Ojos Dr. Nano, Centro Panamericana, Buenos Aires, Argentina

References

[1] The AREDS Research Group, Indaram M, Agrón E, Clemons TE, Sperduto RD, Wong WT, Ferris FL III, Emily Y. Chew changes in lens opacities on the age-related eye disease study

grading scale predict progression to cataract surgery and vision loss: Age-related eye disease study (AREDS) report #34. Ophthalmology. 2015;**122**:888-896. DOI: 10.1016/j.ophtha.2014.12.037

[2] Bourne RR, Stevens GA, White RA, et al. Causes of vision loss worldwide, 1990–2010: A systematic analysis. The Lancet Global Health. 2013;**1**:e339-e349. DOI: 10.1016/S2214-109X(13)70113-X

[3] Pascolini D, Mariotti SP. Global estimates of visual impairment: 2010. The British Journal of Ophthalmology. 2012;**96**:614-618. DOI: 10.1136/bjophthalmol-2011-300539

[4] Khairallah M, Kahloun R, Bourne R, et al. Number of people blind or visually impaired by cataract worldwide and in world regions, 1990 to 2010. Investigative Ophthalmology & Visual Science. 2015;**56**:6762-6769. DOI: 10.1167/iovs.15-17201

[5] Groessl EJ, Liu L, Sklar M, Tally SR, Kaplan RM, Ganiats TG. Measuring the impact of cataract surgery on generic and vision-specific quality of life. Quality of Life Research. 2013;**22**:1405-1414. DOI: 10.1007/s11136-012-0270-z

[6] Lundstrom M, Goh PP, Henry Y, et al. The changing pattern of cataract surgery indications: A 5-year study of 2 cataract surgery databases. Ophthalmology. 2015;**122**:31-38. DOI: 10.1016/j.ophtha.2014.07.047

[7] Weikel KA, Garber C, Baburins A, Taylor A. Nutritional modulation of cataract. Nutrition Reviews. 2014;**72**:30-47. DOI: 10.1111/nure.12077

[8] Christen WG, Glynn RJ, Michael Gaziano J, Darke AK, Crowley JJ, Goodman PJ, Lippman SM, Lad TE, Bearden JD, Goodman GE, Minasian LM, Thompson IM Jr, Blanke CD, Eric A. Klein age-related cataract in a randomized trial of selenium and vitamin E in men: The SELECT Eye Endpoints (SEE) Study. JAMA Ophthalmology. 2015;**133**:17-24. DOI: 10.1001/jamaophthalmol.2014.3478

[9] Kyei S, Koffuor GA, Ramkissoon P, Afari C, Asiamah EA. The claim of anti-cataract potential of *Heliotropium indicum*: A myth or reality? Ophthalmology and Therapy. 2015;**4**:115-128. DOI: 10.1007/s40123-015-0042-2

[10] Bissen-Miyajima H. Ophthalmic viscosurgical devices. Current Opinion in Ophthalmology. 2008;**19**:50-54

[11] Higashide T, Sugiyama K. Use of viscoelastic substance in ophthalmic surgery—Focus on sodium hyaluronate. Clinical Ophthalmology. 2008;**2**:21-30

[12] Chawla HB, Adams AD. Use of the anterior chamber maintainer in anterior segment surgery. Journal of Cataract and Refractive Surgery. 1996;**22**:172-177

[13] Wright M, Chawla H, Adams A. Results of small incision extracapsular cataract. Surgery using the anterior chamber maintainer without viscoelastic. The British Journal of Ophthalmology. 1999;**83**:71-75

[14] Blumenthal M, Moissiev J. Anterior chamber maintainer for extracapsular cataract extraction and intraocular lens implantation. Journal of Cataract and Refractive Surgery. 1987;**13**:204-206

[15] Jain K, Mallik KP, Gupta S. Corneal status following modified Blumenthal technique of manual small incision cataract surgery (MSICS) compared to phacoemulsification in treatment of grade III or more nuclear sclerosis-cohort study. Nepalese Journal of Ophthalmology. 2015;**7**:47-51. DOI: 10.3126/nepjoph.v7i1.13166

[16] Shingleton BJ, Mitrev PV. Anterior chamber maintainer versus viscoelastic material for intraocular lens implantation: Case-control study. Journal of Cataract and Refractive Surgery. 2001;**27**:711-714

[17] Ravalico G, Botteri E, Baccara F. Long-term endothelial changes after implantation of anterior chamber intraocular lenses in cataract surgery. Journal of Cataract and Refractive Surgery. 2003;**29**:1918-1923

[18] Liesegang TJ. Viscoelastic substances in ophthalmology. Survey of Ophthalmology. 1990;**34**:268-293

[19] Chang DF, Campbell JR. Intraoperative floppy iris syndrome associated with tamsulosin. Journal of Cataract and Refractive Surgery. 2005;**31**:664-673

[20] Sihota R, Saxena R, Agarwal HC. Intravitreal sodium hyaluronate and secondary glaucoma after complicated phacoemulsification. Journal of Cataract & Refractive Surgery. 2003;**29**:1226-1227

[21] Chang DF, Packard RB. Posterior assisted levitation for nucleous retrieval using Viscoat after posterior capsule rupture. Journal of Cataract and Refractive Surgery. 2003;**29**: 1860-1865

[22] Bissen-Miyajima H. In vitro behavior of ophthalmic viscosurgical devices during phacoemulsification. Journal of Cataract and Refractive Surgery. 2006;**32**:1026-1031

[23] Sholohov G, Levartovsky S. Retained ophthalmic viscosurgical device material in the capsular bag 6 months after phacoemulsification. Journal of Cataract and Refractive Surgery. 2005;**31**:627-629

[24] Altıntaş AK, Ciritoğlu MY, BeyazyıldıZ Ö, Can ÇÜ, Polat S. Toxic anterior segment syndrome outbreak after cataract surgery triggered by viscoelastic substance. Middle East African Journal of Ophthalmology. 2017;**24**:43-47. DOI: 10.4103/meajo.MEAJO_226_15

[25] Schulze SD, Bertelmann T, Manojlovic I, Bodanowitz S, Irle S, Sekundo W. Changes in corneal endothelium cell characteristics after cataract surgery with and without use of viscoelastic substances during intraocular lens implantation. Clinical Ophthalmology. 2015;**9**:2073-2080. DOI: 10.2147/OPTH.S90628

[26] Oksuz H, Daglioglu MC, Coskun M, Ilhan O, Tuzcu EA, Ilhan N, Ayıntap E, Keskin U, Taşkın I. Vacuum-assisted continuous circular capsulorhexis using bimanual irrigation and aspiration system of Phaco machine in immature cataract. Journal of Ophthalmology. 2013;**2013**:921646. DOI: 10.1155/2013/921646

[27] Sallet G. Viscoless microincision cataract surgery. Clinical Ophthalmology. 2008;**2**:717-721

[28] Galan A. Phaco-emulsification without the use of visco-elastic devices. Ocular Surgery News. Europe/Pacific Edition. 2005

[29] Bianchi GR. Phacoemulsification cataract surgery without viscoelastic substance. 2017; **4**(5):555646. DOI: 10.19080/JOJO.2017.04.555646

12

Trabecular Meshwork and Intraocular Pressure Dynamics: Oxidative Stress-Induced Changes

Bettina Hohberger,

Ulrich-Christoph Welge-Lüßen and Alice Yu

Abstract

Glaucoma is known as progressive neurodegenerative disease with irreversible loss of vision. Next to perimetric visual field defects, morphological alterations of the optic nerve and an increased intraocular pressure (IOP) occur. IOP is a fine regulated, complex homeostasis of production of aqueous humor (AH) in the non-pigmented ciliary body and its outflow. About 80% of AH is drained throughout the trabecular meshwork (TM). Any outflow resistance, with consecutive increase in IOP, can be generated by a decreased pore size or any other alterations of TM, making it more rigid. Oxidative stress, a disbalance of oxidants and antioxidants, is one mechanism, causing an altered extracellular matrix (ECM), and seems to play a key role in the pathogenesis of glaucomatous nerve atrophy. Damage of DNA, caused by oxidative stress, was shown in TM cells of glaucoma patients. This chapter gives a review about oxidative stress and its pathological alterations in the main outflow pathway—the trabecular meshwork—in glaucoma patients.

Keywords: glaucoma, trabecular meshwork, intraocular pressure, oxidative stress

1. Introduction

Glaucoma is known as a progressive neurodegenerative disease with irreversible loss of vision. Next to perimetric visual field defects, morphological alterations of the optic nerve and an increased intraocular pressure (IOP) occur. Additionally, special examinations were investigated in the last years for glaucoma diagnosis and follow-up [1–4].

IOP is a fine regulated, complex homeostasis of production of aqueous humor (AH) in the non-pigmented ciliary body and its outflow. About 80% of AH is drained throughout the trabecular meshwork (TM) [5], a sponge-like network of TM cells with glycoproteins, hyaluronic acid, elastic fibers, collagen and extracellular matrix (ECM). Any outflow resistance can be generated by a decreased pore size or any other alterations of TM, making it more rigid, resulting in an increased IOP. TM cells have the ability of different functions. Up to date it is not known, if cellular or intracellular disturbances are the origin of the altered TM in glaucoma. It is also conceivable that both mechanisms are impaired.

Oxidative stress is one mechanism, causing an altered extracellular matrix (ECM) [6] due to a disbalance of oxidants (free radicals, ROS) and antioxidants. If there is any imbalance between both with preponderance of oxidants, an irreversible cell loss is induced. Oxidative stress seems to have a key role in the pathogenesis of glaucomatous nerve atrophy [7, 8]. Damage of DNA, caused by oxidative stress, correlates significantly with IOP as well as with visual field defects [9, 10], and could be shown in TM cells in glaucoma patients [11]. Additionally, an increased lipid peroxidation, being the result of a ROS-induced cell damage, was noticed [12] as well as an impairment of metalloproteinases-2 (MMP-2) expression, resulting in an accumulation of ECM [13]. This accumulation (i.e., 'plaques') in TM could be seen several years before by electron microscopy studies [14, 15]. Additionally, actin expression can be induced by oxidative stress [16, 17], which is responsible for the rigidity of TM—the more amount of actin, the more rigid the TM [18].

In which way is oxidative stress induced, especially in glaucoma patients? Certainly, endogenous and exogenous factors contribute together. For example, daylight (especially ultraviolet light) can induce ROS in AH [19, 20]. Further on a vascular dysregulation [21] is discussed in glaucoma pathogenesis. An impaired blood flow with decreased nutritive supply can result in hypoxia, the main factor of inducing oxidative stress [22]. This hypothesis is supported by an increased concentration of vascular endothelial growth factor (VEGF) and erythropoietin in samples of AH in glaucoma patients [23, 24].

2. Oxidative stress and glaucoma

2.1. Oxidative stress: ROS and RNS

Oxidative stress was first described by Sies [25]. It is the result of an imbalance between oxidant (free radicals, reactive oxygen species and ROS) and antioxidant agents. Commonly, it is assumed that an excess of ROS, which follows from an increased production or decreased depletion, is the main reason for oxidative stress. Furthermore, a reduced antioxidant level can cause elevated ROS levels [26]. This imbalance with a preponderance of ROS results in a cytotoxicity with an irreversible cell loss.

The molecular basic for this damage can be found the reactivity of ROS. Free radicals are very aggressive molecules due to their unpaired electron [27]. They are generated under aerobic conditions. Excessive physical activities, infections or toxicity (e.g. cigarette smoke, UV radiation), are only some of the ROS causing agents. Even microwave radiation was found to induce oxidative stress [28]. ROS production can be found mainly in mitochondria [29]. Electrons (e^-) and protons (H^+), which were released by oxidation of fats and carbohydrates, enter the 'electron transfer chain.' In this chain, several consecutive reactions transfer electrons from NAPH to O_2 (oxygen) via respiratory enzyme complexes [30]. 'NADH dehydrogenase complex' transfers the electrons from NADH via flavin and iron-sulfur centers to ubiquinone. At this point, the second complex 'cytochrome b-c1' passes the electrons to cytochrome c, containing the 'cytochrome oxidase complex'. This step forwards the electrons to react with O_2 [30]. Almost 98% of O_2 is reduced to H_2O. The remaining 2% were reduced only incompletely, resulting in the production of ROS [31]. Considering this fact, it is of interest that not only the biochemical alterations of free radicals, but also the cellular energy level (redox status) is important, when talking about oxidative stress [32].

Several molecules are subsumed in the ROS group, which are all intermediate products, originated from O_2: hydrogen peroxide (H_2O_2), singlet oxygen (½ O_2), hydroxyl radical (HO) and superoxide (O_2^-). Molecular O_2 reacts with a single electron, followed by the uptake of several protons. This reaction produces the reactive oxygen species [33]:

$$O_2 + e^- \rightarrow \mathbf{O_2\cdot^-} \quad (1)$$

$$O_2\cdot^- + H^+ \rightarrow HO_2 \quad (2)$$

$$HO_2\cdot + e^- + H^+ \rightarrow \mathbf{H_2O_2} \quad (3)$$

$$H_2O_2 + e^- + H^+ \rightarrow \mathbf{HO\cdot} + H_2O \quad (4)$$

$$HO\cdot + e^- + H^+ \rightarrow H_2O \quad (5)$$

If iron reacts with ROS, the production of further ROS is catalyzed (Fenton reaction, [33]).

$$H_2O_2 + Fe^{2+} \rightarrow OH^- + FeO^{2+} + H^+ \rightarrow \mathbf{HO\cdot} + HO^- + Fe^{3+} \quad (6)$$

The hydroxyl radical is the most powerful radical, which is known up to now. It can cause membrane peroxidation and protein carbonylation [33], dectract or add electrons and hydrogen to the DNA, resulting in further radicals [34–36].

Organisms show diverse cellular escape mechanisms against ROS, which eliminates superoxide under normal conditions [29, 33, 37–39]:

$$2\mathbf{O}_2{\cdot}^{-} \rightarrow \tfrac{1}{2}\, O_2 \tag{7}$$

$$2\mathbf{O}_2{\cdot}^{-} + SOD \rightarrow H_2O_2 + O_2 \tag{8}$$

$$\mathbf{H_2O_2} + \mathbf{O_2}^{-} \rightarrow O_2 + HO{\cdot} + HO^{-} \tag{9}$$

$$\mathbf{H_2O_2} + Katalase \rightarrow H_2O + \tfrac{1}{2}\, O_2 \tag{10}$$

$$\mathbf{H_2O_2} + 2\ GSH + GSH - Peroxidase \rightarrow GSSG + 2\ H_2O \tag{11}$$

SOD superoxide dismutase

GSH glutathione

GSSG glutathione disulfide

At 'normal' ROS levels, these free radicals are interacting with other cellular molecules in cell regulation, transcription and cell proliferation. Additionally, they are very important as protective mechanism against distinct bacteria or fungi [26, 29, 33]. However with increasing amounts, ROS changes its function from defensive to aggressive.

Next to ROS, N-containing radical molecules were known to have oxidative power [40, 41]. Reactive nitrogen species (RNS) are derived from the nitric oxide (NO). Free radicals react rapidly with NO, forming RNS [42, 43]:

$$O_2{\cdot}^{-} + NO{\cdot} \rightarrow \mathbf{ONOO^{-}} \tag{12}$$

$ONOO^-$ peroxynitrite

Superoxide can be built by diverse reactions (see above) under different conditions. High concentrations of lipoproteins disturb the NOS pathway, which cause an increased amount of superoxide [25]. Peroxynitrite is not a stable molecule. It reacts very fast with almost all classes of biomolecules, thus being a potential cytotoxic agent [42]. It works similar to hydroxyl radicals, thus inducing DNA damages with breaks, nitrations and oxidations [36]. Unlike H_2O_2 peroxynitrite can be degraded without metal ions by inducing radicals [44, 45]:

$$ONOO^{-} + H^{+} \rightarrow OH{\cdot} + {\cdot}NO_2 \tag{13}$$

Peroxynitrite can react with several molecules. Next to molecules with aromatic structures (e.g. alpha-tocopherol [46]), thiols [47] can be modified. These reactions generate further radicals, which can induce themselves peroxidation in lipids [48].

In which way does ROS or RNS accumulate? Is there an alteration at the protein or even gene level, which results in this imbalance? Which external factors induce this 'program?' The final answer to all these questions is open up to now. There are evident hints that several transcription factors are involved in this complex network (e.g. p53, [49]).

2.2. Oxidative stress: molecular interactions

ROS and RNS can react with even each biochemical molecule (e.g. lipids, proteins). Cell membranes, containing a high amount of phospholipids and triglycerides, are one of the targets [50, 51]. After peroxidation of the lipids, bond arrangement and nonenzymatic Hock cleavage start. The produced α, β polyunsaturated lipid aldehydes act as radicals in turn [52]. Thus, a reaction chain is triggered. Additionally, the membrane structure and integrity are disturbed [53]. In particular, nerve structures are even more sensitive for oxidative stress as showing a large amount of lipids and high energy requirement [54].

Additionally, free radicals attack the ion channels within the cellular [55] as well as intracellular membranes [56]. The conductance is significantly altered, resulting in an altered excitability of the membranes. After free radical attacks proteins change their backbone and/or side chain structure in that way, that it reacts itself with other amino acid side chains to build carbonyl chains. Unfolding, misfolding and consecutive loss of activity remains [57].

As third target, ROS/RNS attack DNA by purine or pyridine bases structure changes. Yet, protein cross-linking and breaks in the DNA string were detected [39, 58]. These mutations can concern nuclear as well as mitochondrial DNA (mtDNA). However, in particular, mitochondrial DNA is affected, resulting in an impaired energy production [59, 60].

Why are mutations more dangerous, when affecting mitochondrial than nuclear DNA? Several hypotheses were discussed in this context. It is assumed that because of the local closeness of the enzyme complexes, which are involved in the electron transfer chain, next to the mitochondrial DNA, the produced ROS can attack the mtDNA more severe [61–63]. Additionally, mtDNA can replicate independently of the S-Phase, thus being more sensitive for oxidative agents, when the redox level is more oxidative [64], and free nucleotides are low [65]. Recent reports even suggest that hPrimpol1/CCDC111 (human primase-polymerase 1) is involved in DNA reparation due to its primase and DNA polymerase activity [66].

2.3. Oxidative stress: glaucoma

The influence of oxidative stress is discussed in the pathogenesis of several neurodegenerative diseases, like Morbus Parkinson or Morbus Alzheimer, as well as ophthalmic disorders, for example, glaucoma. The pathogenesis of glaucoma, being the second cause for blindness [67], is unknown up to now.

Glaucoma seems to be a multifactorial disorder. The most important risk factor for converting to glaucoma or glaucoma progression can be seen in the IOP [68, 69]. However, not all patients show a stable glaucoma disease after IOP regulation, and thus, several other factors seem to be involved. 'Vascular dysregulation' [21], glutamate exotoxicity [70], an interrupted retrograde transport of neutrophins [71] as well as ocular ischemia [72–74] and oxidative stress [7, 8, 75–77] are established in this discussion.

Glaucoma is characterized by an altered optic disc, visual field defects and an elevated intraocular pressure (IOP). As consequence of the increased IOP, retinal ganglion cells (RGC) and axons will die and cause the typical optic nerve appearance with glaucomatous excavation. Free radicals are known to induce oxidative stress in retinal ganglion cells, resulting in apoptosis of these cells [78]. Trapping ROS/RNS with NF-E2 related factor 2 (Nrf2), the death of RGC, seems to be prevented [79]. Several studies have been performed to investigate the potential influence of oxidative stress in glaucoma patients. It was shown that the L-arginine/nitric oxide system is altered in patients with glaucoma [80]. Increased concentrations of superoxide dismutase, malondialdehyde and glutathione peroxidase could be detected in aqueous humor of patients with primary open-angle glaucoma (POAG) [81, 82]. Additionally, antioxidant activity was shown to be decreased in POAG [82]. If systemic antioxidant reserve is low, more severe perimetric defects occurred [83, 84]. Further on the DNA damage, caused by oxidative stress, correlates significantly with glaucomatous visual field defects and IOP [9, 10].

Up to now, there are evident hints for a critical role of oxidative stress in the pathogenesis of glaucoma, yet there are several questions unanswered. However, oxidative stress induces change within different ocular structures, whereas alterations in tissues, influencing IOP, are of special interest.

3. Intraocular pressure

Intraocular pressure is the result of aqueous humor (AH) production and outflow through trabecular meshwork and uveoscleral. This circular flow is regulated until a steady state arises. The production of AH starts at the non-pigmented ciliary body. Plasma of the vascular plexus is filtrated by diffusion, ultrafiltration and active secretion to build the AH. First of all, lipid-soluble molecules diffuse according to a gradient. Second, water and water-soluble molecules are ultrafiltrated because of an osmotic gradient and hydrostatic pressure [85]. Active secretion completes the process of AH production [86]. Electrolytes flow due to an electrochemical gradient [87] into the interstitial space, whereas protein transporters, ion channels, aquaporins and enzymes work together to pass molecules, ions or ascorbic acid through the blood-aqueous barrier [88–91]. Liquid diffusion is a consecutive result of the movement of electric charge [92], which is completed by the work of aquaporins.

The produced AH is similar to plasma, yet proteins are 200× less and ascorbic acid 20× higher than in plasma [93]. Additionally, endothelin-1 [94], several growth factors [95], enzymes (collagenase) [96] or Immunoglobulin G [97], intrinsic glycoproteins [98] and transferrin [99] can be detected.

After production in the posterior part of the eye, AH flows through the pupil. Convection effectuates the movement of AH in the anterior chamber. AH circulates with an upward trend at the cornea and downstream flow at the iris [100]. The outflow of AH is provided by two pathways: The trabecular meshwork in the anterior chamber angle drains off the AH into the Schlemm's canal. The fluid passes multiple intrascleral collector canals until drainage into episcleral veins, ciliary veins and veins of the extraocular muscles [101, 102]. The second draining pathway is the uveoscleral outflow. Through the uveal meshwork and the anterior parts of the ciliary muscle, AH flows toward suprachoroidal space and sclera, where it is resorbed by several veins [103–105].

To generate the IOP distinct, resistance factors have to be considered: the conventional outflow pathway via trabecular meshwork with resistance of 3–4 mmHg/μl/min and the episcleral vein pressure of 8–10 mmHg [106–108] results in IOP of about 15.5 ± 2.57 mmHg in normals [109–111].

Because the outflow through the trabecular meshwork (TM) is dependent on resistance of the trabecular meshwork, the factors, influencing resistance in TM, are of special interest in IOP.

4. Trabecular meshwork

In patients with POAG, the trabecular meshwork is characterized by an increased outflow resistance leading to an elevated IOP. It is assumed that the increased outflow resistance is attributed to various morphological and biochemical alterations of the TM of glaucomatous eyes. So have electron microscopic and immunohistochemical studies of TM cells demonstrated an increased accumulation of extracellular matrix, the so-called plaque material, in the juxtacanalicular region of the TM [112, 113]. An increased accumulation of fibronectin was found in the TM of glaucomatous donor eyes as compared to the TM of control eyes [114]. In addition, TM cells showed an increased cell loss as compared to age-matched control TM cells [115]. Later, Liton et al. have also demonstrated an accelerated senescence of TM in comparison with age-matched control donors [116].

The reasons for these changes are still not clear. One factor, which may play an important role in the pathogenesis of POAG, is oxidative stress [117]. Patients with POAG showed mutations in the mitochondrial genome and a reduced mitochondrial respiratory activity compared to control groups [118]. Also the antioxidative capacity in the aqueous humor of patients with POAG was found to be reduced by more than 50% compared to non-glaucomatous eyes [119]. Furthermore, an increased level of 8-hydroxy-2′-deoxyguanosine, a molecular biomarker for oxidative damage, was detected in TM samples collected from glaucoma patients undergoing standard filtration surgery [10]. The oxidative damage in these cells correlated with the visual field defects of these operated glaucoma patients [10]. Besides that, oxidative stress can also induce inflammation of the TM cells [8] and alter their mobility [120], which leads to contractile dysfunction and damage of the TM cells. Thus, these studies suggest that oxidative stress may be involved in the pathogenesis of POAG.

The human TM is a highly sensitive tissue to oxidative stress, since it is equipped with few antioxidant defense mechanisms [121, 122]. *In vitro* studies showed that increased levels of hydrogen peroxide stimulated the migration of TM cells, which lead to trabecular thickening and enlargement or collapse [123]. Furthermore, hydrogen peroxide could also cause endothelial cell loss and thus a disruption and collapse of the TM [124]. It is assumed that TM cell loss is caused by oxidative stress-induced apoptosis via inflammation, mitochondrial damage, hypoxia and endothelial dysfunction [125]. We could demonstrate that oxidative stress in form of hydrogen peroxide was able to induce cell death, extracellular matrix production, and accelerated senescence in cultured human TM cells. Based on these studies, it was postulated that oxidative stress may play a role in cell death, release of inflammatory markers, extracellular matrix accumulation, advanced senescence and disarrangement of the cytoskeleton of TM cells. These oxidative stress-induced TM changes may be responsible for a reduced outflow facility and thus an increased IOP.

Author details

Bettina Hohberger[1*], Ulrich-Christoph Welge-Lüßen[1] and Alice Yu[2]

*Address all correspondence to: Bettina.hohberger@uk-erlangen.de

1 Department of Ophthalmology, Friedrich-Alexander-Universität Erlangen-Nürnberg (FAU), Erlangen, Germany

2 Ophthalmology Center-Stachus, Munich, Germany

References

[1] Brehmer K, Rutrecht P, Mißlinger S, Jünemann A, Horn FK, Kremers J, Hohberger B. 25 Hz adaptation: influence on recovery time in glaucoma. Ophthalmol J 2016;1:1–9.

[2] Rutrecht P, Brehmer K, Kremers J, Horn FK, Jünemann A, Hohberger B. Temporal contrast sensitivity: a potential parameter for glaucoma progression, especially in advanced stages. Ophthalmol J 2016;1:10–17.

[3] Kara K, Jünemann A, Redjak R, Hohberger B. Glaucoma: confrontation visual field test using Bagolini striated glasses—a new screening method for detecting visual field defects. Ophthalmol J 2016;1:18–23.

[4] Horn FK, Scharch V, Mardin CY, Lämmer R, Kremers J. Comparison of frequency doubling and flicker defined form perimetry in early glaucoma. Graefes Arch Clin Exp Ophthalmol. 2016;25:937–946.

[5] Gabelt BT, Kaufman PL. Changes in aqueous humor dynamics with age and glaucoma. Prog Retin Eye Res 2005;24:612–637.

[6] Dumont P, Burton M, Chen QM et al. Induction of replicative senescence biomarkers by sublethal oxidative stresses in normal human fibroblast. Free Radic Biol Med 2000;28:361–373.

[7] Tezel G. Oxidative stress in glaucomatous neurodegeneration: mechanisms and consequences. Prog Retin Eye Res 2006;25:490–513.

[8] Aslan M, Cort A, Yucel I. Oxidative and nitrative stress markers in glaucoma. Free Radic Biol Med. 2008;45:367–376.

[9] Gupta N, Yucel YH. Glaucoma as a neurodegenerative disease. Curr Opin Ophthalmol 2007;18:110–114.

[10] Sacca SC, Pascotto A, Camicione P et al. Oxidative DNA damage in the human trabecular meshwork: clinical correlation in patients with primary open-angle glaucoma. Arch Ophthalmol 2005;123:458–463.

[11] Izzotti A, Cartiglia C, De Flora S, Sacca S. Methodology for evaluating oxidative DNA damage and metabolic genotypes in human trabecular meshwork. Toxicol Mech Methods 2003;13:161–168.

[12] Babizhayev MA, Bunin AYa. Lipid peroxidation in open-angle glaucoma. Acta Ophthalmol 1989b;67(4):371–377.

[13] Welge-Lüssen U, Eichhorn M, Bloemendal H et al. Classification of human scleral spur cells in monolayer culture. Eur J Cell Biol 1998;75:78–84.

[14] Babizhayev MA, Brodskaya MW. Fibronectin detection in drainage outflow system of human eyes in ageing and progression of open-angle glaucoma. Mech Ageing Dev 1989a;47:145–157.

[15] Rauhut D, Rohen JW. Electron microscopic study of the trabecular meshwork in alphachymotrypsin glaucoma. Albrecht Von Graefes Arch Klin Exp Ophthalmol 1972;184:29–41.

[16] Zhu J, Zhou K, Hao JJ et al. Regulation of cortactin/dynamin interaction by actin polymerization during the fission of clathrin-coated pits. J Cell Sci 2005;118:807–817.

[17] Dalle-Donne I, Rossi R, Giustarini D et al. Actin carbonylation: from a simple marker of protein oxidation to relevant signs of severe functional impairment. Free Radic Biol Med 2001;31:1075–1083.

[18] Tan JC, Peters DM, Kaufman PL. Recent developments in understanding the pathophysiology of elevated intraocular pressure. Curr Opin Ophthalmol 2006;17:168–174.

[19] Balansky RM, Izzotti A, D'Agostini F et al. Systemic genotoxic effects produced by light, and synergism with cigarette smoke in the respiratory tract of hairless mice. 2003;24(9): 1525–1532.

[20] Wei H, Ca Q, Rahn R et al. DNA structural integrity and base composition affect ultraviolet light-induced oxidative DNA damage. Biochemistry 1998;37:6485–6490.

[21] Flammer J. The vascular concept of glaucoma. Surv Ophthalmol 1994;38:3–6.

[22] Nakabayashi M. Review of the ischemia hypothesis for ocular hypertension other than congenital glaucoma and closed-angle glaucoma. Ophthalmologica 2004;218:344–349.

[23] Alge CS, Priglinger SG, Neubauer AS et al. Retinal pigment epithelium is protected against apoptosis by alphaB-crystallin. Invest Ophthalmol Vis Sci 2002;43:3575–3582.

[24] Cumurcu T, Bulut Y, Demir HD et al. Aqueous humor erythropoietin levels in patients with primary open-angle glaucoma. J Glaucoma 2007;16:645–648.

[25] Sies H. Oxidative stress: from basic research to clinical application. Am J Med 1991;91:31–38.

[26] Poljsak B, Suput D, Milisav I. Achieving the balance between ROS and antioxidants: when to use the synthetic antioxidants. Oxid Med Cell Longev 2013;2013:Article ID 956792.

[27] Riley PA. Free radicals in biology: oxidative stress and the effects of ionizing radiation. Int J Radiat Biol 1994;65:27–33.

[28] Chauhan P, Verma HN, Sisodia R, Kesari KK. Microwave radiation (2.45 GHz)-induced oxidative stress: whole-body exposure effect on histopathology of Wistar rats. Electromagn Biol Med 2017;36(1):20–30.

[29] Dröge W. Free radicals in the physiological control of cell function. Physiol Rev 2002;82:47–95.

[30] Alberts B, Johnson A, Lewis J, et al. Molecular Biology of the Cell. 4th edition. New York: Garland Science; 2002. Electron-Transport Chains and Their Proton Pumps. Available from: http://www.ncbi.nlm.nih.gov/books/NBK26904/

[31] Pinazo-Durán MD, Zanón-Moreno V, Gallego-Pinazo R, García-Medina JJ. Oxidative stress and mitochondrial failure in the pathogenesis of glaucoma neurodegeneration. Prog Brain Res. 2015;220:127–153.

[32] Lopez-Alarcona C, Denicola A. Evaluating the antioxidant capacity of natural products: a review on chemical and cellular-based assays. Anal Chim Acta 2013;763:1–10.

[33] Imlay JA. Pathways of oxidative damage. Annu Rev Microbiol 2003;57:395–418.

[34] Hutchinson F. Chemical changes induced in DNA by ionizing radiation. Prog Nucleic Acid Res. 1985;32:116–154.

[35] Dizdaroglu M, Rao G, Halliwell B, Gajewski E. Damage to the DNA bases in mammalian chromatin by hydrogen peroxide in the presence of ferric and cupric ions. Arch Biochem Biophys 1991;285:317–324.

[36] Kohen R, Nyska A. Oxidation of biological systems: oxidative stress phenomena, antioxidants, redox reactions, and methods for their quantification. Toxicol Pathol 2002;30:620–650.

[37] Forth W, Henschler D, Rummel W, Starke K. General and Specific pharmacology and toxicology, 7th version, 1998. Heidelberg: Spektrum Akademischer Verlag.

[38] Miao L, Clair DKS. Regulation of superoxide dismutase genes: implications in disease. Free Radic Bio Med 2009;47:344–356.

[39] Gandhi S, Abramov AY. Mechanism of oxidative stress in neurodegeneration. Oxid Med Cell Longev 2012;2012:428010.

[40] Rubbo H, Darley-Usmar V, Freeman BA. Nitric oxide regulation of tissue free radical injury. Chem Res Toxicol 1996;9:809–820.

[41] McAndrew J, Patel RP, Jo et al. The interplay of nitric oxide and peroxynitrite with signal transduction pathways: implications for disease. Semin Perinatol 1997;21:351–366.

[42] Beckman JS, Beckman TW, Chen J et al. Apparent hydroxyl radical production by peroxynitrite: implications for endothelial injury from nitric oxide and superoxide. Proc Natl Acad Sci USA. 1990;87:1620–1624.

[43] Crow JP, Beckman JS. The importance of superoxide in nitric oxide-dependent toxicity: evidence for peroxynitrite-mediated injury. Adv Exp Med Bio 1996;387:147–161.

[44] Green SJ, Mellouk S, Hoffman SL et al. Cellular mechanisms of nonspecific immunity to intracellular infection: cytokine-induced synthesis of toxic nitrogen oxides from L-arginine by macrophages and hepatocytes. Immunol Lett 1990;25:15–19.

[45] Hou YC, Janczuk A, Wang PG. Current trends in the development of nitric oxide donors. Curr Pharm Des 1999;5:417–441.

[46] Hogg N, Joseph J, Kalyanaraman B. The oxidation of alpha-tocopherol and trolox by peroxynitrite. Arch Biochem Biophys 1994;314:153–158.

[47] Quijano C, Alvarez B, Gatti RM et al. Pathways of peroxynitrite oxidation of thiol groups. Biochem J 1997;322:167–173.

[48] Radi R, Beckman JS, Bush KM, Freeman BA. Peroxynitrite-induced membrane lipid peroxidation: the cytotoxic potential of superoxide and nitric oxide. Arch Biochem Biophys 1991;288:481–487.

[49] Szczepanek K, Lesnefsky EJ, Larner AC. Multi-tasking: nuclear transcription factors with novel roles in the mitochondria. Trends Cell Biol. 2012;22:429–437.

[50] Bielski BH, Arudi RL, Sutherland MW. A study of the reactivity of HO2/O2- with unsaturated fatty acids. J Biol Chem 1983 Apr 25;258:4759–4761.

[51] Gardner HW. Oxygen radical chemistry of polyunsaturated fatty acids. Free Radic Biol Med. 1989;7:65–86.

[52] Benedetti A, Comporti M, Esterbauer H. Identification of 4-hydroxynonenal as a cytotoxic product originating from the peroxidation of liver microsomal lipids. Biochim Biophys Acta 1980;620:281–296.

[53] Zhong H, Yin H. Role of lipid peroxidation derived 4-hydroxynonenal (4-HNE) in cancer: focusing on mitochondria. Redox Biol 2015;4:193–199.

[54] Pearson JN, Patel M. The role of oxidative stress in organophosphate and nerve agent toxicity. Ann N Y Acad Sci 2016;1378(1):17–24.

[55] Evans JR, Bielefeldt K. Regulation of sodium currents through oxidation and reduction of thiol residues. Neuroscience 2000;101:229–236.

[56] Coronado R, Morrissette J, Sukhareva M, Vaughan DM. Structure and function of ryanodine receptors. Am J Physiol 1994;266:1485–1504.

[57] Headlamand HA, Davies MJ. Markers of protein oxidation: different oxidants give rise to variable yields of bound and released carbonyl products. Free Radic Biol Med 2004;36:1175–1184.

[58] Pisoschi AM, Pop A. The role of antioxidants in the chemistry of oxidative stress: a review. Eur J Med Chem 2015;97:55–74.

[59] Krishnan KJ, Reeve AK, Samuels DC et al. What causes mitochondrial DNA deletions in human cells? Nat genet 2008;40:275–279.

[60] Schon EA, DiMauro S, Hirano M. Human mitochondrial DNA: roles of inherited and somatic mutations. Nat Rev Genet 2012;13:878–890.

[61] Wallace DC, Ye JH, Neckelmann SN et al. Sequence analysis of cDNAs for the human and bovine ATP synthase beta subunit: mitochondrial DNA genes sustain seventeen times more mutations. Curr Genet 1987;12:81–90.

[62] Yakes FM, Van Houten B. Mitochondrial DNA damage is more extensive and persists longer than nuclear DNA damage in human cells following oxidative stress. Proc Natl Acad Sci U S A 1997;94:514–519.

[63] Rajala N, Gerhold JM, Martinsson P et al. Replication factors transiently associate with mtDNA at the mitochondrial inner membrane to facilitate replication. Nucleic Acids Res 2014;42:952–967.

[64] Klevecz RR, Bolen J, Forrest G, Murray DB. A genomewide oscillation in transcription gates DNA replication and cell cycle. Proc Natl Acad Sci U S A 2004;101:1200–1205.

[65] Borst P, Kroon AM. Mitochondrial DNA: physicochemical properties, replication, and genetic function. Int Rev Cytol 1069;26:107–190.

[66] Wan L, Lou J, Xia Y et al. hPrimpol1/CCDC111 is a human DNA primase-polymerase required for the maintenance of genome integrity. EMBO Rep 2013;14:1104–1112.

[67] Kass MA, Heuer DK, Higginbotham EJ et al. The ocular hypertensin treatment study: a randomized trial determines that topical ocular hypotensive medication delays or prevents the onset of primary open-angle glaucoma. Arch Ophthalmol 2002;120:701–713.

[68] Sommer A. Intraocular pressure and glaucoma. Am J Ophthalmol 1989;107:186–188.

[69] Garrat S. Primary Open Angle Glaucoma. Preferred Practice Pattern. San Francisco: American Academy of Ophthalmology; 1996.

[70] Vorwerk CK, Lipton SA, Zurakowski D et al. Chronic low-dose glutamate is toxic to retinal ganglion cells. Toxicity blocked by memantine. Invest Ophthalmol Vis Sci 1996;37:1618–1624.

[71] Quigley HA. Ganglion cell death in glaucoma: pathology recapitulates ontogeny. Aust N Z J Ophthalmol 1995;23:85–91.

[72] Begg IS, Drance SM. Progress of the glaucomatous process related to recurrent ischaemic changes at the optic disc. Exp Eye Res 1971;11:141.

[73] Hayreh SS. Posterior ciliary arterial occlusice disorders. Trans Ophthalmol Soc UK 1971;91:291–303.

[74] Cioffi GA. Care guidelines and optic nerve assessment. J Glaucoma 1996;5:A12.

[75] Levin L. Direct and indirect approaches to neuroprotective therapy of glaucomatous optic neuropathy. Surv Ophthalmol 1999;43:98–101.

[76] Osborne NN. Pathogenesis of ganglion "cell death" in glaucoma and neuroprotection: focus on ganglion cell axonal mitochondria. Prog Brain Res 2008;173:339–352.

[77] Kong GY, Van Bergen NJ, Trounce IA, Crowston JG. Mitochondrial dysfunction and glaucoma. J Glaucoma 2009;18:93–100.

[78] Yokoyama Y, Maruyama K, Yamamoto K et al. The role of calpain in an *in vivo* model of oxidative stress-induced retinal ganglion cell damage. Biochem Biophys Res Commun 2014;451:510–515.

[79] Himori N, Yamamoto K, Maruyama K et al. Critical role of Nrf2 in oxidative stress-induced retinal ganglion cell death. J Neurochem 2013;127:669–680.

[80] Polak K, Luksch A, Berisha F, Fuchsjaeger-Mayrl G, Dallinger S, Schmetterer L. Altered nitric oxide system in patients with open-angle glaucoma. Arch Ophthalmol 2007;125:494–498.

[81] Ghanem AA, Arafa LF, El-Baz A. Oxidative stress markers in patients with primary open-angle glaucoma. Curr Eye Res 2010;35:295–301.

[82] Zanon-Moreno V, Marco-Ventura P, Lleo-Perez A et al. Oxidative stress in primary open-angle glaucoma. J Glaucoma 2008;17:263–268.

[83] Tanito M, Kaidzu S, Takai Y, Ohira A. Correlation between systemic oxidative stress and intraocular pressure level. PLoS One 2015;10:e0133582.

[84] Tanito M, Kaidzu S, Takai Y, Ohira A. Association between systemic oxidative stress and visual field damage in open-angle glaucoma. Sci Rep 2016;6:25792.

[85] Civan MM, Macknight AD. The ins and outs of aqueous humour secretion. Exp Eye Res 2004;78:625–31.

[86] Cole DF. Secretion of aqueous humor. Exp Eye Res 1977;25:161–176.

[87] Gabelt BT, Kaufman PL. Aqueous Humor Hydrodynamics. In: Adler's Physiology of the Eye, 9th ed. 2003a.

[88] Reddy VN. Dynamics of transport systems in the eye. Friedenwald Lecture. Invest Ophthalmol Vis Sci 1979;18:1000–1018.

[89] Coca-Prados M, Sanchez-Torres J. Molecular approaches to the study of the Na+-K+-ATPase and chloride channels in the ocular ciliary epithelium. In: Civan MM, editor. The eye's aqueous humor. San Diego: Academic Press 1998.

[90] Tsukaguchi H, Tokui T, Mackenzie B et al. A family of mammalian Na+-dependent L-ascorbic acid transporters. Nature 1999;399:70–75.

[91] Yamaguchi Y, Watanabe T, Hirakata A, Hida T. Localization and ontogeny of aquaporin-1 and -4 expression in iris and ciliary epithelial cells in rats. Cell Tissue Res 2006;325:101–109.

[92] Tornquist P, Alm A, Bill A. Permeability of ocular vessels and transport across the blood-retinal-barrier. Eye 1990;4:303–309.

[93] Gabelt BT, Kaufman PL. Aqueous Humor Hydrodynamics. In: Adlers's Physiology of the Eye. 10th ed. 2003.

[94] Lepple-Wienhues A, Becker M, Stahl F et al. Endothelin-like immunoreactivity in the aqueous humour and in conditioned medium from cultured ciliary epithelial cells. Curr Eye Res 1992;11:1041–1046.

[95] Cousins SW, McCabe MM, Danielpour D, Streilein JW. Identification of transforming growth factor-beta as an immunosuppressive factor in aqueous humor. Invest Ophthalmol Vis Sci 1991;32:2201–2211.

[96] Vadillo-Ortega F, Gonzalez-Avila G, Chevez P, Abraham CR, Montano M, Selman-Lama M. A latent collagenase in human aqueous humor. Invest Ophthalmol Vis Sci 1989;30:332–335.

[97] McClellan BH, Whitney CR, Newman LP, Allansmith MR. Immunoglobulins in tears. Am J Ophthalmol 1973;76:89–101.

[98] Haddad A, Laicine EM, de Almeida JC. Origin and renewal of the intrinsic glycoproteins of the aqueous humor. Graefes Arch Clin Exp Ophthalmol 1991;229:371–379.

[99] Tripathi RC, Borisuth NS, Tripathi BJ, Gotsis SS. Quantitative and qualitative analyses of transferrin in aqueous humor from patients with primary and secondary glaucomas. Invest Ophthalmol Vis Sci 1992;33:2866–2873.

[100] Heys JJ, Barocas VH. A boussinesq model of natural convection in the human eye and the formation of Krukenberg's spindle. Ann Biomed Eng 2002;30:392–401.

[101] Worthen DM. Scanning electron microscopic study of the interior of Schlemm's canal in the human eye. Am J Ophthalmol 1972;74:35–40.

[102] Tenner A, Jaeger W, Koch W. Demonstration of aqueous veins through injection of fluorescein into the anterior chamber in rabbits. Klin Monatsbl Augenheilkd 1974;164:628–632.

[103] Bill A, Hellsing K. Production and drainage of aqueous humor in the cynomolgus monkey (*Macaca irus*). Invest Ophthalmol 1965;4:920–926.

[104] Bill A, Phillips CI. Uveoscleral drainage of aqueous humour in human eyes. Exp Eye Res 1971;12:275–281.

[105] Johnson M, Erickson K. Mechanisms and routes of aqueous humor drainage. In: Albert DM, Jakobiec FA, Eds. Principles and practice of ophthalmology. Philadelphia: WB Saunders; 2000.

[106] Brubaker RF. Determination of episcleral venous pressure in the eye. A comparison of three methods. Arch Ophthalmol 1967;77:110–114.

[107] Brubaker RF. The effect of intraocular pressure on conventional outflow resistance in the enucleated human eye. Invest Ophthalmol 1975;14:286–292.

[108] Phelps CD, Armaly MF. Measurement of episcleral venous pressure. Am J Ophthalmol 1978;85:35–42.

[109] Leydhecker W, Akiyama K, Neumann HG. Intraocular pressure of normal human eyes. Klin Monatsbl Augenheilkd 1958;133:662–670.

[110] Schottenstein EM. Intraocular pressure. In: Ritch R, Shields MB, Krupin T, Eds. The glaucomas. St. Louis: Mosby 1989;301–317.

[111] Millar C, Kaufman PL. Aqueous humor: secretion and dynamics. In: Tasman W, Jaeger EA, Eds. Duane's foundations of clinical ophthalmology. Philadelphia: Lippincott-Raven; 1995.

[112] Rohen JW, Witmer R. Electron microscopic studies on the trabecular meshwork in glaucoma simplex. Albrecht Von Graefes Arch Klin Exp Ophthalmol 1972;183:251–266.

[113] Lütjen-Drecoll E. Morphological changes in glaucomatous eyes and the role of TGFbeta2 for the pathogenesis of the disease. Exp Eye Res 2005;81:1–4.

[114] Babizhayev MA, Brodskaya MW. Fibronectin detection in drainage outflow system of human eyes in ageing and progression of open-angle glaucoma. Mech Ageing Dev 1989;47:145–157.

[115] Alvarado J, Murphy C, Juster R. Trabecular meshwork cellularity in primary open-angle glaucoma and nonglaucomatous normals. Ophthalmology 1984;91(6):564–79.

[116] Liton PB, Challa P, Stinnett S, Luna C, Epstein DL, Gonzalez P. Cellular senescence in the glaucomatous outflow pathway. Exp Gerontol 2005;40:745–748.

[117] Izzotti A, Bagnis A, Sacca SC. The role of oxidative stress in glaucoma. Mutat Res 2006;612:105–114.

[118] Abu-Amero KK, Morales J, Bosley TM. Mitochondrial abnormalities in patients with primary open-angle glaucoma. Invest Ophthalmol Vis 2006;47:2533–2541.

[119] Ferreira SM, Lerner SF, Brunizini R, Evelson PA, Liesuy SF. Oxidative stress markers in aqueous humor of glaucoma patients. Am J Ophthalmol 2004;137:62–69.

[120] Nathanson JA, McKee M. Alterations of ocular nitric oxide synthase in human glaucoma. Invest Ophthalmol Vis Sci 1995;36(9):1774–1784.

[121] Izzotti A, Saccà SC, Longobardi M, Cartigl C. Sensitivity of ocular anterior chamber tissues to oxidative damage and its relevance to the pathogenesis of glaucoma. Invest Ophthalmol Vis Sci 2009;50(11):5251–5258.

[122] Nita M, Grzybowski A. The role of the reactive oxygen species and oxidative stress in the pathomechanism of the age-related ocular diseases and other pathologies of the anterior and posterior eye segments in adults. Oxid Med Cell Longev 2016;2016:3164734.

[123] Hogg P, Calthorpe M, Batterbury M, Grierson I. Aqueous humor stimulates the migration of human trabecular meshwork cells *in vitro*. Invest Ophthalmol Vis Sci 2000;41(5):1091–1098.

[124] Zhou L, Li Y, Yue BYJT. Oxidative stress affects cytoskeletal structure and cell-matrix interactions in cells from an ocular tissue: the trabecular meshwork. J Cell Physiol 1999;180(2):182–189.

[125] Saccà SC, Gandolfi S, Bagnis A, Manni G, Damonte G, Traverso CE, Izzotti A. From DNA damage to functional changes of the trabecular meshwork in aging and glaucoma. Ageing Res Rev 2016;29:26–41.

13

Optimizing Outcome of Cataract Surgery in Resource Scarce Sub-Saharan Africa

Lawan Abdu

Abstract

Background: Sub-Saharan Africa disproportionately accounts for high number of avoidably blind largely caused by cataracts.

The blindness burden: Limitation in human and material resource for delivery of cataract surgical services, cost, gender, distance to hospital, time off for the care giver, fear of surgery, uncultured behavior of eye care personal, poor visual outcome, general governments neglect of health care, lack of health insurance for vast majority of the population, healthcare funded by individuals as out of pocket despite grinding poverty, reliance on poorly coordinated and unsustainable outreach program, malpractices of quacks and traditional eye healers amongst other reasons.

More than just a cataract: Cataract services require systematic evaluation of the patients' general condition as well as the eye. Appropriate counseling is required to understand the goal and expectation of treatment. Adequate planning of surgery includes ocular biometry and provision of the appropriate intra ocular lens. The management protocol must ensure adequate measures are taken to prevent/ manage critical incidents whenever such a need arises.

Conclusion: Cataract surgical services need to be patient centered with the goal of optimizing resources for quality outcome without compromising safety.

Keywords: cataract, surgery, resource, outcome, patients, safety

1. Introduction

Age-related cataract is the leading cause of avoidable blindness [1–4]. While Africa hosts 11.9% of the World population, it also disproportionately accounts for about 15% of those avoidably blind. Sub-Saharan Africa carries the worse burden with 4.8 million blind partly due to 66% population growth [5]. Other factors accounting for this include scarcity of eye care personnel, limitation in technology and training for eye care, lack of local production of eye medicine, and other consumables leading to dependency on importation in the presence of limited foreign exchange availability, unrestrained and unregulated malpractices of quacks, and traditional eye care providers. It is not unusual for such unregistered practitioners to be patronized by the political class resulting in wide-scale eye couching with all the related complications. In Sub-Saharan African region where human and material resources are scarce, health care is on a free fall as health insurance is largely inaccessible to the vast majority of the population [6].

Unfavorable health indicators such as high maternal mortality, high infant and under five mortality [7], high morbidity and mortality from both communicable [8] and noncommunicable diseases [9], and reduced life expectancy are the norm [10]. The poor people pay for health care as out-of-pocket expenses. Whenever health personnel knock on their door to administer vaccines, they become suspicious, considering the fact that they have to wait long hours to be attended to at government hospitals and clinics and most times they buy drugs from unprofessional vendors in pharmacy shops. Clerics and community leaders who should have been carried along are uninformed and often unsupportive of such programs. As such "free" healthcare programs are shunned by some communities who are made to believe they are aimed at subtly curtailing their population.

Local eye care advocacy groups can spend months to years hoping to see government officials to suggest ways forward to no avail. Expatriate eye care teams who surface once or twice in a year to do a few hundred cataract surgeries are received almost immediately by the local authorities. Such teams are treated with care and concern providing a photo opportunity for the politicians and giving the impression that all the eye problems of the community have been solved. Dependence on inconsistent external outreach services by authorities lead to further complacency and neglect.

Inappropriate appointment of members into district, state and national blindness prevention committees is such that technocrats hardly have a say in decision making. Such committees hardly meet, and when they do, decisions are hardly transformed into action. Often there is no time scale for implementation, no mechanism for self-audit, and no follow-up on programs, and the roles of members are hardly clearly stated. Most eye care teams are bedeviled with lingering rivalry and leadership crisis, which tend to be prolonged and incapacitating causing inability to achieve the goal of the team. There is need for models of leadership capacity building to address the need for core technical and management competencies [11].

There are unlimited barriers to eye care, which include distance to facility, transportation cost, time off for the care giver to accompany the patient, gender, cost of cataract surgery, rude behavior of some eye care workers, cost of investigations (blood sugar level, hepatitis, HIV, etc.), multiple visits, long bookings for surgery, and poor outcome as perceived by those who preceded the index patient [12–18]. The need to optimally use available materials and human resource to ensure that patients get the best outcome of surgery despite the existing limitations is of paramount importance.

2. More than just a cataract

Cataract surgery is considered one of the most rewarding medical interventions. Suffice it to say that sight is restored almost immediately thus improving the patients' quality of life [19, 20]. This observation may result in considering the procedure so casually without taking meticulous steps that ensure that there is quality in terms of postoperative visual acuity and patient's safety. Removing the cataractous lens and inserting an intraocular lens no matter how fast and quick this is achieved are not synonymous with obtaining good postoperative vision and ensuring patient's safety.

Good clinical practice starts with obtaining reliable history. The ophthalmologist should be courteous and willing to listen to the patients' complaints. There should be no indication, behavior, or action to make the client feel he is in a police station facing interrogation or a courtroom on trial for what he did or should have done about his eye condition. Rural folks constitute majority of the population in the region and often tend to fear such formal interactions with unfamiliar personalities in an unusual environment. When the patient becomes fearful and suspicious, reliable history may not be obtained, thus heralding the first step toward not obtaining quality outcome.

Ordinarily, patients present with painless progressive loss of vision over a time frame often in months to years. Additional information related to pain could arise from a number of factors including secondary glaucoma from intumescent cataract, inflammation, and/or panophthalmitis due to infection from attempted couching. A positive history of application of (harmful) traditional eye medication (TEM) could be obtained by gentle probing. TEM use is not unusual despite its harmful effect [21, 22]. This may require making a suggestive comment such as "losing one's sight is quite disturbing, please were you able to obtain traditional medicine that someone has tried in your community in the hope that your eye will open?" Compare this statement with "did you apply damaging traditional eye medication instead of coming to see us here in the eye clinic where we can offer you the best treatment?" Some TEMs are potentially contaminated and may contain substances that can damage the cornea.

In other instances, patients could have had surgery elsewhere with improper guidance on follow-up or the postoperative medication has finished and nowhere/no means to buy. Postoperative inflammation tends to last more than 6 weeks perhaps due to environmental and genetic factors. Complain of pain should warrant careful probing of possible preexisting ocular and systemic diseases. There is need to ask for presence of discharge from orifices, skin, and other body parts. This is relevant to treat any source of infection before surgery. This will reduce the risk of transmission of microbes to the raw eye postsurgery.

The clinician needs to enquire whether the patient is a known hypertensive, diabetic, or living with HIV. This is necessary in order to ensure control of the preexisting medical conditions for the safety of the patient, the staff, and other clients. Patients with hypertension or cardiac disease could have exacerbations with adrenaline-containing local anesthetic injection. Centers must have dedicated instruments set for those with hepatitis virus infection and HIV as these diseases are found among patients undergoing eye surgery [23]. Fore knowledge of these diseases will ensure taking measures to safe guard the health of all those attended to in the facility. A positive history of previous drug reactions and the type of medication must be solicited. Reaction can occur with both orthodox and traditional medications [24].

Knowledge of musculoskeletal diseases is important to ascertain that the patient can lie down properly in the supine position during the procedure. It is unforgiving to miss such crucial information from the history and/or during general clinical examination and make such discoveries while the patient is on the table.

History of urinary frequency must be obtained in older male patients to exercise caution in administration of carbonic anhydrase inhibitors pre-op as this may push them into acute retention. Similarly, patients with bladder outlet obstruction tend to have urinary frequency and may go into urge incontinence while on the operating bed. Thus, appropriate measures are taken to limit such distress during surgery.

2.1. Ocular examination

Visual acuity is measured at 6 m with good illumination. Illuminated charts are more helpful; where electricity supply is irregular, vision could be tested in the open. Snellen chart is for literate patients and Landolt C or "E" chart is for the nonliterate ones. Vision can be as low as perception of light (PL). Cataract no matter how dense should not lead to no perception of (NPL) vision. Presence of NPL vision should make the clinician curios to search for additional cause of ocular morbidity co-existing with the cataract. The lids are examined for position and alignment as cicatricial trachoma is still prevalent leading to entropion/trichiasis [25]. Periocular vascular congestion is a pointer of intraocular inflammation and/or infection. The superior limbus should be examined for tale-tell scar from possible previous surgery. A bleb indicates the patient had previous glaucoma surgery [26]. This knowledge is important in counseling the patient on visual outcome before surgery for cataract.

The cornea should be clear. Dot opacity may indicate transcorneal couching [27]. Couching is associated with worse vision outcome [28]. Cornea should be examined for climatic droplet keratopathy or calcific band keratopathy in patients with prolonged ocular surface disease. Pseudophakic bullous keratopathy could be seen in cases of previous cataract surgery that had endothelial damage. If present in one eye, this should warrant additional precaution in operating the index eye by limiting unnecessary entry of instruments into the open eye, cushioning the endothelium with viscoelastic material, and reducing operating time. Such surgery should not be performed by a trainee on the learning curve. Similar advice is advocated for patients with an only eye. The anterior chamber (A/C) should be deep and quite even with pen light inspection. Shallow a/c with corneal edema may result from a swollen cataractous lens; in this instance, the intraocular pressure (IOP) is elevated. It is not unusual to observe cortical matter or nucleus in the A/C from previous couching. Fresh keratic precipitates (KPs) are indicative of active anterior uveitis and thus such cataract could be secondary to the inflammation that requires treatment before any surgical intervention is considered.

The pupillary reaction should be brisk. Abnormal pupillary reaction should lead the clinician to evaluate for signs of gross retinal or optic nerve disease such as retinal detachment or optic atrophy from glaucoma or other causes. Direct fundal examination may not reveal even a red reflex with fully matured cataracts. Immature cataracts could allow examination of the posterior pole particularly with the binocular indirect ophthalmoscope (BIO). A normal optic disk and retina are expected in age-related cataract in the absence ocular comorbidity. Gross retinal function could be assessed by using four-quadrant like projection. In the light projection test, the patient should be able to point in the direction of the light accurately when presented from above, below, and to the left and right sides of the index eye. Other techniques include shining two bright light spots on the index eye after occluding the contra lateral eye. The patient should be able to discern the 2 light sources apart at 5, 7, and 12 cm for visual acuity of counting finger, hand motion, and light perception, respectively. B mode ocular ultrasound scan can be used to rule out retinal detachments or intraocular mass particularly where there are equivocal clinical findings.

The intraocular pressure (IOP) is measured with Goldman's (or other tonometer where available) and should be within the normal limits. A normal IOP measurement does not rule out glaucoma. Noncontact and minimal contact tonometer such as Pulse air and Rebound are more tolerated albeit available in few eye centers. They are more expensive in the presence of lean health budget in the region. Low IOP may indicate retinal detachment warranting further investigation. Slit lamp bio-microscopy is done to inspect the cornea, anterior chamber (a/c), lens and iris, this may be with associated with pupillary dilatation to detect presence of synaechia, to determine morphologic appearance and grading of the cataract. Specular microscopy is performed to assess the endothelial cell density; low density is associated with the risk of corneal decompensation after surgery, although measures are always taken to prevent such occurrence. Less expensive handheld slit lamps could serve the same purpose.

2.2. Preparing the patient for cataract surgery

Eye care teams in the region must ensure that there is appropriate preoperative assessment of patients, proper counseling, and informed consent administration. Basic eye and general examination is essential in planning for good outcome of surgery. This does not necessarily have to be expensive. Preparation includes measurement of the pre operative visual acuity, the state of the corneal clarity, pupillary reaction and intra ocular pressure measurement. The anterior segment is assessed with slit lamp to identify age related degenerative changes, other ocular co-morbidity, presence of posterior synaechia, dislocated lens from possible attempted couching, and anterior uveitis. Four quadrant light projection test is performed to grossly assess state of the retina.

Systemic examination is necessitated to ensure the safety of the patient. It includes blood pressure measurement and fasting blood glucose level estimation. The packed cell volume should be no less than 10 mg/dl. Patients with diabetes mellitus must have adequate control where necessary and available 3-month sugar level pattern can be ascertained by determining the glycosylated hemoglobin (HbA_1c level 7.2% or less is considered normal) [29]. Diabetic eye complications are potentially blinding and can coexist with the cataract [30]. Cataract surgery is also known to exacerbate diabetic retinopathy, making proper counseling on projected visual expectation and the need for further treatment related to the underlying disease important. Cataract surgery is known to improve vision and vision-related quality of life in patients with diabetes [31, 32].

At this stage, it is worthy to ascertain clinically clear respiratory system, a normal cardiac examination consisting of blood pressure, regular normal volume peripheral pulse, undisplaced cardiac apex position, and first and second heart sounds. An electrocardiogram maybe requested for when needed and a cardiologist can be asked to review and stabilize the patient. The central nervous system is examined to rule out obvious cranial nerve palsy and motor dysfunction, and the patient should be in a stable mental state to understand and cooperate during the procedure.

An abdominal examination is needed to detect suprapubic distension caused by a full bladder in patients with suspected urinary outflow obstruction. The general physical examination protocol will determine the presence of any musculoskeletal anomalies that can interfere with positioning of the patient on the operating table.

Other investigations include screening for hepatitis and HIV for the safety of the patient, the eye care team, and other patients. Trimming of bushy lashes will make the eye neater intraoperatively and during postoperative dressing. Oral carbonic anhydrase inhibitor such as acetazolamide is administered the night before and on the morning of surgery. Tropicamide is used to dilate the eye. Consent to undergo surgery is obtained from the patient in the presence of the care giver. As much as can be allowed, day-case surgery should be encouraged. The advantages include reduced/abolished cost of admission to the patient and circumventing the issue of limited bed space, which will otherwise reduce the number of surgeries performed in a session. Perhaps, this is even more desirable particularly in hospitals where ophthalmic and other potentially septic surgical patients share common ward space.

2.3. Ocular biometry

This consists of A-mode ultrasound scan to determine the axial length of the eye and keratometry to obtain corneal power in the two principal meridians. IOL Master gives error message and is not useful in patients with fully matured cataract. The two values are factored into calculating the intraocular lens power. Various formulae are incorporated into determining the IOL power. To prevent obtaining postoperative refractive deficits, there is a need to obtain accurate IOL power [33]. The practice of using standard power IOL perhaps based on experiences on most frequently used power in parts of the region can be adopted out of necessity. Such patients depending on their visual needs may turn out to need further spectacle correction, an unnecessary additional out-of-pocket expense that could have been avoided. Ideally, all patients should and must have the best, as residual refractive errors may manifest later. Manual keratometry will suffice where automated ones are unavailable though these are not as user-friendly.

2.4. The operating room (OR)

Standard requirement includes wall, floor, and ceiling that will not retain dirt and germs. There should be wall and floor tiling that can easily be washed and mopped. The windows need to be kept closed and ventilation provided by room air conditioning. Floor, wall, or ceiling fan will sprinkle dirt and other contaminants into the opened eye. Where grid energy is unavailable, a portable generator can be used. There should be no thoroughfare in the operation room. There should be a red line beyond which unauthorized persons are not allowed. Bidirectional swing doors are preferred to enable the surgical team move in and out of the operating suite without the need to handle the door. Patients have to substitute their clothes with the theater gown before going into the operating room (OR). The scrubbing area should be in an adjacent room. Where such an arrangement is not possible, moveable wash pans can be used on a stand. The changing room is adjacent to the theater. Windows should be cleaned regularly and kept closed. Open floor drains should as much as possible be avoided. Staff must not bring food items into the OR as this may encourage pests. Regular fumigation is advocated to improve sterility.

A simple examination couch can serve as operating bed. Where space allows, two couches can be placed. This will reduce transit time wasting in between cases. Two surgeons can man each station or one surgeon can alternatively switch between the stations. There should be a minimum of four cataract sets, whereby two can be sterilized alternating for patients with no identifiable communicable disease, in addition to one set dedicated for patients with HIV and the other for those with hepatitis. Boilers are ineffective in sterilization. Hot air oven does not blunt sharp instruments and is preferred to steam autoclave. A minimal of two trolleys is required to set the instruments. Trolleys are routinely washed and cleaned with appropriate disinfectant solution. Aluminum drip stands with tray are used to hang irrigation fluid and cannula. Cannula needs to be washed, flushed, and sterilized with activated glutaraldehyde solution not forgetting to flush again with saline before use on the patient. Plastic microscope handles and other control covers should be similarly treated. To ensure safety, a separate cannula should be used for each patient and sterilized in between cases. At the end of the session, unused fluids must be discarded.

A sharp box is required to dispose of used needles, whereas other used items can be thrown into the kick about bucket for conveyance to the incinerator later. There should be separate drape for each patient. Bilateral simultaneous cataract extraction must be avoided to limit morbidity in the event of postoperative endophthalmitis. There are low-cost ophthalmic microscopes from Far East countries, which despite having less versatility (stereopsis/zoom/camera attachment, etc.) can serve adequately.

The surgeon and assistant (ideally a trained ophthalmic nurse) should be properly scrubbed and gowned. Separate pair of gloves is to be used for each patient. An idle team should consist of the surgeon(s) and two assistants, one to stay with the surgeon and the other to circulate ensuring used instruments are promptly removed and replaced by sterilized ones. An attendant should serve the role of bringing in the patients with their folder and appropriate power IOL. The surgeon can dictate critical incident to be recorded by the circulating assistant before full documentation in the patient's record note at the end of the session. The notes could be designed with tick boxes that the attendant can fill easily as dictated by the surgeon during the procedure.

2.5. Regional anesthesia

Cataract surgery is performed under local anesthesia unless there are indications to do otherwise. More often, lignocaine with adrenaline 1:100,000 dilutions is administered. This may be mixed with hyaluronidase to improve local spread with less amount of anesthetic. Retro bulbar block is preferred to periocular and topical anesthesia as patients tend to have a low pain threshold. Facial block is administered around the neck of the mandible (O'Brien), under the periosteum of the lateral orbital rim (Van Lint), or in between these two locations (Atkinson). Systemic absorption could result in tachycardia and elevation of blood pressure. Retro bulbar bleeding could give rise to instant proptosis, if significant it may be wiser to postpone and reschedule the surgery. Where possible, periocular regional anesthetic block should be administered outside the OR.

Extra capsular cataract extraction (ECCE) is widely practiced as transition to manual small incision (MSICS) and to phaco surgery spread gradually in the region. Trainers guide trainees to acquire surgical skills in that order. Sutures contribute significantly to the overall cost of surgery, thus MSICS provides some relief in cost [34]. Proper suture placement is essential with ECCE to reduce postoperative astigmatism, thus avoiding the use of high-power cylindrical correction on the pseudophakic eye. However, MSICS requires the use of keratome, crescent blades, and side port lance. These maybe used once and discarded in developed countries, and in resource-scarce regions, they are resterilized up to five times such that six patients can benefit from each one. Phaco services are available in few centers perhaps due to high cost of the equipment and limited training opportunity. Some studies have shown no statistically insignificant difference in visual outcome between phaco and ECCE in the long term. Patients who can afford should have a choice. Public-private partnership could be a solution to obtaining expensive equipment and training in this part of the world.

2.6. Extra capsular cataract extraction

The periocular skin is cleaned with 10% povidone iodine and a head towel is placed under and tied around the patient's head. A drape with appropriate widow is applied covering the rest of the face excluding the index eye. A speculum wire is placed to part the lids open. Povidone iodine 5% is applied onto the conjunctiva and a cotton tip applicator is used to clean as saline irrigation is performed simultaneously. A toothed forceps is used to pick the superior rectus muscle and bridle silk suture is passed under it. This is then stabilized by fixing the suture with artery forceps to the face drape. The surgeon has numerous options of accessing the anterior chamber. A stab limbal incision can be made before filling the A/C with viscoelastic material and subsequent anterior capsulotomy. A superior corneal incision with razor fragment can be performed and extended with scissors. Alternatively, a keratome can be used to make a bevel stab corneal incision, which is later extended with scissors. There are various techniques of capsulotomy; can opener or continuous curvilinear capsulorhexis is appropriate. The nucleus is manipulated into the A/C and delivered with vectis while applying counter pressure with a muscle hook. The A/C is cleared of cortical matter using irrigation aspiration cannula. More viscoelastic material is injected into the eye, thus deepening the posterior capsule. The IOL is removed from the package, flushed with normal saline inserted, rotated, and dialed into position. When properly placed, the pupil appears round, regular, and central. Depending on the surgeon's choice, interrupted or continuous monofilament silk sutures are applied to close the wound. Sutures have to be well aligned to reduce/limit/ prevent postoperative astigmatism. The bite length should be a third on the corneal and two-thirds on the sclera sides and the bite depth is two third of the cornea/scleral thickness. Burying the suture on either of the two ends is advised as this limits irritation. Any remaining viscoelastic material is aspirated. Intracameral and subconjunctiva antibiotic is administered. In addition, subconjunctival steroid is administered and an eye shield is placed over the eye. Some studies obtained good visual outcome of ECCE in 47.5, 78.8, and 94.3%, respectively [35–37]. Biometric IOL power determination partly accounts for those with better outcome.

2.7. Manual small incision cataract surgery

Preliminary cleaning, draping, and bridle suture placement are similar to that in ECCE. The superior rectus muscle insertion ends about 7.5 millimeters from the limbus. A fornix-based conjunctiva flap is raised, and the underlying sclera is exposed. Limited bipolar wet field cautery may be applied to close bleeders. A horizontal incision of 6.5 to 7.0 millimeters is made 3 millimeters away from the limbus. A frown-shaped sclera incision produces less astigmatism. The proximal sclera lip is gently lifted to allow using the crescent blade to construct a tunnel into the A/C. Thin tunnel roof can lead to button hole and a thick roof may lead to premature entry into the A/C. The tunnel is widened with a keratome as it enters the A/C. The internal opening should be 30% wider than the entrance wound. After administering viscoelastic material into the A/C, a lance is used to make a side port. Anterior capsulotomy is then performed. Nucleus is separated from the cortex by hydrodissection and maneuvered into the A/C by gentle rotation and subsequent delivery with vectis. In some instance, the surgeon may prefer to break the nucleus into halves using a pair of forceps before delivery. Viscoelastic material is used to cushion the endothelium and allow insertion, rotation, and dialing of the lens into position. The side port can be used toward this aim. With the IOL in position, any residual cortical matter and viscoelastic material are aspirated. Lens matter at the sclera tunnel entrance into the A/C is approached via the side port. Any residual viscoelastic material is aspirated. Antibiotic and steroid administration is similar to that of ECCE. MSICS was demonstrated to show better uncorrected postoperative vision when compared to ECCE [38]. Even when final visual recovery is similar in MSICS and ECCE, eyes in the small incision group tend to have significantly faster recovery [39].

2.8. Phaco surgery

After routine cleaning and draping, a superior rectus bridle suture is applied and the globe stabilized. A 3.2 mm keratome is used to make a stab bevel incision into the anterior chamber followed by viscoelastic material administration and side port stab incision. An A/C maintainer is placed to maintain stability of the intraocular pressure during the procedure. Continuous curvilinear capsulotomy is done minding that a well-delineated margin is required. Femto second laser for making corneal incision, capsulotomy, and lens fragmentation is largely unavailable in the region. A 25G cannula mounted on a syringe is used for hydrodissection by gently injecting saline in each quadrant with the aim of separating and lifting the nucleus away from the cortex. The surgeon has the option of cracking the nucleus into two halves at this stage. It appears easier to completely displace the nucleus into the anterior chamber. For those on the continuous learning process, this limits the risk of posterior capsular tear and drop nucleus. When the nucleus is fully in the A/C, a golden ring sign appears around it. The nucleus can be cracked in half with a fragmenter. The A/C is deepened to keep the postcapsule away during fragmentation/aspiration and to protect the corneal endothelium. The phaco tip is inserted through the keratome incision and a phaco spatula through the side port to stabilize the nucleus as it is fragmented and aspirated. Any remaining cortical matter is aspirated with simcoe double cannula. The A/C is further deepened with viscoelastic material in preparation for foldable IOL insertion. Preloaded lens tend to be more expensive when unavailable. Where such is unavailable, the lens is loaded onto the syringe, which contains viscoelastic material. The tip is inserted into the eye and with gentle pressure on the stylus the IOL glides into the posterior capsular sac (in the bag). Dialing maybe required infrequently. A miotic agent is administered to narrow the pupil. Any residual viscoelastic material is aspirated. Saline is injected to swell off the stab corneal wound site as suturing is not required. Phaco surgery has been demonstrated to give good postoperative visual acuity in the immediate and intermediate postoperative period [40].

2.9. Intraoperative challenges

Each procedure is unique and every patient is special and deserves to get the best. Despite adequate training and experience, challenges could arise during surgery that require diligence in decision making and appropriate action to ensure that the goal of safety and quality outcome is realized. Posterior capsular rent could occur with any of the three procedures described earlier. Minimal tears may not require derailment from completing the surgery as planned. Larger tears could interfere with the placement and stability of the IOL. Often times, such big tears are associated with vitreous in the A/C. This will require manual and where available phacovitrectomy. This may necessitate the need to use an anterior chamber or iris claw IOL instead.

The other disturbing scenario is when the nucleus drops into the vitreous. Where combined phacovitrectomy machine is available, this is used to clear lens remnants from the vitreous. Manual attempt to do so could lead to retinal detachment. Where material and human resource to assure appropriate intervention is lacking, it is imperative to immediately refer the patient to the few centers where such services are available.

2.10. Care after surgery

Patients are advised to lie on their back or on the side of the nonoperated eye perhaps to limit undue position-related pressure on the raw eye. Postoperative medications include topical antibiotic-steroid combination eye drops, a mydriatic agent with moderate cycloplegic effect, oral broad-spectrum antibiotic, and nonsteroidal anti-inflammatory agent. It is of importance to obtain drugs from a reliable source due to preponderance of fake and substandard makes.

Admitted and day-case patients are reviewed a day after surgery. The routine should start from asking the patient if there are any complaints. The visual acuity is then determined unaided and with pin hole, followed by careful inspection of the wound site for any leakages/iris prolapse. The IOP should be within limits. The cornea is examined for clarity. Presence of corneal edema and/or striate keratopathy is noted and these usually improve with medication. The pupil should be regular, central, and round. Any peaking is a sign of iris entrapment in the wound edge or improper IOL placement. Open wound will give rise to shallow A/C with low IOP and a positive Seidel's test may require secondary suturing. Cortical remnants may be observed with slit lamp in the A/C or behind the IOL and may require aspiration. Tilted or decentered IOL is to be redialed into position.

2.11. Postoperative infective endophthalmitis

Postoperative bacterial endophthalmitis is arguably the most dreaded complications of intraocular surgery, although relatively rare with some reports indicating an incidence of 0.6% [40], 0.13–0.7% [41]. The commonest agents are conjunctival commensals like Staph epidermidis 70%, Staph aureus 10%, Strep species 2%, and occasionally the devastating *Pseudomonas aeruginosa* [42]. This can arise within 48–72 hours after surgery. Typically, the patient develops ocular pain and drop in vision after initial postoperative improvement. On examination, the lids appear tense and tender, with periocular congestion. The cornea is cloudy and there are signs of intraocular inflammation, a hypopyon may be seen in the anterior chamber. Inflammatory reaction in the anterior vitreous is noticed with slit lamp examination. The posterior segment is poorly visible. This is an emergency and the patient requires admission. Appropriate intraoperative intracameral antibiotic administration has been demonstrated to reduce the incidence [43, 44].

Endophthalmitis management protocol involves preparing intravitreal injection of vancomycin 2 mg and ceftazidime 2 mg (or 0.5 mg amikacin). A vitreous tap is performed and aspirate is sent to the laboratory for gram staining, microscopy, culture, and sensitivity. The prepared intravitreal antibiotic is administered. In addition, subconjunctival ivancomycin 50 mg and ceftazidime 125 mg (or amikacin 50 mg in those with penicillin allergy) is administered. Topical ceftazidime 5% and vancomycin 5% eye drops are to be instilled hourly. Topical 1% atropine drop is used six hourly to relieve ciliary spasm. The patient's clinical condition is monitored. A reduction in ocular pain/inflammation is indicative of improvement. Treatment is continued as the patient is monitored. If there is no improvement, repeat vitreous tap and antibiotics. The choice of antibiotics maybe modified based on the culture results/clinical improvement. Topical or systemic steroids can be administered when there is indication that the infection is under control based on clinical parameters such as pain reduction, fibrin contracting, and hypopyon reducing. The treatment is tapered based on the patient's response and culture results [45].

Posterior capsular opacity: This is a cause of intermediate and long-term reduction in postoperative visual acuity. Nd:Yag capsulotomy is performed to restore vision. Open capsulotomy may be considered where laser services are unavailable.

2.12. Identifying recording and limiting critical incident

Critical incidents are events or incidents that cause harm to the patient [46]. There is hardly any documentation on prevalence of such events in sub-Saharan African countries. Such incidents may include failing to make the right diagnosis, faulty assessment and preparation of the patient, mislabeling of the index eye, theater-related mishaps comprising defective sterilization, contaminated irrigation fluids, intraoperative and postoperative complications, use of substandard medications, etc. Documenting such incidents and reviewing the patient's management protocol in order to forestall future occurrence is very important. Linking such events to individual is counterproductive as isolated blame game does not solve systemic failures [47].

2.13. Steps toward preventing critical incidents, obtaining successful visual outcome, and ensuring the patient's safety

Gaining trust of the patient and care giver by creating an enabling environment to make them believe they're not in a court under cross examination is essential in obtaining a reliable ocular and systemic history. The ophthalmologist must perform careful and purposeful ocular and systemic assessment to determine the correct diagnosis and identify any ocular co-morbidity. Prompt and appropriate management of underlining ocular and or systemic diseases will ensure the patient condition is optimal for obtaining a predictable favorable cataract surgical outcome. Patient should be counseled on the cause of vision loss (cataract), the preparations for surgery, the cost, logistics, the need to buy and use prescribed medications, the visual expectations after surgery and the symptoms that should alert the patient of potential complications. Ocular biometry must be done routinely to determine the correct IOL power is available and used for each patient. Similarly, consumables and post operative medications are to be obtained from a certified and reliable source. Obtaining and maintaining a conducive and safe operating environment is essential in securing favorable surgical outcome. Basic minimum eye clinic and theater equipments have to be provided as well as purpose built operating room. The clinician must ensure that correct medication in appropriate dose is given to the patient. Obtaining and maintaining the basic minimum eye clinic and theater equipments necessary to getting good surgical outcome. Use of appropriate not necessarily purpose built operating space.

While in the operating room: Ensure the patient has bathed/is clean before coming to the O.R. The patient must exchange personal clothes with theater gown. Ensure that the correct eye is labeled by double checking and comparing with the patient's notes. Ensure all instruments are cleaned and sterilized. Ensure all drapings are washed and sterilized. Ensure separate and sterilized instruments are used for each patient. Use separate irrigation/aspiration cannula for each case. Resterilize all reusable instruments in between cases. The surgeon and assistant are to be properly gowned. Install purpose made water taps with long handle that are elbow controlled in the scrubbing area. Where unavailable, an assistant can pour water with a bowel for the person scrubbing. Appropriate scrubbing of the surgical team with antiseptic lotion. Trim dirty nails before surgery and ensure wrist watches, rings, and bangles are removed before scrubbing. Take meticulous and purposeful steps toward successful completion of the procedure. Avoid impulsive and erratic moves that can cause tissue damage leading to critical incident. Record all critical incidents for the purpose of internal audit and rectification of any short comings while avoiding individual blame. Provide dedicated instrument sets for patients with hepatitis and/or HIV. Ensure correct and appropriate eye medications are applied as the eye is padded. A perforated eye shield is better than a gauze pad. Provide dedicated instrument set for patients living with HIV/hepatitis.

Maintaining a committed and motivated eye care team. Timely and strategic training of the eye care team. Provision of refraction services. Ensuring staff and patient's safety in the operating room and at all times. Prompt documentation of procedure including critical incidents. Arranging follow-up visits till postoperative ocular status is stable.

2.14. Good visual outcome and safety-centered cataract outreach service

Cataract outreach entails an eye care team leaving the base hospital to provide services in locations within or even outside national boundaries. Often times, there is inadequate and improper planning of such programs with suboptimal preparation for the conduct of the camp services and patient monitoring till full recuperation. There is need to change from appearing, operating, and disappearing without proper arrangement on who cares for the patient when the outreach team is gone.

Guide toward successful cataract surgical outreach:

- There should be an advance team to evaluate the facility were the outreach will be conducted ensuring that basic minimal infrastructure is available without compromising patient safety.
- The advance team should liaise with and co-opt local eye care team in order to ensure joint participation in the conduct of the program.
- Any prior advocacy visit must include the local eye care team and their relevance highlighted to ensure continuity and success of the program.

- Proper screening and documentation of the selected patients are conducted by the joint advance and local team. This should include appropriate tests to detect communicable diseases such as hepatitis and HIV.
- Venue and date are agreed upon with the approval of relevant local health authorities.
- Biometry is performed on all the patients so that the correct power of IOL is determined and provided.
- Where possible, counselors are involved in discussing all issues related to the cause of the patient's blindness, the proposed intervention, the expected visual recovery, the use of medications, and postoperative follow-up. Patients must be given opportunity to ask questions.
- There has to be informed individual consent administration.
- The correct eye is labeled appropriately.
- Staggered scheduling is advised to reduce overcrowding, thus ensuring that the patients arrive and are operated and dispatched in manageable batches.
- Patient records must be kept at the facility used for reference whenever required and not be carried away by the outreach team.
- The local team is to continue the patients' care when the outreach team is gone.
- The philosophy is quality visual outcome based on integrated eye care team without compromising the patient's safety. The care is patient centered not client's eye.
- Collaborative long-term partnership, strengthening of local eye care teams, and sustained intervention program appear to yield better cataract prevention services in sub-Saharan African setting [48].

2.15. The big question and the final answer

Ophthalmologist and other eye care personnel need to ask themselves if they are willing to have cataract surgery in the centers they work. If the answer is not an affirmative "Yes," such institutions are not good enough to provide cataract surgery with favorable outcome and may not be safe for patients to patronize!

Author details

Lawan Abdu

Address all correspondence to: lawal1966@yahoo.com

Department of Ophthalmology, Faculty of Clinical Sciences, College of Health Sciences, Bayero University Kano, Nigeria

References

[1] Abdu L. Prevalence and causes of blindness and low vision in Dambatta local government area of Kano state Nigeria. Nigerian Journal of Medicine. 2002 Sept;**11**(3):108-112

[2] Lee CM, Afshari NA. The global state of cataract blindness. Current Opinion in Ophthalmology. 2017 Jan;**28**(1):98-103

[3] Mohammed MA, Selvaraj S, Gudlavalleti VS, et al. Causes of blindness and visual impairment in Nigeria: The Nigeria national blindness and visual impairment survey. Investigative Ophthalmology & Visual Science. 2009 Sept;**50**(9):4114-4120

[4] Vonor K, Amedome KM, Dzidzinyo K, et al. Cataracts in rural areas in Togo: Awareness and attitudes. The British Journal of Ophthalmology. 2016 Sep;**100**(9):1157-1162. DOI: 10.1136/bjophthalmol-2015-308328

[5] Nadoo K, Gichuhi S, Mario-Gloria B, et al. Prevalence and causes of vision loss in sub-Saharan Africa: 1990-2010. The British Journal of Ophthalmology. 2014;**98**:612-618

[6] www.who.int/bulletin/volume/86/3/07-042135/en/ [Accessed 12th September 2017]

[7] https://www.unicef.org/Nigeria/children_1926.html [Accessed 12th September 2017]

[8] www.worldbank.org/en/news/2013/09/09/global-burden-of-diseases-findings-for-sub-saharan-africa [Accessed 13th September 2017]

[9] BeLue R. The role of family in non-communicable diseases prevention in sub-Saharan Africa. Global Health Probelems. 2017 Sep;**24**(3):71-74. DOI: 10.1177/1757975915614190

[10] Misganaw A, Haregu TN, Deribe KN, et al. National mortality burden due to communicable, non-communicable, and other diseases in Ethiopia, 1990-2015: Findings from the Global Burden of Disease Study 2015. Population Health Metrics. 2017 Jul 21;**15**:29. DOI: 10.1186/s12963-017-0145-1

[11] Leslie C, Lauren T, Peggy GC, et al. Experiences of leadership in health care in sub-Saharan Africa. Human Resources for Health. 2012;**10**:33

[12] Shaheer A, Paul C. Barriers to cataract surgery in Africa: A systematic review. Middle East African Journal of Ophthalmology. 2016 Jan-Mar;**23**(1):145-149

[13] Joackim PK, Susan L. Poverty as a barrier to accessing cataract surgery: A study from Tanzania. The British Journal of Ophthalmology. 2007 Sep;**91**(9):1114-1116

[14] Susan L, Elena S, Emma J, et al. Factors affecting cataract surgical coverage and outcomes: A retrospective cross-sectional study of eye health systems in sub-Saharan Africa. BMC Ophthalmology. 2015;**15**:67. DOI: 10.1186/s12886-015-0063-6

[15] Rabiu M. Cataract blindness and barriers to uptake of cataract surgery in a rural community of northern Nigeria. The British Journal of Ophthalmology. 2001 Jul;**85**(7):776-780. DOI: 10.1136/bjo.85.7.776

[16] Nazaradden I, Francisco PM, Clare G. Direct non-medical costs double the total direct costs to patients undergoing cataract surgery in Zamfara state, Northern Nigeria: A case series. BMC Health Services Research. 2015;**15**:163. DOI: 10.1186/s12913-015-0831-2

[17] Zelalem AM, Redda THZ, Fitsum BG. Barriers to cataract surgical uptake in central Ethiopia. Middle East African Journal of Ophthalmology. 2013 Jul-Sep;**20**(3):229-233

[18] Ojo PO, Caleb DM, Muhammad R, et al. Cataract blindness, surgical coverage, outcome, and barriers to uptake of cataract services in Plateau State, Nigeria. Middle East African Journal of Ophthalmology. 2012 Jul-Sep;**19**(3):282-288. DOI: 10.4103/0974-9233.97925

[19] Javed U, McVeigh K, Scott NW, et al. Cataract extraction and patient vision-related quality of life: A cohort study. Eye (London). 2015 Jul;**29**(7):921-925. DOI: 10.1038/eye.2015.70

[20] Robert PF, David GK, Eva F. The impact of successful cataract surgery on quality of life, household income and social status in South India. PLoS One. 2012;**7**(8):e44268. DOI: 10.1371/journal.pone.0044268

[21] Boniface IE, Chimdi MC, Judith NU. Traditional eye medicine use by newly presenting ophthalmic patients to a teaching hospital in south-eastern Nigeria: Socio-demographic and clinical correlates. BMC Complementary and Alternative Medicine. 2009;**9**:40. DOI: 10.1186/1472-6882-9-40

[22] Catherine UU, Nanaiashat M. Incidence and complications of traditional eye medications in Nigeria in a teaching hospital. Middle East African Journal of Ophthalmology. 2010 Oct-Dec;**17**(4):315-319. DOI: 10.4103/0974-9233.71596

[23] Alhassan MB, Unung P, Adejor GO. HIV and HBsAg sero positivity amongst patients presenting for ocular surgery at a tertiary eye care hospital in Nigeria. The Open Ophthalmology Journal. 2013;**7**:18-19. DOI: 10.2174/1874364101307010018

[24] Bernard KF, Clovis F. Adverse drug reactions in some African herbal medicine: Literature review and stakeholders' interview. Integrative Medicine Research. 2014 Sep;**3**(3):126-132. DOI: 10.1016/j.imr.2014.05.001

[25] Mpyet C, Muhammad N, Adamu MD. Prevalence of trachoma in Kano State, Nigeria: Results of 44 local government area-level surveys. Ophthalmic Epidemiology. 2017 Jun;**24**(3):195-203. DOI: 10.1080/09286586.2016.1265657

[26] Abdu L. Pattern of presentation and outcome of surgical management of primary open angle in Kano, northwestern Nigeria. Annals of African Medicine. 2007;**6**(4):181-186

[27] Isawumi MA, Kolawole OU, Hassan MB. Couching techniques for cataract treatment in Osogbo, South West Nigeria. Ghana Medical Journal. 2013 Jun;**47**(2):64-69

[28] Gilbert CE, Murthy GVS, Sivasubramaniam S, et al. Couching in Nigeria: Prevalence, risk factors and visual acuity outcomes. Ophthalmic Epidemiology. 2010;**17**:269-275

[29] Adebisi SA, Oghahon EK, Akande TM, et al. Glycated hemoglobin and glyceamic control of diabetes in Ilorin. Nigerian Journal of Clinical Practice. 2009 Mar;**12**(1):87-91

[30] Abdu L, Tijjani BM. Pattern of diabetic retinopathy in Kano, Nigeria. Annals of African Medicine. 2012 Apr-Jun;**11**(2):75-79

[31] Onakpoya OH, Bekibele CO, Adegbeingbe SA. Cataract surgical outcome in diabetic patients: Case control study. Middle East African Journal of Ophthalmology. 2009 Apr-Jun;**16**(2):88-91

[32] Bijun Z, Yingyan M, Senlin L, et al. Vision related quality of life and visual outcome from cataract surgery in patients with vision threatening diabetic retinopathy: A prospective observational study. Health and Quality of Life Outcomes. 2017;**15**:175

[33] Nick M. Accurate IOL power determination is very important in preventing post operative refractive surprises. Journal of Cataract & Refractive Surgery. 2003;**29**(1):1-3

[34] Gogate PM, Deshpande M, Wormald RP. Is manual small incision cataract surgery affordable in developing countries? A cost comparison with extra capsular cataract extraction. The British Journal of Ophthalmology. 2003;**87**(7):843-846

[35] Isawumi MA, Soetan EO, Adeoye AO, et al. Evaluation of cataract surgery outcome in western Nigeria. Ghana Medical Journal. 2009 Dec;**43**(4):169-174

[36] Olawoye DA, Ashaye AO, Bekibeli CO, et al. Visual outcome after cataract surgery at the University College Hospital Ibadan. Annals of Ibadan Postgraduate Medicine. 2011 Jun;**9**(1):8-13

[37] Tilahun Y, Sisay A. Audit of exracapsular cataract extraction with posterior chamber intraocular lens implantation in a tertiary eye care center in Ethiopia. Ethiopian Medical Journal. 2006;**44**(1):61-66

[38] Gogate PM, Deshpande M, Wormald RP, et al. Extra capsular cataract surgery compared with manual small incision cataract surgery in community eye care setting in western India: A randomized control trial. The British Journal of Ophthalmology. 2003;**87**(6):667-672

[39] Guzek JP, Ching A. Small incision manual extra capsular cataract surgery in Ghana, West Africa. Journal of Cataract and Refractive Surgery. 2003;**29**(91):57-64

[40] Abdulsalam S. Visual outcome of phacoemulsification cataract surgery. Nigerian Journal of Ophthalmology. 2013;**21**(1):1-3

[41] Mamalis N, Kearsly L, Birintu E. Post operative endophthalmitis. Current Opinion in Ophthalmology. 2002;**13**:14-18

[42] Buzard K, Liapis S. Prevention of endophthalmitis. Journal of Cataract and Refractive Surgery. 2004;**70**:1953-1959

[43] Hesam H, Reza M, Melidi K, et al. Post cataract surgery endophthalmitis: Brief literature review. Journal of Current Ophthalmology. 2016 Sept;**78**(3):101-105

[44] Lee PS, Margaret AS. Post cataract endophthalmitis prophylaxis using irrigation, incisional hydration and eye pressurization with vancomycin. Clinical Ophthalmology. 2015;**9**:1337-1345

[45] Nuwan N, Nick D. Endophthalmitis: Controlling infection before and after cataract surgery. Community Eye Health Journal. 2008 Mar;**21**(65):9-10

[46] https://www.who/feature/factfile/patient_safety/en/ [Accessed 20th September 2017]

[47] Robert L. patient safety in low income countries. Community Eye Health Journal. 2016;**29**(94):21-22

[48] Muhammad N, Adamu MD, Caleb M, et al. Changing patterns of cataract services in North-West Nigeria: 2005-2016. PLoSOne 2017 Aug 17;**12**(8):e0183421. DOI: 10.1371/journal.pone.0183421 eCollection 2017

14

Glaucoma Surgery and Aqueous Dynamics

Parul Ichhpujani

Abstract

Reduction in intraocular pressure is the only proven method to treat glaucoma. When medical treatment does not achieve adequate intraocular pressure reduction with acceptable adverse effects, laser or incisional surgeries are introduced. In this chapter, we discuss the physiological basis for the established surgical procedures as well as the newer surgical procedures. Most new surgical innovations have been designed according to natural physiology by routing aqueous as nature intended, through the Schlemm's canal. This has been possible because of better understanding of the outflow system and the availability of micro-technology to manipulate it.

Keywords: trabeculectomy, glaucoma drainage device, minimally invasive glaucoma surgery, outflow resistance

1. Introduction

Glaucoma is defined as a group of disorders that result in death of ganglion cells due to axonal damage at the level of the lamina cribrosa of the optic nerve.

Intraocular pressure (IOP) is considered to be the only alterable risk factor for diagnosis and treatment of glaucoma. IOP reduction is attained either by increasing outflow or by reducing aqueous humor production [1]. Therefore, basic understanding of aqueous humor circulation is important for successful management of glaucoma. Aqueous humor pathways have been discussed in detail in a prior chapter in the book. This chapter focuses on the various surgical modalities available to reduce or bypass the outflow resistance.

2. Site of outflow resistance

Evidence suggests that the majority of outflow resistance in the trabecular meshwork is generated in the inner wall endothelium of Schlemm's canal and its underlying matrix in the juxtacanalicular trabecular meshwork [2]. Rosenquist et al. has shown that following trabeculotomy, close to half (49%) of outflow resistance is eliminated at a perfusion pressure of 7 mm Hg [3]. In another study, Grant has shown that nearly two-third (71%) resistance is eliminated at a perfusion pressure of 25 mm Hg [4]. Schuman et al. have shown that 35% of resistance is eliminated at a perfusion pressure at 10 mm Hg, when 1 O'clock hour of the tissue from the outer wall of Schlemm's canal was ablated using the excimer laser [5]. These studies suggest that one-third to half of the outflow resistance lies distal to the inner wall of Schlemm's canal at normal pressure and partly outflow resistance is related to pressure-dependent changes in the outflow pathway. As the intraocular pressure increases, Schlemm's canal collapses and reduces outflow and effective filtration.

3. Restoration of the outflow facility

Excision of sites causing increased outflow resistance would result in restoration of outflow. It is not possible for a surgeon to precisely pinpoint the area which needs to be excised for an individual patient, therefore, logically, surgeons would like to address all aspects of the outflow system.

The current gold standard, trabeculectomy, has done well for many medically refractory glaucoma patients. Despite its efficacy in lowering IOP, ease of the surgical procedure, it is fraught with potential sight threatening issues. Glaucomatologists and bioengineers are leaving no stone unturned to find a better alternative to address the flaws of trabeculectomy.

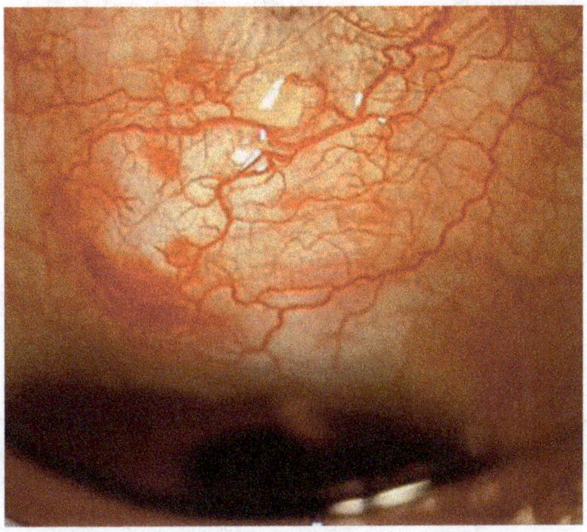

Figure 1. Failing trabeculectomy bleb with corkscrewing of conjunctival vessels secondary to scarring.

3.1. Surgeries addressing trabecular meshwork

- *Trabeculectomy:* Opening a pathway through the meshwork, either by removing tissue or punching a hole (trabeculectomy) encourages aqueous outflow into Schlemm's canal.

  Despite modulation of the subconjunctival space into a porous matrix, the procedure is **not** a physiological bypass and remains dependent on the size of the ostium, tension in the sclera flap, as well as wound healing and its modulation [6].

  A decrease in the hydraulic conductivity of the bleb capsule results in an increase in fluid pressure within the bleb, altering its mechanical and biochemical environment resulting in progressive scarring (**Figure 1**) and consequent bleb failure [7].

  In addition, these incisional surgeries can result in decreased quality of life due to bleb-related foreign body sensation, induced astigmatism, and secondary cataracts.

- *Trabeculectomy with collagen implants:* The development of tissue engineering has offered a plausible solution to reduce postoperative fibrosis and scarring. The use of collagen-glycosaminoglycan copolymers leads to random and relatively loose reorganization of regenerating myofibroblasts, fibroblasts, and the secreted extracellular collagen matrix, resulting in reduced scar formation [8]. These implants offer a potential alternative to antifibrosis agents as they produce more loosely organized, yet more abundant bleb tissue than a bleb created without antimetabolites.

  Ologen (Aeon Astron Corporation, Taipei, Taiwan) (also named iGen) is the commonly available collagen implant, which consists of >90% lyophilized porcine atelocollagen and <10% lyophilized porcine glycosaminoglycan. This implant also acts as a spacer to mechanically separate the subconjunctival and episcleral tissues to prevent fibrosis. The implant is placed subconjunctivally over the scleral flap posteriorly and only a small portion covers the scleral flap (**Figure 2**), else the implant would act as a mechanical tamponade and prevent outflow from the subscleral space [9].

- *iStent:* Trabecular bypass devices such as iStent reduce IOP by bypassing the thin layer of juxtacanalicular tissue, without the need for creating a hole in the sclera and a filtration bleb. iStent bypasses the meshwork, creating a direct route from the anterior chamber into Schlemm's canal (**Figure 3**).

  There is also a second-generation model called the iStent inject (Glaukos Corporation), which has been CE marked for use in Europe. It contains a head facing the anterior chamber that is 230 μm in width with four inlets for the passage of aqueous into the device and out through Schlemm's canal.

  Zhou and Smedley have shown in their cultured autopsy eye perfusion experiments that adding successive bypass shunts produces a step-wise increase in outflow. The first shunt has the maximum IOP reducing effect, reducing IOP from 21.4 ± 3.8 to 12.4 ± 4.2 mm Hg, successive addition of up to four stents placed into SC produced step-wise reduction in system pressure [10].

Hunter et al. showed in anterior segment perfusion models with the iStent inject that outflow facility increases from 0.16 ± 0.05 μL/min/mm Hg to 0.38 ± 0.23 ($P < 0.03$, $n = 7$), and then an additional iStent inject further increased outflow facility to 0.78 ± 0.66 ($n = 2$) [11].

- *Ex-PRESS:* The Ex-PRESS device relies on nonphysiologic subconjunctival flow as its mechanism of IOP lowering. In eyes with prior failed trabeculectomies, Ex-PRESS can help to reestablish the aqueous flow without having to repeat the original procedure [12]. The Ex-PRESS fits easily in the middle ground between a repeat trabeculectomy and a larger glaucoma drainage device like a Baerveldt, Molteno, or an Ahmed tube shunt.

- *Viscocanalostomy:* In viscocanalostomy, inner wall of the endothelium is disrupted and communication is established between the lumen of the canal and the juxtacanalicular space. Bed of canal is scraped with a forceps or trabecular aspiration. This leads to the removal of a homogenous external trabecular membrane in one coherent plane that allows aqueous humor to egress through the remaining inner trabecular layers [13].

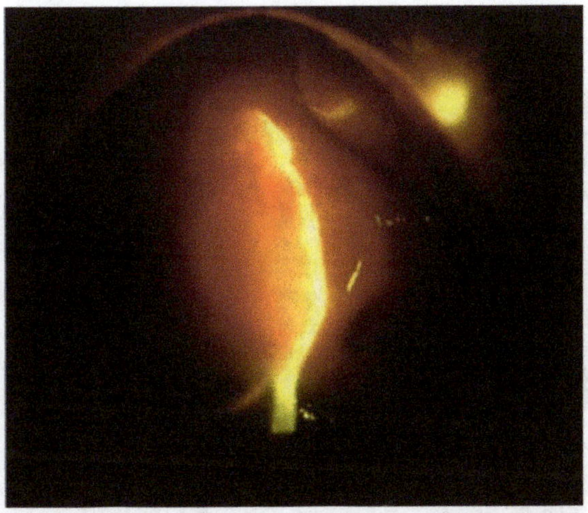

Figure 2. Ologen implant in subconjunctival space.

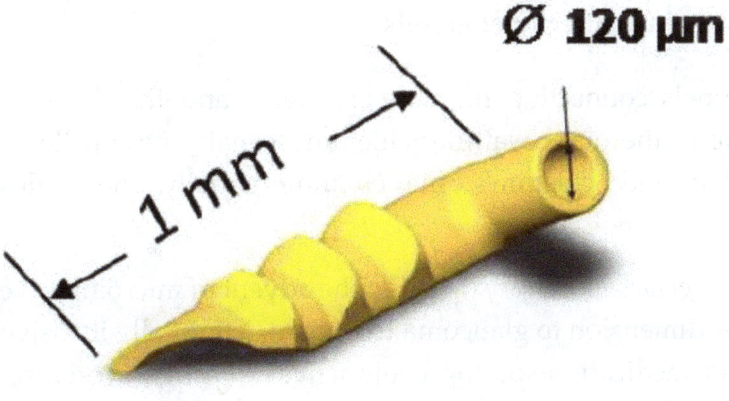

Figure 3. First-generation iStent.

3.2. Surgeries addressing Schlemm's canal

The detailed mechanism of aqueous humor dynamics across the endothelial lining of Schlemm's canal from the Juxtacanalicular trabecular meshwork (JCT) via giant vacuoles and pores has been discussed in detail in a prior chapter. The number of giant pores and vacuoles is less in glaucomatous eyes as compared to normal eyes, thus accounting for the increase in outflow resistance [14].

- *Viscocanalostomy:* Dilating Schlemm's canal with viscoelastic material may remove the stenosis-related resistance, as discussed earlier.
- *Canaloplasty:* Canaloplasty is an ab externo procedure that entails 360° intubation of Schlemm's canal (**Figure 4**), along with suture-assisted distension of the canal in order to restore physiologic outflow via the conventional pathway without the formation of a fistula or bleb. Potentially, the suture tension may increase TM permeability, similar to the action of pilocarpine [15] as well as help to maintain a patent canal lumen, similar to the intraocular tensioning suture [16].

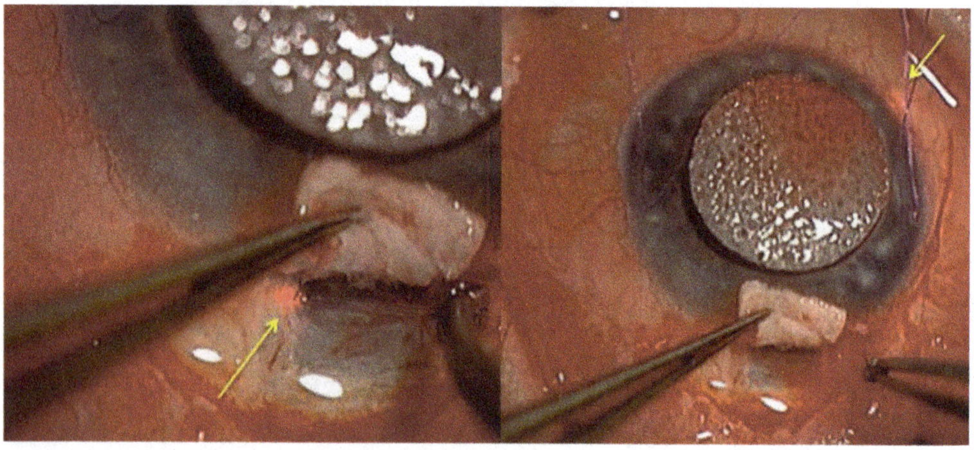

Figure 4. Nonpenetrating Schlemm's canaloplasty using the iScience cannula.

3.3. Surgeries addressing collector channels

The collector channels connecting the aqueous veins and the distal part of the outflow pathways originate in the outer wall of Schlemm's canal. These collector channels are not evenly distributed around Schlemm's canal circumferentially. The outflow is closer to areas with larger collector channels.

- *Minimally invasive glaucoma surgery (MIGS):* The advent of microinvasive glaucoma surgery has brought new dimension to glaucoma treatment. Minimally invasive glaucoma surgery is likely to provide medication-sparing, conjunctival-sparing, ab interno, more physiological approach to IOP reduction for patients with mild-to-moderate glaucoma that is safer than traditional incisional glaucoma surgery.

MIGS stents, e.g., iStent, Hydrus, give better results when positioned close to a patent collector channel, thus increasing the possibility of surgical success.

- *Canaloplasty:* Schuman et al. have shown that when the IOP is elevated, trabecular meshwork herniates into the ostia of collector channels and reduces the passage for aqueous outflow. Cannulating the whole of Schlemm's canal, as in canaloplasty, and injecting viscoelastic material may "pop" open these herniations and enable 360° access to collector channel ostia for the egressing aqueous [17].

3.4. Surgeries addressing episcleral venous system

Theoretically, IOP should directly correlate with the episcleral venous pressure (EVP). However, when the entire TM is removed, 25% of total resistance still remains, underscoring the importance of EVP measurement in an accurate and reproducible way [18]. Episcleral venous pressure is highly variable and may range from 3 to 14 mm Hg. In addition, if the pressure gradient differential is low and resistance is also located distally in the episcleral venous system, restorative outflow surgery has less chance of being effective than if the pressure gradient differential is high.

In cases with elevated episcleral venous pressure, incisional filtration surgery can help lower the IOP, but it is associated with a high incidence of choroidal effusion or hemorrhage.

Preoperative IOP reduction may be attained by intravenous mannitol and other systemic antiglaucoma medications. Additionally, the flow through the scleral flap may be adjusted to allow for a higher IOP in the early postoperative period. Using a releasable suture allows controlled reduction of IOP. Drainage implants may also be a good choice if the flow through the implant is kept to a minimum in the early postoperative period.

Another way of classifying various surgical procedures depends on how the procedure influences the aqueous dynamics.

3.4.1. Surgeries that bypass conventional aqueous outflow pathway

- Trabeculectomy
- Nonpenetrating deep sclerectomy
- Glaucoma drainage devices:

  Most conventional shunts consist of a tube designed to shunt aqueous from the anterior chamber to a distal plate via a tube to the posterior subconjunctival space, from where aqueous is directly absorbed into the sclera and episcleral vasculature to enter the orbital circulation, bypassing both the conventional and uveoscleral pathways. The primary tube-plate junction includes a rim through which the tube empties onto the explant plate surface to avoid closure of the tube orifice following eventual encapsulation of the device by fibrosis [19].

- Viscocanalostomy, canaloplasty

- Trabeculotomy
- Goniotomy
- Ab interno trabeculotomy or Trabectome surgery:

  Selective removal of the TM and inner wall of SC is performed using the Trabectome; while leaving the rest of the outflow system (outer wall of SC, collector channels, and aqueous veins) relatively intact. A strip of TM and inner wall of SC spanning 80–100° is ablated and removed under direct gonioscopic visualization. The simultaneous aspiration of tissue debris reduces the inflammatory stimuli and opportunity for scarring among shards of incised or ruptured tissues remaining after traditional goniotomy or trabeculotomy [20].

3.4.2. Surgeries that increase the uveoscleral outflow

- ExPRESS shunt
- iStent
- Suprachoroidal gold SOLX shunt:

  This shunt is an ab externo suprachoroidal trans-limbal shunt and works as a "controlled" cyclodialysis, draining aqueous into the suprachoroidal space. The anterior end of this 24-karat gold device is placed into the anterior chamber over the sclera spur via a scleral incision and the posterior end positioned in the suprachoroidal space (**Figure 5**). It includes several channels through its body. Aqueous flows both through the channels in the body of the shunt and around its body [21].

- Cypass:

  This mini shunt is placed in the supraciliary and suprachoroidal space to increase uveoscleral outflow by creating a small cyclodialysis (**Figure 6**) [22].

  Along the length of the stent are microholes that allow for circumferential egress of aqueous into the suprachoroidal space and the distal end of the stent allows longitudinal egress of fluid.

- Hydrus:

  Hydrus is implanted using s a preloaded injector via a clear corneal incision and is inserted into and sits within Schlemm's canal, wherein it extends 3 clock hours. It does not block the collector channel ostia in the posterior portion of Schlemm's canal as it has a scaffold design, and it has a 1 mm inlet portion, which resides within the anterior chamber. As a standalone procedure, it can be inserted through a 1–1.5 mm corneal incision. Once inserted into Schlemm's canal, it can dilate it by four to five times the natural width of the canal [23].

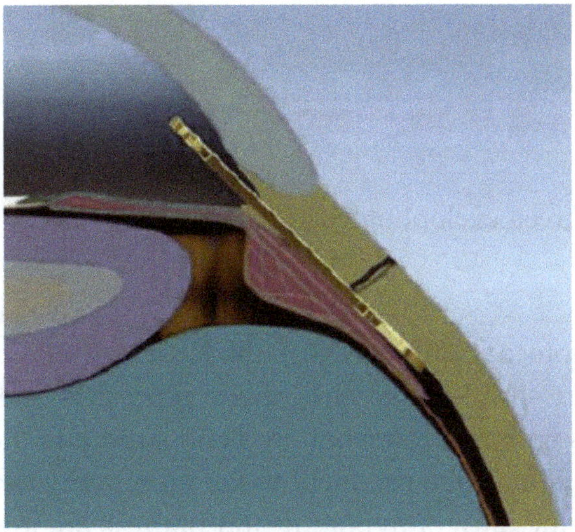

Figure 5. Gold SOLX shunt in suprachoroidal space.

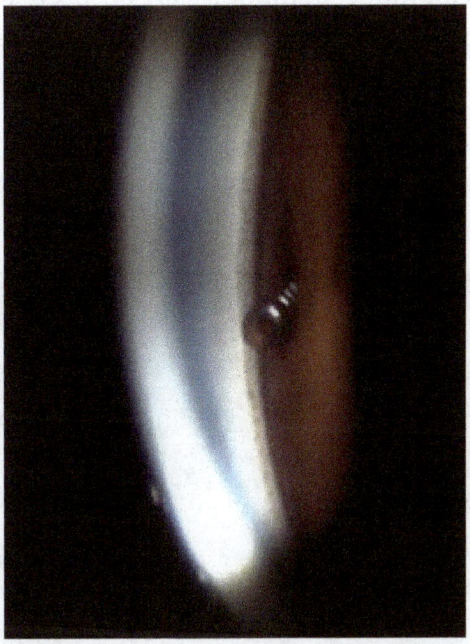

Figure 6. CyPass shunt *in situ*.

3.4.3. *Surgeries that decrease aqueous production*

Cycloablative procedures reduce IOP by destroying the ciliary body epithelium that produces aqueous humor. Modalities include:

- Contact (transscleral) cycloablation
  - Cyclocryotherapy [24]

    - Diode/Nd:YAG [25]

- Noncontact cycloablation

    - Nd:YAG/Diode

- Transpupillary argon green cyclophotocoagulation

- Endoscopic ablation

  In endoscopic cyclophotocoagulation (ECP), the laser is applied under direct endoscopic view causing localized shrinkage of the ciliary processes due to thermal coagulation (**Figure 7**). This causes an initial reduction in blood supply to the ciliary processes, and a consequent reduction in aqueous production. Partial reperfusion of the ciliary body over 4–6 weeks means that the rates of hypotony and phthisis are lower than those associated with other methods of cyclodestruction.

  Earlier cycloablative procedures were reserved only for refractory cases, but recent studies have shown that endocyclophotocoagulation can be used for the treatment of mild-to-moderate glaucoma. It is conjunctival-sparing, blebless, and can be combined with cataract surgery [26, 27].

Despite all the aforementioned advances, the quest for a perfectly predictable and physiological glaucoma procedure with rapid recovery and a greater margin of safety is ongoing.

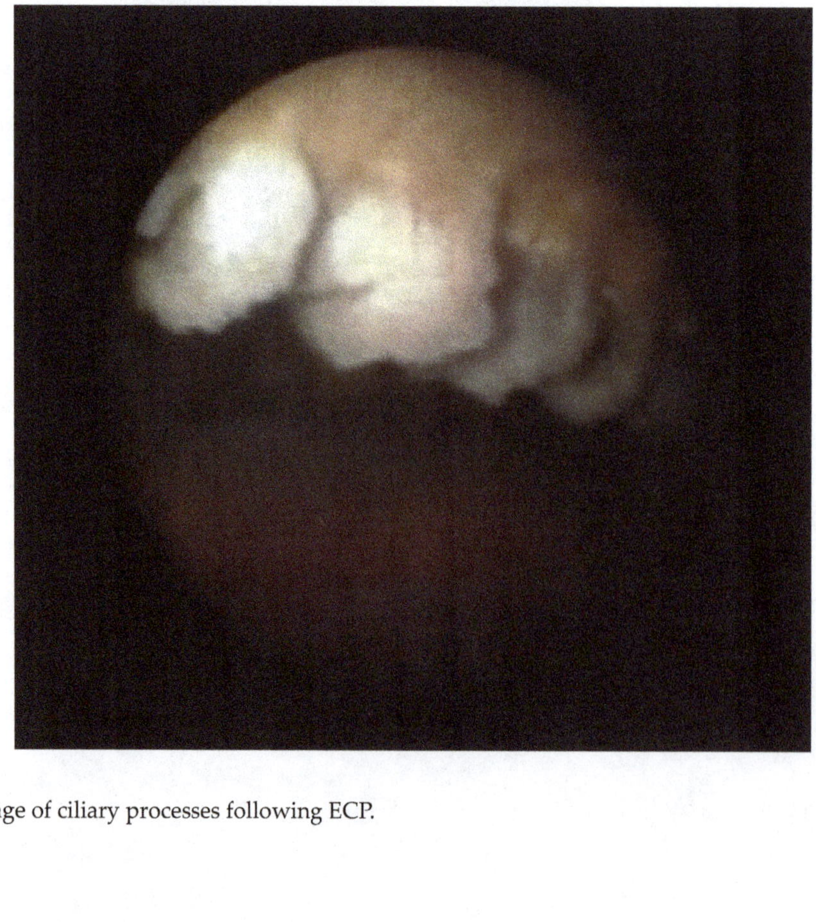

Figure 7. Shrinkage of ciliary processes following ECP.

Author details

Parul Ichhpujani

*Address all correspondence to: itsdrparul@gmail.com

Department of Ophthalmology, Glaucoma Services, Government Medical College and Hospital, Chandigarh, India

References

[1] Ritch R, Shields M, Krupin T. *The Glaucomas: Clinical Science*. 2nd ed. St. Louis: Mosby; 1996.

[2] Goel M, Picciani RG, Lee RK, Bhattachary SK. Aqueous humor dynamics: a review. Open Ophthalmol J. 2010; 4:52–59.

[3] Rosenquist R, Epstein D, Melamed S, et al. Outflow resistance of enucleated human eyes at two different perfusion pressures and different extents of trabeculotomy. Curr Eye Res. 1989; 8:1233–1240.

[4] Grant WM. Experimental aqueous perfusion in enucleated human eyes. Arch Ophthalmol. 1963; 69:783–801.

[5] Schuman JS, Chang W, Wang N, de Kater AW, Allingham RR. Excimer laser effects on outflow facility and outflow pathway morphology. Invest Ophthalmol Vis Sci. 1999; 40(8):1676–1680.

[6] Jea SY, Francis BA, Vakili G, Filippopoulos T, Rhee DJ. Ab interno trabeculectomy versus trabeculectomy for open-angle glaucoma. Ophthalmology. 2012; 119(1):36–42.

[7] Rossier A, Uffer S, Mermoud A. Aqueous dynamics in experimental ab externo trabeculectomy. Ophthalmic Res. 2000; 32:165–171.

[8] Hsu WC, Spilker MH, Yannas IV, Rubin PA. Inhibition of conjunctival scarring and contraction by a porous collagen-glycosaminoglycan implant. Invest Ophthalmol Vis Sci. 2000; 41:2404–2411.

[9] Cillino S, Casuccio A, Di Pace F, Cagini C, Ferraro LL, Cillino G. Biodegradable collagen matrix implant versus mitomycin-C in trabeculectomy: five-year follow-up. *BMC Ophthalmology*. 2016;16:24. doi:10.1186/s12886-016-0198-0.

[10] Zhou J, Smedley G. A trabecular bypass flow hypothesis. J Glaucoma. 2005; 14:74–83.

[11] Hunter KS, Fjield T, Heitzmann H, Shandas R, Kahook MY. Characterization of micro-invasive trabecular bypass stents by ex vivo perfusion and computational flow modeling. Clin Ophthalmol. 2014; 8:499–506.

[12] Buys YM. Trabeculectomy with Ex-PRESS: weighing the benefits and cost. Curr Opin Ophthalmol. 2013; 24(2):111–118.

[13] Smit BA, Johnstone MA. Effects of viscoelastic injection into Schlemm's canal in primate and human eyes: potential relevance to viscocanalostomy. Ophthalmology, 2002; 109(4): 786–792.

[14] Maepea O, Bill A. Pressures in the juxtacanalicular tissue and Schlemm's canal in monkeys. Exp Eye Res 1992; 54:879–883.

[15] Flocks M. The anatomy of the trabecular meshwork as seen in tangential section. AMA Arch Ophthalmol 1956; 56(5):708–718.

[16] Ashton N, Brini A, Smith R. Anatomical studies of the trabecular meshwork of the normal human eye. Br J Ophthalmol 1956; 40(5):257–282.

[17] Lewis RA, von Wolff K, Tetz M, et al. Canaloplasty: circumferential viscodilation and tensioning of Schlemm's canal using a flexible microcatheter for the treatment of open-angle glaucoma in adults: interim clinical study analysis. J Cataract Refract Surg. 2007; 33:1217–1226.

[18] Linner E, Rickenbach C, Werner H. Comparative measurements of the pressure in the aqueous veins and the conjunctival veins using different methods. Acta Ophthalmol (Copenh). 1950; 28:469–478.

[19] Minckler DS, Francis BA, Hodapp EA, Jampel HD, Lin SC, Samples JR, Smith SD, Singh K. Aqueous shunts in glaucoma. A report by the American Academy of Ophthalmology. Ophthalmology 2008; 115:1089–1098.

[20] Minckler DS, Mosaed S, Dustin L, Francis BA. Trabectome (trabeculectomy-internal approach): additional experience and extended follow-up. Trans Am Ophthalmol Soc. 2008; 106:1–12.

[21] Mastropasqua L, Agnifili L, Ciancaglini M, et al. In vivo analysis of conjunctiva in gold micro shunt implantation for glaucoma. Br J Ophthalmol. 2010; 94(12):1592–1596.

[22] Helmut H, Ahmed IK, Grisanti S, et al. Early postoperative safety and surgical outcomes after implantation of a suprachoroidal micro-stent for the treatment of open-angle glaucoma concomitant with cataract surgery. J Cataract Refract Surg. 2013; 39(3): 431–437.

[23] Grover DS, Godfrey DG, Smith O, Feuer WJ, Montes de Oca I, Fellman RL. Gonioscopy-assisted transluminal trabeculotomy, ab interno trabeculotomy: technique report and preliminary results. Ophthalmology. 2014; 121:855–861.

[24] Bellows AR, Grant WM. Cyclocryotherapy in advanced inadequately controlled glaucoma. Am J Ophthalmol. 1973; 75:679–684.

[25] Egbert PR, Fiadoyor S, Budenz DL, et al. Diode laser transscleral cyclophotocoagulation as a primary surgical treatment for primary open-angle glaucoma. Arch Ophthalmol. 2001; 119:345–350.

[26] Siegel MJ, Boling WS, Faridi OS, et al. Combined endoscopic cyclophotocoagulation and phacoemulsification versus phacoemulsification alone in the treatment of mild to moderate glaucoma. Clin Experiment Ophthalmol. 2015; 43:531–539.

[27] Francis BA, Berke SJ, Dustin L, Noecker R. Endoscopic cyclophotocoagulation combined with phacoemulsification versus phacoemulsification alone in medically controlled glaucoma. J Cataract Refract Surg. 2014; 40:1313–1321.

Permissions

All chapters in this book were first published in DCS, by InTech Open; hereby published with permission under the Creative Commons Attribution License or equivalent. Every chapter published in this book has been scrutinized by our experts. Their significance has been extensively debated. The topics covered herein carry significant findings which will fuel the growth of the discipline. They may even be implemented as practical applications or may be referred to as a beginning point for another development.

The contributors of this book come from diverse backgrounds, making this book a truly international effort. This book will bring forth new frontiers with its revolutionizing research information and detailed analysis of the nascent developments around the world.

We would like to thank all the contributing authors for lending their expertise to make the book truly unique. They have played a crucial role in the development of this book. Without their invaluable contributions this book wouldn't have been possible. They have made vital efforts to compile up to date information on the varied aspects of this subject to make this book a valuable addition to the collection of many professionals and students.

This book was conceptualized with the vision of imparting up-to-date information and advanced data in this field. To ensure the same, a matchless editorial board was set up. Every individual on the board went through rigorous rounds of assessment to prove their worth. After which they invested a large part of their time researching and compiling the most relevant data for our readers.

The editorial board has been involved in producing this book since its inception. They have spent rigorous hours researching and exploring the diverse topics which have resulted in the successful publishing of this book. They have passed on their knowledge of decades through this book. To expedite this challenging task, the publisher supported the team at every step. A small team of assistant editors was also appointed to further simplify the editing procedure and attain best results for the readers.

Apart from the editorial board, the designing team has also invested a significant amount of their time in understanding the subject and creating the most relevant covers. They scrutinized every image to scout for the most suitable representation of the subject and create an appropriate cover for the book.

The publishing team has been an ardent support to the editorial, designing and production team. Their endless efforts to recruit the best for this project, has resulted in the accomplishment of this book. They are a veteran in the field of academics and their pool of knowledge is as vast as their experience in printing. Their expertise and guidance has proved useful at every step. Their uncompromising quality standards have made this book an exceptional effort. Their encouragement from time to time has been an inspiration for everyone.

The publisher and the editorial board hope that this book will prove to be a valuable piece of knowledge for researchers, students, practitioners and scholars across the globe.

List of Contributors

Humberto D. Silva and Eduardo D. Silva
Universidade Federal de Pernambuco, Recife, Brazil

Maria Tamires D. Silva, Cristiana P. Dória and Cristiane P. Dória
Independent Professional, Recife, Brazil

Maria Letizia Salvetat
Department of Ophthalmology, Azienda Ospedaliero-Universitaria "Santa Maria degli Angeli", Pordenone, Italy

Marco Zeppieri
Department of Ophthalmology, Azienda Ospedaliero-Universitaria "Santa Maria della Misericordia", Udine, Italy

Paolo Brusini
Glaucoma Unit, "Città di Udine" Health Center, Udine, Italy

Umit Yolcu, Abdullah Ilhan and Ahmet Tas
Mevki Military Hospital, Ophthalmology Service, Ankara, Turkey

Baris Komur
Haseki Education and Research Hospital, Istanbul, Turkey

Joanna Jabłońska, Katarzyna Lewczuk and Marek Rękas
Department of Ophthalmology, Military Institute of Medicine, Warsaw, Poland

Bleau Anne-Marie, Vargas Beatriz, Jiménez Ana Isabel and Pañeda Covadonga
Sylentis c/Santiago Grisolía, Tres Cantos, Madrid, Spain

Jesús Jiménez-Román, Carolina Prado-Larrea and Luis Laneri-Pusineri
Glaucoma Department, Asociación para Evitar la Ceguera, Mexico City, Mexico

Roberto Gonzalez-Salinas
Research Department, Asociación para Evitar la Ceguera, Mexico City, Mexico

Iva Dekaris, Nikica Gabrić, Ante Barišić and Adis Pašalić
Department of Ophthalmology, Specialty Eye Hospital 'Svjetlost', University of Rijeka, Zagreb, Croatia

Alejandro Rodriguez-Garcia
Tecnológico de Monterrey, Escuela de Medicina y Ciencias de la Salud, Institute of Ophthalmology and Visual Sciences, Ocular Immunology and Uveitis Service, Monterrey, Mexico

C. Stephen Foster
Massachusetts Eye Research and Surgery Institute, Waltham, MA, USA
Ocular Immunology and Uveitis Foundation, Weston, MA, USA
Department of Ophthalmology, Harvard Medical School, Boston, MA, USA

Adrian E. Rendon-Nava and Luis Nino-de-Rivera
National Polytechnic Institute, Mexico City, Mexico

Alejandro Díaz-Méndez
National Institute of Astrophysics, Optics and Electronics, Puebla, Mexico

Germán R. Bianchi
Clínica de Ojos Dr. Nano, Centro Panamericana, Buenos Aires, Argentina

Bettina Hohberger and Ulrich-Christoph Welge-Lüßen
Department of Ophthalmology, Friedrich-Alexander-Universität Erlangen-Nürnberg (FAU), Erlangen, Germany

Alice Yu
Ophthalmology Center-Stachus, Munich, Germany

Lawan Abdu
Department of Ophthalmology, Faculty of Clinical Sciences, College of Health Sciences, Bayero University Kano, Nigeria

Parul Ichhpujani
Department of Ophthalmology, Glaucoma Services, Government Medical College and Hospital, Chandigarh, India

Index

CPSIA information can be obtained
at www.ICGtesting.com
Printed in the USA
LVHW060158060222
710369LV00002B/52